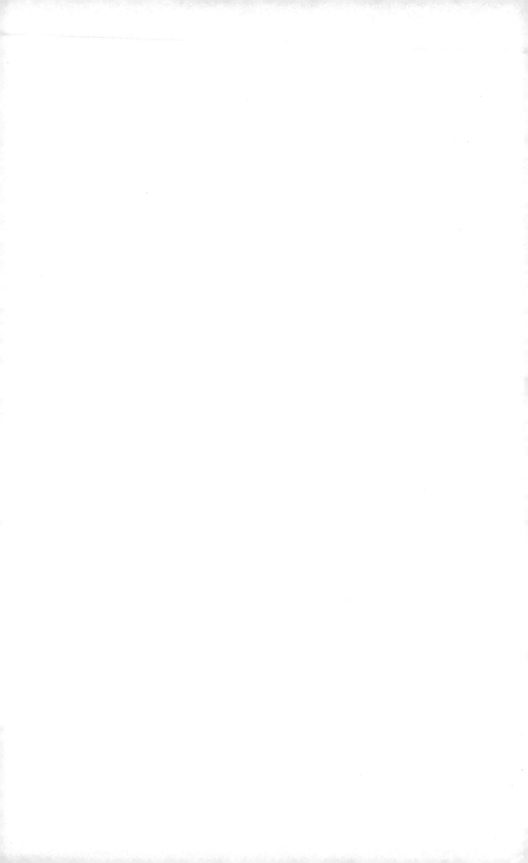

Regulating Abortion

REGULATING
ABORTION

The Politics of US Abortion Policy

DEBORAH R. MCFARLANE
and
WENDY L. HANSEN

Johns Hopkins University Press
Baltimore

Johns Hopkins University Press
2715 North Charles Street
Baltimore, Maryland 21218
www.press.jhu.edu

Library of Congress Cataloging-in-Publication Data

Names: McFarlane, Deborah R., 1951– author. | Hansen, Wendy L., author.
Title: Regulating abortion : the politics of US abortion policy /
Deborah R. McFarlane, Wendy L. Hansen.
Description: Baltimore : Johns Hopkins University Press, 2024. | Includes
bibliographical references and index.
Identifiers: LCCN 2023028587 | ISBN 9781421448701 (hardcover ; alk. paper)
| ISBN 9781421448718 (ebook)
Subjects: MESH: Abortion, Legal | Government Regulation |
Health Policy—legislation & jurisprudence | Legislation, Medical |
United States
Classification: LCC HQ767.5.U5 | NLM WQ 33 AA1 | DDC
362.1988/800973—dc23/eng/20231214
LC record available at https://lccn.loc.gov/2023028587

A catalog record for this book is available from the British Library.

Special discounts are available for bulk purchases of this book. For more information,
please contact Special Sales at specialsales@jh.edu.

To our mothers

Bette Jean (Bastian) McFarlane (1928–2017)
Rosa Theresia (Brandl) Hansen (1930–2021)

CONTENTS

FIGURES

TABLES

When we began this book project, we had no idea that American abortion policy would be completely upended before we finished. We were struck by the variation in state regulation of abortion and the focus on extreme regulations even as the incidence and risks of abortion decreased. We decided to take the long view beginning in the late '80s, when NARAL issued its first annual report, *Who Decides?* (1989). We started with two questions: Why do the states treat abortion so differently, and what difference do these state actions make?

In the course of completing this project, we have had a great deal of help. At the University of New Mexico, we would especially like to thank Eve Espey, Distinguished Professor and chair of the Department of Obstetrics and Gynecology, and Ernesto Longa, professor of law and law librarian. They both listened to our questions, provided research materials, and read drafts of this book without delay, despite holidays, sabbaticals, and heavy responsibilities.

In the initial stages of this project, the late James Trussell of Princeton University helped us gain access to the full series of NARAL Pro-Choice America's annual reports. Andrzej Kulczycki at the University of Alabama at Birmingham School of Public Health read our manuscript drafts and encouraged us to analyze the politics of this important issue. Susan Newcomer, formerly at the National Institutes of Health, suggested reviewers and other resources. Carol Weissert at Florida State University encouraged us to pursue this research and recommended Hopkins Press as a publisher. At the Press, we thank acquisitions editor Robin Coleman for his enthusiastic response to our proposal, as well as the patient and nimble copyeditors who helped us as we tried to keep up with the rapidly changing abortion landscape. Thanks also to Carlos Castillo-Salgado for his support and to our anonymous reviewers for their suggestions.

We also want to thank Joan Lamunyon Sanford, executive director of the New Mexico Religious Coalition for Reproductive Choice, and Maggie Toulouse Oliver, New Mexico's Secretary of State, for explaining abortion politics in the Land of Enchantment. Thank you to Warren Hern for sharing his experiences as a longtime provider of abortion services.

On the home front, we thank our husbands—Juan Javier Carrizales (Deborah) and Philip Ashkenazy (Wendy)—for being there, keeping abreast of new developments in abortion policies, passing on news stories, and offering boundless encouragement.

Regulating Abortion

On June 24, 2022, the US Supreme Court ruled on *Dobbs v. Jackson Women's Health Organization.*[1] At issue was Mississippi's Gestational Age Act, which prohibited induced abortions after 15 weeks of pregnancy, with no exceptions for rape or incest. Based on longstanding precedents, two lower federal courts had already struck down this Mississippi statute. Nonetheless, the State of Mississippi appealed to the US Supreme Court on June 15, 2020, asking the high court to reconsider the case.

On average, it takes six weeks for the Supreme Court to act once a petition has been filed (Supreme Court of the United States 2022). In *Dobbs,* however, the Court waited 11 months before agreeing to take the case. During that unusually long interval, liberal Justice Ruth Bader Ginsberg died and was replaced by conservative Justice Amy Coney Barrett (Liptak 2021a).

Tossing aside the principle of *stare decisis,* the 6–3 *Dobbs v. Jackson* decision upheld the Mississippi statute. In so doing, the Court explicitly overturned almost a half century of "settled law" (Goldman 2021, 115) established by *Roe v. Wade* in 1973 and reaffirmed by *Planned Parenthood of Southeastern Pennsylvania v. Casey* in 1992. Writing for the majority, Justice Samuel Alito stated, "It is time to heed the Constitution and re-

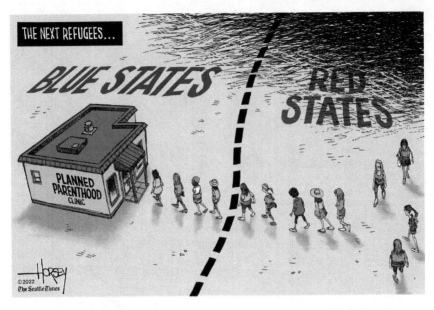

FIGURE I.1. The Next Refugees. *Source:* © 2022 David Horsey, published in the *Seattle Times*. Reprinted with permission of the artist.

turn the issue of abortion back to the people's elected representatives" (597 U.S. _____ (2022) 6).

Almost overnight, states were free to prohibit the practice of abortion within their borders. While *Dobbs* was a monumental change, states were already regulating abortion in very different ways. Figure I.1 depicts that, even before this decision, women in states that heavily restricted abortions crossed state lines for abortion care far more than did women living in states less hostile to abortion rights (Kaiser Family Foundation 2020).

The majority opinion was scathing in its interpretation of past legal reasoning. It dismissed "*Roe* as an 'elaborate scheme' that was 'concocted' to divine a constitutional right." It assailed "the 1973 decision with adverbial abandon, calling it 'egregiously wrong,' 'exceptionally weak' and 'deeply damaging'" (Lozada 2022). The majority opinion concluded that "the right to abortion was not deeply rooted in the country's history and traditions," and it rejected Roe's extensive historical analysis of abortion practice as "constitutionally irrelevant" and "plainly incorrect." The *Dobbs* decision, however, made selective use of US history and tradition,[2] and it took refuge in portions of the very rulings it overturned (Lozada 2022; 597 U.S. ____ (2022)).

The majority opinion showed little civility for different viewpoints, including the concurrence by Chief Justice John Roberts; the dissent signed by Justices Stephen Breyer, Elena Kagan, and Sonia Sotomayor; or the amicus briefs filed by scores of professional groups (Center for Reproductive Rights 2022a). Although Chief Justice Roberts concurred with the *Dobbs* majority in upholding Mississippi's 15-week limit on abortions, he stopped short of overturning *Roe* and *Casey*. Instead of respectfully recognizing the chief justice's position, the majority opinion stated, "the most fundamental defect [in the concurrence] is its failure to offer any principled basis for its approach" (597 U.S. ____ (2022) 73). Regarding the dissent's treatment of abortion history, the majority opinion simply asserted that "the dissent's failure to engage with this long tradition is devastating to its position" (597 U.S. ____ (2022) 35–36). Suggesting that its historical interpretations were faulty, the majority also dismissed the amicus brief of the American Historical Association[3] (597 U.S. ____ (2022) 28).

The editorial boards of both the *New York Times* and the *New England Journal of Medicine* decried this decision. Specifically, the *New York Times* stated, "For the first time in history, the Supreme Court has eliminated an established constitutional right involving the most fundamental of human concerns: the dignity and autonomy to decide what happens to your body." This change in course will be "devastating, throwing America into a new era of struggle over abortion laws—an era that will be marked by chaos, confusion and human suffering" (*New York Times* 2022b). The *New England Journal of Medicine* called the *Dobbs* decision "a stunning reversal of precedent that inserts government into the personal lives and health care of Americans." Pointing out that "maternal mortality due to induced abortion is 0.41 per 100,000 procedures compared to 23.8 per 100,000 live births," the editors remarked that "experience around the world has demonstrated that restricting access to legal abortion care does not substantially reduce the number of procedures, but it dramatically reduces the number of *safe* procedures, resulting in increased morbidity and mortality" (*New England Journal of Medicine*, The Editors, 2022, 367–368).

Regardless of its tone, content, or reasoning, the *Dobbs* opinion imposed a new order on what was already one of the most regulated health services in the country. But this new regulatory order did not come as a surprise. After all, President Donald J. Trump had vowed to nominate anti-abortion justices, and he kept that promise. Due to the maneuvering of Senate Majority Leader Mitch McConnell (*New York Times* 2022b), three of Trump's nominees sat on the Court by November 2020, and the Court agreed to hear the *Dobbs* case on May 17, 2021. A year later, *Politico* leaked Alito's draft opinion striking down both *Roe* and *Casey* (Gerstein and Ward 2022).

The changing composition of the Court, however, made this outcome predictable. Recent Supreme Court decisions, especially regarding the delivery of abortion services during the COVID-19 pandemic (Liptak 2021b), signaled the Court's changing stance toward abortion.

On January 12, 2021, just eight days before the inauguration of President Joe Biden, the US Supreme Court (6–3) stayed a federal district court's nationwide injunction in *Food and Drug Administration, et al. v. American College of Obstetricians and Gynecologists, et al.*[4] The debate concerned a federal regulation requiring that women seeking to end their pregnancies through medication abortion had to pick up their pills in person from a hospital or medical office.[5] In light of the coronavirus epidemic, the federal judge issuing the injunction had blocked the in-person requirement, stating that "a needless trip to a medical facility during a health crisis very likely imposed an undue burden on the constitutional right to abortion" (Liptak 2021b).

Chief Justice Roberts wrote the brief order to invalidate the injunction, thus reinstating the in-person requirement. His explanation was short: "Courts owe significant deference to the politically accountable entities with the 'background, competence and expertise to assess public health'" (592 U.S. ____ (2021)). Here, Roberts was referring to the expertise of the US Food and Drug Administration (FDA), which was being sued by the American College of Obstetricians and Gynecology (ACOG), whose 60,000 members deliver much of women's reproductive health services in the country (Liptak 2021b; Litman 2021).

In dissent, "Justice Sonia Sotomayor, joined by Justice Elena Kagan, said that the majority was grievously wrong" (Liptak 2021b). Sotomayor wrote, "This country's laws have long singled out abortions for more onerous treatment than other medical procedures that carry similar or greater risks" (592 U.S. ____ (2021)). Citing the plaintiff's complaint, Sotomayor continued, "Of the over 20,000 FDA-approved drugs, mifepristone [for medication abortion] is the only one that the FDA requires to be picked up in person for patients to take at home" (592 U.S. ____ (2021); ACOG 2020). She noted that the inevitable delays, exacerbated by the COVID-19 pandemic, could be responsible for patients missing the gestational age limit for medication abortion (Blackman 2021).

For affluent women, an in-person requirement may have been inconvenient but was not insurmountable. For many low-income women, disproportionately women of color and those lacking access to reliable transportation and affordable childcare, the in-person requirement was prohibitively burdensome. Poor women are much more likely to face an unintended pregnancy than their higher income counterparts, largely because they often lack access to effective contraception. During the COVID-19 pandemic, the in-person requirement added another obstacle to an already medically underserved population (American College of Obstetricians and Gynecologists 2020a).

On April 12, 2021, the FDA temporarily rescinded its two-decade-old requirement that medication abortion pills had to be picked up in person. The FDA's temporary decision nullified the US Supreme Court's ruling in *Food and Drug Administration, et al. v. American College of Obstetricians and Gynecologists, et al.* (Fox and Cole 2021), but this suspension permitted patients to get mifepristone by mail only for the duration of the pandemic. The FDA then launched a scientific review to see whether or not the in-person requirement and other restrictions should be lifted permanently (McGinley and Shepherd 2021).

Until December 2021, "the original in-person requirements for medication abortion were on track to be restored" (Fox and Cole 2021).[6] On December 16, the FDA sent a letter to ACOG saying that "it was dropping the in-person dispensing requirement 'to minimize the burden on the health care delivery system' and 'to ensure that the benefits of the drug outweigh the risks'" (McGinley and Shepherd 2021). The FDA's internal scientific review had concluded that the ban against medication abortions obtained through telemedicine was unwarranted (McGinley and Shepherd 2021).

Neither the FDA's temporary nor permanent reprieve applied to all American women of reproductive age. State regulations in 19 states already mandated that physicians must be in the physical presence of the patients when prescribing medication abortion, thus precluding prescribing through telemedicine. For now, these state laws are in effect, although future lawsuits may address questions about "federal preemption of these state laws and the extent to which states may impose requirements on medication abortion drugs that are subject to FDA regulation" (Staman and Shimabukuro 2022, 3). This in-person requirement, originally upheld by *FDA, et al. v. ACOG, et al.* and negated by the FDA's reversal on the in-person dispensing requirement, is emblematic of all abortion regulation in the United States—widespread, ever-changing, partisan, gendered, racialized, and often having a dubious medical or scientific basis (Daniels et al. 2016).

Abortion regulation is consequential because induced abortion is prevalent in the United States. Although its incidence has decreased in recent years, pregnancy termination is still common. If current age-specific abortion rates persist, nearly one in four American women will have an abortion by age 45. The risk of unintended pregnancy, however, is not uniformly distributed: low-income and women of color face a much higher than average likelihood of having an abortion (Jones and Jerman 2017c).

Although prevalent, abortion is among the most regulated health services in the nation (Cheung 2018; NAS 2018). The constitutional basis for these regulations emanates from the US Supreme Court, which has handed down more than 40 decisions related to abortion since *Roe v. Wade*.[7] That 1973 landmark decision legalized abortion throughout the United States, but *Roe* also permitted considerable state discretion. Subsequent decisions, notably, *Webster v. Reproductive Health Services* (1989) and *Planned Parenthood of Southeastern Pennsylvania v. Casey* (1992), upheld and expanded state latitude in abortion policymaking (Patton 2007). Now, the *Dobbs v. Jackson* decision has vacated both *Roe* and *Casey*, ushering in a new era in abortion regulation.

Notwithstanding the Supreme Court's primacy in interpreting abortion laws, states are the key players in developing abortion regulations (Halva-Neubauer 1990). Since 1988, states have enacted nearly 500 restrictions on access to abortion and over 100 protections of that access. Even in the midst of the COVID-19 epidemic, states continued to issue new abortion regulations (Jones et al. 2020). Fueled by partisanship, this trend shows no signs of abating.

Long before the *Dobbs* decision, the configuration of abortion policies differed greatly among states. By 2017, the year before the *Dobbs* case began, only 17 states were funding abortion for low-income women; 33 states and the District of Columbia were not. Thirty-two states mandated specific counseling, often medically inaccurate (Daniels et al. 2016), for women seeking abortion; 18 states and the District of Columbia did not. Twenty-six states required waiting periods between the time an abortion was requested and the procedure performed or medication dispensed. Twenty-four states and the District of Columbia had no such requirement. As of 2017, 43 states imposed parental consent or notification regulations on minors seeking abortion; seven states and the District of Columbia did not.

Before *Dobbs*, state abortion laws also regulated providers and payers. By 2017, 44 states and the District of Columbia had stricter regulations for abortion clinics than for other medical providers. Fourteen states even regulated private physicians' offices that offered abortion services, and 18 states had mandates for clinical sites dispensing only medication (pharmacological) abortion (Guttmacher Institute 2017). Eleven states required abortion providers to have an affiliation with a local hospital, and one state, Mississippi, required the clinician to be either a board-certified obstetrician-gynecologist or eligible for certification (Guttmacher Institute 2017). Twenty-four states prohibited state health insurance exchanges from offering plans with abortion coverage, and 11 states forbade any abortion coverage in their private insurance markets.

Before *Dobbs*, states also enacted laws to protect a woman's right to choose abortion. By 2017, 17 states and the District of Columbia had laws defending abortion patients and providers from harassment and anti-choice violence. Ten states had expanded the scope of practice for advanced-practice clinicians (e.g., nurse practitioners) to include medication and/or surgical abortion. Similarly, 17 states and the District of Co-

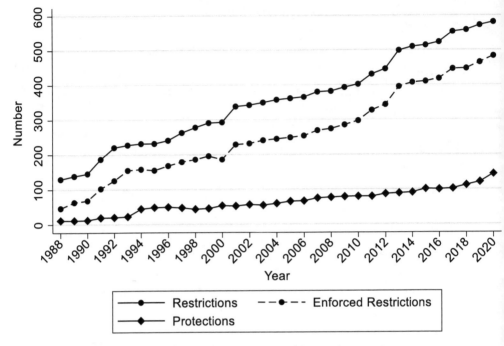

FIGURE I.2. Total State Abortion Restrictions and Protections, 1988–2020.
Note: The solid line shows enacted restrictions; the dashed line shows enforced restrictions.

lumbia had enacted laws or policies protecting access to emergency contraception, which can curtail the need for abortion. During the midst of the COVID-19 pandemic, 12 states codified the right to choose (Capello 2020; Jones et al. 2020).

The annual total number of state abortion restrictions and protections through 2020, the most recent year for which complete data are available, are shown in figure I.2. Clearly, restrictions are more numerous and long-standing than abortion protections. Few protections were in place before 1994, and until very recently, they were growing at a slower rate than restrictions (NARAL 2020). In many states, courts had enjoined specific abortion restrictions, prohibiting their enforcement.

Less than six months after the *Dobbs* decision, 13 American states (Alabama, Arkansas, Idaho, Kentucky, Louisiana, Mississippi, Missouri, Oklahoma, South Dakota, Tennessee, Texas, West Virginia, and Wisconsin) had already banned abortion. An additional state (Georgia) had a six-week LMP (first day of last menstrual period) gestational limit, effectively banning abortion because many women do not realize they are pregnant at that point. Five more states (Arizona, Indiana, North Dakota, Utah, and Wyoming) had near total abortion bans, but various courts had temporarily blocked them. Many of these states were already heavily restricted in terms of abortion regulations (Kaiser Family Foundation 2022a).

For years, the intensity of abortion regulation has been greatly disproportionate to its risks. For example, the National Academy of Sciences reported that the risks associated with medication abortion were low and "similar in magnitude to the reported risks of serious adverse effects of commonly used prescription and over-the-counter medications" (NAS 2018, 58). Moreover, there was no difference in patient outcomes between in-person and telemedicine visits (NAS 2018).

In terms of morbidity, less than a quarter of one percent of all legal abortions, both medication and surgical, results in major complications (NAS 2018; Upadhyay et al. 2012). The risk of death for abortion patients is also low; induced abortion is 14 times safer than childbirth (Raymond and Grimes 2012). In many states, however, more stringent regulations apply to abortion providers than to other ambulatory surgical facilities performing procedures with far higher complication risks (Jones et al. 2018).

Despite its safety, the abortion issue has had great staying power in American politics. For example, abortion nearly derailed the 2010 Patient Protection and Affordable Care Act (ACA). Not a single Republican in either chamber of Congress voted in support of the ACA, so passage of the final House bill required solid Democratic support—a formidable undertaking within such a diverse political party. The party platform had a pro-choice position, but Democratic members of Congress represented the full spectrum of abortion opinion (Burgin and Bereznyak 2013).

In order to garner enough votes, the Democratic House leadership had to make concessions to anti-abortion Democrats who refused to commit their votes until there was a pledge not to fund abortions (Benson 2010) The resulting interparty compromise reinforced and even extended the existing Hyde Amendment that prohibits the expenditure of any federal funds for abortion, except in the rare case of rape, incest, or life endangerment of the pregnant woman. To seal this endgame compromise, President Barack Obama promised to issue a specific executive order following the House vote; this order would reinforce bans on public abortion funding already in the pending legislation. Consequently, the day after signing the ACA with great fanfare, the president quietly penned Executive Order 13535, Ensuring Enforcement and Implementation of Abortion Restrictions in the Patient Protection and Affordable Care Act, doubly ensuring that the new law would prohibit federally funded abortions (McFarlane 2015).

As often is the case with abortion regulations, carrying out this Executive Order occurred at the state level. Twenty-four states enacted laws banning health insurance plans available through their marketplaces from including abortion coverage. Of these, 11 states banned *any* abortion coverage in all private insurance plans (Salganicoff and Sobel 2015). Among states permitting abortion coverage, marketplace insurance plans offering this protection had to create separate accounts for abortion coverage premiums and premiums for all other health services. Women opting for abortion coverage have had to write a separate check for that eventuality (Ranji and Salganicoff 2015). The ACA required that at least one plan within each state insurance exchange must not offer abortion coverage beyond the narrow exceptions of rape, incest, and life of the pregnant woman (Salganicoff et al. 2014). No other health service was singled out and regulated in this manner.

Our original purpose in writing this book was twofold: (1) to examine how and why abortion is regulated in the United States, and (2) to assess the impact of these regulations. In addressing this important policy area, we spent several years coding state abortion restrictions and protections over the last three decades. We wanted to understand how and why states make abortion decisions as well as what difference these regulatory policies make.

Toward the end of this project, the *Dobbs* decision upended the entire regulatory framework for American abortion policy. Consequently, most of the analyses in this book show the state of the US legal and political situation through the very end of *Roe* and on the eve of its overthrow. We also glance into the future of the new regulatory regime. We hope that this work provides a vital benchmark for the reproductive rights field going forward as researchers begin to document the fallout from this decision.

The first chapter, Abortion Services in the United States and Theoretical Approaches to Their Regulation, introduces the intersection of regulation and abortion. We first address abortion in the United States, considering the prevalence of abortion since 1973. We also examine characteristics of abortion patients and providers over time. Next, we focus on regulation and regulatory politics. We examine how various types of regulation and different theoretical approaches (regulatory politics, morality politics, and gender politics) apply to abortion regulation. Then, we present three myths surrounding abortion regulation that obfuscate policymaking.

Chapter 2, Setting the Parameters for State Abortion Policies: Historical Background and US Supreme Court Decisions, provides a brief history of abortion prior to 1973 and covers US Supreme Court rulings on abortion since 1973. This chapter begins with colonial America, when abortion was available, risky, and minimally regulated, and goes on to juxtapose abortion practices and policies through 1972. The chapter then covers US Supreme Court rulings on abortion from *Roe v. Wade* (1973) to *Dobbs v. Jackson* (2022). Throughout the chapter, we consider how the composition of the court influences decisions about abortion.

Chapter 3, Weakening *Roe*: The Proliferation of Abortion Regulations in US States, describes the types of and volume of state abortion regulations, both enacted and enforced, over the last three decades. Of these regulations, abortion restrictions, which curtail access to abortion, far exceed abortion protections, which protect access to abortion. Even in the face of the COVID-19 pandemic, abortion regulation has accelerated, precipitating more state abortion restrictions as well as protections.

Chapter 4, Politics across the States: Explaining State Differences in Abortion Regulation, examines reasons why states' regulation of abortion differs so widely. Using an original data set that spans more than three decades, we consider political, religious, and socioeconomic factors. Political factors include the stated abortion positions of state politicians, the partisanship of state governments (both governors and legislatures), the representation of women, and interest group spending. State religious composition is shown with particular attention to pro-life or anti-abortion religious adherents. We also consider state differences in levels of education, employment, and income. We analyze factors that predict aggregate state abortion restrictions and protections, respectively, followed by examining whether or not different forces explain the enactment and enforcement of specific types of restrictions.

Chapter 5, After the Policymakers Go Home: Effects of State Abortion Regulations, examines the impact of state abortion regulations on abortion rates. We examine the differential effects of demand-side restrictions versus supply-side restrictions. We also report and explain racial and ethnic differences in the effects of abortion regulation.

Chapter 6, How Abortion Is Regulated in Western Europe: A Comparison with the United States, compares abortion regulation in US states with abortion regulation in 18 Western European countries. We examine the relationship between the different types of abortion regulations with abortion rates across these Western European countries, and we compare that relationship to the effects of abortion regulation in the US states. We also consider how COVID-19 affected the delivery of abortion services in this region compared with the United States.

Chapter 7, The *Dobbs* Decision and Beyond, describes the short-term aftermath of overturning Roe in both red and blue states. We also explain the frenzy of state abortion policymaking while the Dobbs decision was pending, and we discuss the likelihood that this ruling will exacerbate racial and class divides among US women.

The book concludes by revisiting the three myths about abortion regulation that are introduced in Chapter 1. We explain how they deter realistic and compassionate abortion regulation. We end by discussing post-*Dobbs* polls and elections as well as pending legislation and judicial cases.

Our use of language regarding abortion and its politics follows the lead of Ehrlich and Doan (2019, xi); they note that the choice of words in any discussion of abortion is "highly freighted." Their preferred term for discussing groups or individuals who are opposed to abortion is *anti-abortion*, but they note that at times, they use the term pro-life "to clearly and accurately convey expressed ideas and beliefs" (Ehrlich and Doan 2019, x–xi). In this book, we have chosen to hyphenate anti-abortion, pro-life, and pro-choice.

Abortion Services in the United States and Theoretical Approaches to Their Regulation

Abortion is "among the most regulated medical procedures in the nation" (NAS 2018, 6). This high level of state control is not due to the riskiness of surgical procedures or medications used for pregnancy terminations. "Abortion is now one of the safest procedures in medicine," if performed by a trained professional in hygienic conditions using modern methods (Kulczycki 2015, 171). Medication[1] or pharmacologic abortion is similarly low risk (Nippita and Paul 2018; Paul and Stein 2011). To put its safety record in perspective, Table 1.1 shows that induced abortion is less dangerous than childbirth, colonoscopy, or even wisdom tooth extraction (NAS 2018, 75). Nevertheless, abortion remains far more stringently regulated than other health services.

Reliable abortion data for the United States have been available since before 1973, when *Roe v. Wade* legalized abortion throughout the country.[2] Abortion rates[3] increased throughout the 1970s, topping off at 29.3 per 1,000 women of reproductive age in 1981.[4] The total number of abortions crested in 1990, with an estimated 1,608,600 abortions (Henshaw 1998a; Jones et al. 2022a). From 1990 to 2017, annual abortion numbers declined despite a steady increase in total population.[5] By 2017, the number of abortions had decreased to 862,320, and the abortion rate dropped

TABLE 1.1

*Comparison of US Mortality Rates for Abortion, Childbirth,
Colonoscopy, Dental Procedures, Plastic Surgery, and Tonsillectomy*

Procedure	Mortality rate (number of deaths per 100,000 procedures)
Abortion (1988–2010)	0.7
Childbirth (1988–2005)	8.8
Colonoscopy (2001–2015)	2.9
Dental procedures (1999–2005)	0.0 to 1.7
Plastic surgery (2000–2012)	0.8 to 1.7
Tonsillectomy (1968–1972)	2.9 to 6.3

Source: Table 2.4 in National Academies of Sciences, Engineering, and Medicine
(2018). *The Safety and Quality of Abortion Care in the United States.* Washington, DC:
National Academies Press. Used with permission.

to 13.5 abortions per 1,000 women, less than half its peak rate (Jones et al. 2019). After 2017, however, annual abortion rates began to increase, along with the total number of abortions. From 2018 to 2020, the total number of abortions increased by 8 percent, and the US abortion rate increased by 7 percent. Even with this increase, both the number of abortions (930,160) and the abortion rate (14.4 per 1,000 women of reproductive age 15–44) in 2020 were far lower than they had been in 1990. Nonetheless, abortion remains common. In 2020, about one in five pregnancies ended in abortion (Jones et al. 2022c).

As abortion rates fell and the total number of abortions decreased (1991–2017), state abortion regulations continued to mount. Considering these trends, it would be easy to infer that state abortion restrictions were the primary reason for this drop in abortions. But the relationship between abortion rates and abortion restrictions is far more complicated.

A 2018 report from the National Academies of Sciences, Engineering, and Medicine acknowledged this complexity, commenting that the decline in abortion rates is "not fully understood" (NAS 2018, 5). This report pointed out that abortion rates had been going down for more than a decade before state abortion restrictions began to accelerate in the early 1990s. The NAS report concluded that among the factors that caused the decrease in abortions were

the increasing use of effective contraception, especially long-acting reversible methods (e.g., intrauterine devices [IUDs] and implants), historic declines in the rate of unintended pregnancy, and increasing numbers of state regulations that limit the availability of otherwise legal abortion services. (NAS 2018, 5)

Most state abortion regulations are restrictions, which are intended to discourage access to abortion services (and sometimes contraception) (figure 1.1). In any one year, state or federal courts temporarily or permanently enjoin at least 20 percent of these restrictions, which means that these regulations cannot be enforced (discussed more in Chapter 3). Adding to this regulatory complexity are state abortion protections: about half of US states have enacted at least one directive that serves to protect women's access to abortion. Since 2016, these state abortion protections have shown a marked increase.

This chapter introduces the intersection of abortion and regulation. First, the prevalence of abortion, characteristics of abortion patients, current abortion techniques, and types of providers are examined. Then, regulation and regulatory politics in the context of the abortion issue in the United States are addressed. Here, the conception of abortion regulation is interdisciplinary, drawing primarily from political science and public

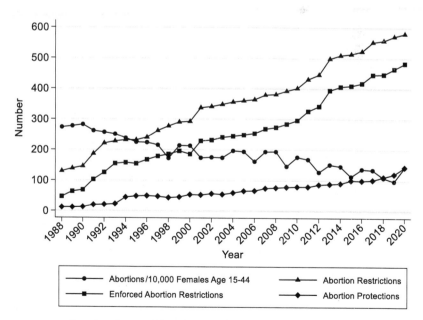

FIGURE 1.1. Abortion Rate and Total State Abortion Restrictions and Protections, 1988–2020

health, but also from demography, economics, history, and law. We integrate concepts and insights from each of these areas to examine abortion regulation and its impact.

Abortion in America

Abortion is a generic term that may refer to spontaneous abortions (miscarriages) or induced abortions (deliberate pregnancy terminations). Spontaneous abortions occur in up to one in four clinically recognized pregnancies. Induced abortions—deliberate pregnancy terminations— occur in about one-fifth of pregnancies in the United States (Kulczycki 2015). Abortion can be induced medically (by pharmacologic means) or procedurally (by surgical means). Throughout this book, *abortion* refers to induced abortion unless otherwise clarified.

In the United States, as in any other country or society, the demand for abortion is predicated on two antecedent events: levels of sexual activity and prevalence of effective contraceptive use. The three steps in the human reproductive process are (1) sexual intercourse, (2) conception, and (3) gestation and parturition (figure 1.2). When sexual abstinence is not practiced consistently, effective contraception is needed for those not trying to become pregnant. If sexually active women not wanting to become pregnant or their partners fail to use effective contraception consistently—or if usually effective contraception fails—then unintended pregnancy is more likely. Higher rates of unintended pregnancy increase the demand for induced abortion[6] (McFarlane 2015; McFarlane and Meier 2001).

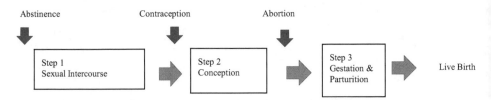

FIGURE 1.2. The Human Reproductive Process. *Source:* Adapted from Davis and Blake (1956); published in Deborah R. McFarlane and Kenneth J. Meier, *The Politics of Fertility Control* (2001), CQ Press (Chatham House Press). Used with permission of the publisher.

Access to Contraception, Unintended Pregnancy, and Abortion

In the United States, many contraceptive methods require a medical prescription (birth control pills) or a clinical intervention (e.g., intrauterine
devices (IUDs)). Ordinarily, women who have health insurance have an
easier time obtaining effective birth control than do those without. Even
when uninsured women have access to clinical services, contraceptive
costs are high.[7] As a result, health insurance often determines access
to contraception. Not surprisingly, unintended pregnancy rates among
women with health insurance are lower than those for uninsured women
(Nearns 2009).

Since the 1980s, unintended pregnancy rates have decreased (table 1.2).
This trend has occurred in all segments of the population, including
teenagers from all income brackets and low-income women of all ages
(Finer and Zolna 2016; Henshaw 1998b). The decrease in rates is due, in
no small part, to the dramatic increase in the availability and use of long-
acting reversible contraception (Richards 2016). Nevertheless, disparities
in unintended pregnancy rates persist.

TABLE 1.2

*Percent of Pregnancies Unintended and Percent of Unintended
Pregnancies Ending in Abortion, Various Years*

Year	Unintended pregnancies (%)	Unintended pregnancies ending in abortion (%)
1981	54.2	53.9
1987	53.5	50.3
1994	48.0	54.0
2001	49.0	48.0
2008	51.0	40.0
2011	45.0	42.0

Sources: Data for years 1981–1994 from Henshaw (1998), data for years 1994–2001 from Finer
and Henshaw (2006), and data for years 2008–2011 from Finer and Zolna (2016).

Who Has Abortions?

Although abortion rates have declined greatly over the last four decades,
abortion is prevalent in the United States. Abortion remains one of the
most common surgical procedures in the country, even with the increasing use of medical or pharmacologic abortion.[8] If current age-specific
abortion rates persist, nearly one in four US women will experience an
induced abortion before she reaches menopause. The likelihood of abor-

tion, however, is far higher for low-income women (Jones and Jerman 2017c).

Low-income women account for an increasingly disproportionate share of abortions. In 2014, women living in households with incomes under the federal poverty level had an abortion rate of 36.6 per 1,000 women aged 15–44. In contrast, women, living in households with incomes at least 200 percent above the poverty level had an abortion rate of 6.0 per 1,000 women aged 15–44 (Jones and Jerman 2017a; Jones and Jerman 2017c).

Differences in unintended pregnancy explain these disparate abortion rates. Low-income women experience higher rates of unintended pregnancy because they have lower rates of health insurance coverage that would pay for birth control, and they use effective contraception less consistently than women with higher incomes. Low-income women also face other structural issues related to poverty and racism, which affect unintended pregnancy rates (Dehlendorf et al. 2013).

Because low incomes and race are intertwined, women of color have considerably higher abortion rates than non-Hispanic white women. Indeed, women of color experience more than half of abortions, far disproportionate to their percentage of the population.[9] Again, unintended pregnancy is the major reason for this disparity. African American women had the highest abortion rate, 27.1 in 2014,[10] followed by 19.1 for Hispanic women, compared with 10.0 for non-Hispanic white women (Jones and Jerman 2017c).

Abortion rates also vary by marital status and age. Unmarried women account for most abortions, clearly a long-standing trend (table 1.3).[11] Women in their early twenties have the highest rates of abortions, followed by women in their upper twenties, but abortion rates for both groups have been declining (Jones and Jerman 2017b; Henshaw and Kost 2008).

Over time, teenagers have accounted for a dwindling percentage of abortions, because adolescent abortion rates have declined more dramatically than for women in their twenties. In 1979, women younger than 20 years of age obtained 30.8 percent of all abortions in the United States; by 2004, that percentage fell to 16.9 percent (Henshaw and Kost 2008, Table 1, 10). This change is due in part to teens' use of long-lasting reversible contraception (Boonstra 2014). With this dramatic decline in teen abortion rates, women in their twenties now account for a higher per-

TABLE 1.3
Abortion Percentages by Select Age Groups and among Unmarried Women,
Various Years

Year	<20 years	20–24 years	25–29 years·	Unmarried (All)
1979	30.8	35.1	19.0	78.5
1989	24.5	32.5	22.1	84.3
2004	16.9	33.2	23.3	86.2
2014	11.7	33.6	26.5	94.5

Sources: Henshaw and Kost (2008) and Jones and Jerman (2017c).

centage of total abortions. Their abortion rates declined, but not as much as the teenage abortion rate.

Most abortions in the United States occur in the first trimester of pregnancy. Early abortion has been the norm since abortion was nationally legalized in 1973. At that time, the majority of abortions occurred before the fourteenth week of gestation. Over time, an increasing proportion of abortions has taken place much earlier in pregnancy. By 2013, 92 percent of abortions occurred before the fourteenth week of pregnancy. Technological advances such as highly sensitive pregnancy tests and medication abortion have allowed pregnancy termination to occur "at increasingly earlier gestational stages" (NAS 2018, 28).

Current Abortion Methods

Four major types of abortion predominate in the United States: medication, aspiration commonly known as dilation and curettage (D&C), dilation and evacuation (D&E), and induction termination (table 1.4). Which method is used depends largely upon gestational age,[12] but also upon "patient preference, provider skill, need and desire for sedation, costs, clinical setting, and state policies and regulations" (NAS 2018, 51). Because more than 90 percent of abortions in the United States occur during the first 13 weeks of pregnancy, medication and aspiration abortions are, by far, the most common methods of pregnancy termination (Centers for Disease Control and Prevention 2021; NAS 2018).

Medication abortion was introduced in Europe in the late 1980s and approved by the US Food and Drug Administration (FDA) in 2000 (Stuenkel and Manson 2021). The use of early medical abortion increased by 120 percent from 2009 to 2018 and by 9 percent from 2017 to 2018

TABLE 1.4
Four Most Common Methods of Induced Abortion in the United States

Method of abortion	Mechanism	Length of gestation
Medication (also called medical abortion)	Involves the use of medications to disrupt implantation and induce uterine contractions that expel the products of conception. The most effective regimens use a combination of mifepristone and misoprostol.	Up to 77 days or 11 weeks
Aspiration (also called surgical or suction curettage)	A hollow tube (curette) is inserted into the uterus. At the other end of the tube, a hand-held syringe or electric device is applied to create suction and empty the uterus.	Up to 14–16 weeks
Dilation and evacuation	"Involves cervical preparation with osmotic dilators and/or medications, followed by suction and/or forceps extraction to empty the uterus. Ultrasound guidance is often used" (NAS 2018, 20).	14 weeks and more
Induction (also called medical abortion)	Involves the use of medications to induce labor and delivery of the fetus. The most effective regimens use a combination of mifepristone and misoprostol (NAS 2018, 20).	14 weeks and more

Sources: Box 1–2, NAS (2018, 20); National Abortion Federation (2022).

(Kortsmith et al. 2020). By 2020, medication abortions accounted for 53 percent of all pregnancy terminations in the United States (Jones et al. 2022b). Substantial medical research has demonstrated the effectiveness of medication abortion during the first trimester of pregnancy (National Abortion Federation 2022; World Health Organization 2022; Kapp et al. 2018).

Most often, two primary medications are used to induce abortion. The first drug, mifepristone, blocks the effects of progesterone, without which the lining of the uterus begins to break down. A second drug, misoprostol, taken 6 to 48 hours later, causes the uterus to contract and expel its contents (Reed 2021; Nippita and Paul 2018). Although mifepristone is safer than Tylenol, "regulatory opposition to mifepristone persists in the form of a special set of burdensome FDA restrictions known as Risk Evaluation and Mitigation Strategy (REMS)" (Reed 2021, 251). When the FDA approved the new drug application for mifepristone in 2000, it imposed certain restrictions, which were approved as a REMS in 2011 (US Food and Drug Administration 2023b). Originally, REMS included three restrictions: (1) the drug could only be dispensed in medical facilities under the supervision of a certified prescriber; (2) health care providers who wanted to prescribe the drug had to be certified by completing and sending a form to the drug distributor; and (3) the patient had to receive an FDA-approved medication guide and sign a patient agreement.

These restrictions have made mifepristone harder for patients to access and more difficult to prescribe. The American College of Obstetricians and Gynecologists (ACOG) has advocated for the removal of REMS restrictions for mifepristone because "these restrictions for mifepristone do not make the care safer, are not based on medical evidence or need, and create barriers to clinician and patient access to medication abortion" (American College of Obstetricians and Gynecologists 2020b). Contrary to the ACOG's recommendation, however, REMS restrictions remain in place. As explained in the Introduction, the FDA permanently dropped the in-person requirement for mifepristone patients in December 2021, and the FDA modified the Mifepristone REMS program again in January 2023 by removing "the restrictions that prevented patients from obtaining medication abortion pills from a retail pharmacy" (Guttmacher Institute 2023c). Now, both health care providers that are certified to prescribe mifepristone and certified pharmacies can dispense mifepristone (US Food and Drug Administration 2023a; US Food and Drug Administration 2023b),[13] but other onerous aspects of REMS remain in place.

These federal changes do not supersede state laws. In states that have a near-total abortion ban, women cannot obtain the medication at a pharmacy or from their doctors (Guttmacher Institute 2023c). In states where abortion is legal, mifepristone remains more heavily regulated than drugs and procedures that are just as safe or riskier (Reed 2021, 252–253).

Clinical experts concur that providing medication abortion does not require specialized facilities, and that these services can be provided safely through telemedicine (NAS 2018). For in-office visits, "a typical medical office with space for private consultation, physical examination, equipment and medication for handling an allergic reaction suffices along with a capacity to arrange for a urine pregnancy test and RH typing" (Nippita and Paul 2018, 794–795). "Medical abortion is well-suited to the scope of practice of primary care providers, including nurse practitioners, nurse midwives, and physicians' assistants" (Nippita and Paul 2018, 794).

However, this scope of practice may not be permitted by state law (Chapter 3).

Aspiration abortion is the second most common abortion procedure in the United States and is a minimally invasive gynecological procedure. It generally takes fewer than 10 minutes; it may be used up to 14 to 16 weeks of gestation. Medical experts concur that "vacuum aspiration using local cervical anesthesia . . . can be provided safely and appropriately in a medical office setting" (Nippita and Paul 2018, 802; Paul and Stein 2011, 716). The office should be equipped with the same emergency back-up and supplies needed to provide injectable medications (drugs and resuscitation equipment to manage an allergic reaction, seizure, or cardiac arrest) (Nippita and Paul 2018; Paul and Stein 2011, 716). Although most states limit abortion provision to physicians, in the few states without such restrictions, advanced practice clinicians (e.g., nurse practitioners) "have provided aspiration abortions for years with an impressive safety record" (Nippita and Paul 2018, 802; Renner et al. 2015; Berer 2009; Weitz et al. 2009). As the use of medical abortion continues to increase, the proportion of abortions performed by aspiration is expected to decline (NAS 2018).

Starting at 16 weeks of gestation, "the most common method for abortion in the United States is dilation and evacuation (D&E), a procedure that combines aspiration with the use of extracting forceps" (Nippita and Stein 2018, 805). Both "the procedure and the concomitant required skills for medical personnel are similar to those for the surgical management of miscarriage after 14 weeks' gestation. D&E requires clinicians with advanced training and/or experience, a more complex set of surgical skills relative to those required for aspiration abortion, and an adequate caseload to maintain these surgical skills" (NAS 2018, 101).

Induction abortion is the termination of pregnancy using medications to induce delivery of the fetus. In the United States, induction abortion is the most infrequently used of all abortion methods, but estimates vary. A 2013 study reported that induction accounted for approximately 2 percent of all abortions at 14 weeks of gestation (NAS 2018, 29). However, calculations by the National Academy of Sciences (2018) showed that induction abortion accounted for only 0.54 percent of all abortions performed at a gestational age of 14 weeks or more.[14]

These rare procedures may be performed because of a lethal fetal abnormality (Hern 2021), a stillbirth, or fetal demise. Because of state gestational bans, many of these procedures can be performed in only a few US states.[15] Therefore, women who face these grave medical situations often must travel great distances to obtain appropriate care or forgo it altogether (Megas 2017).

Abortion Providers

Since the 1980s, both the number and mix of abortion providers have changed. In 1985, there were 2,680 abortion providers in the United States. By 2017, the number of abortion providers had declined more than 40 percent to 1,587. These national totals, however, mask regional declines. The Southern states experienced the biggest decreases, losing 50 clinics from 2011 to 2017, with Texas losing the most. In the same period, the number of abortion providers in the Midwest dropped by 33, whereas the Western states lost a net of seven clinics. By contrast, the Northeast added a net of 59 clinics, the majority of which were in New Jersey and New York (Nash and Dreweke 2019).

From 2017 to 2020, the total number of abortion providers remained about the same at 808 abortion clinics (2017) and 807 (2020). What did change was the regional distribution of abortion clinics. The "number of clinics increased in the Midwest (11%) and in the West (6%) and decreased in the Northeast and in the South (3%)" (Jones et al. 2022a, 134). These regional data, of course, mask state differences. Within individual states, the loss of even one clinic can have substantial impact, a phenomenon discussed in more detail in Chapter 5. Following the *Dobbs* decision, the number of abortion clinics has dropped, particularly in states that have banned abortion altogether (Kirstein et al. 2022).

Types of Abortion Providers

Specialized abortion providers are those for whom at least half of patient visits are for abortion services. Over time, the proportion of total abortion providers that specialize in this service has been consistent: 15 percent in 1985, 16 percent in 2017, and 14 percent in 2020 (table 1.5). Both hospitals and physicians' offices have decreased in overall importance. Nonspecialized clinics have become more prominent, reflecting the shift

TABLE 1.5

Percentages of Abortion Providers by Type of Facility, Various Years

Year	Specialized abortion clinic	Non-specialized medical clinic	Hospital	Physician's office
1985	15	16	44	24
1988	16	18	40	25
1992	19	19	36	27
1996	22	20	34	23
2000	25	21	33	21
2005	21	24	34	21
2008	21	26	34	19
2011	19	30	35	17
2014	16	31	38	15
2017	16	35	33	16
2020	14	36	33	17

Sources: Data for 1985 from Henshaw et al. (1987), data for 1988 from Henshaw and Van Vort (1990), data for 1992 from Henshaw and Van Vort (1994), data for 1996 from Henshaw (1998a), data for 2000 from Finer and Henshaw (2003), data for 2005 from Jones et al. (2008), data for 2008 from Jones and Kooistra (2011), data for 2011 from Jones and Jerman (2014), data for 2014 from Jones and Jerman (2017a), data for 2017 from Jones et al. (2019), and data for 2020 from Jones et al. (2022).

Note: Percentages may not add to 100 because of rounding in the original sources.

toward medication abortion (table 1.5) (Jones et al. 2022a; Jones et al. 2022b; Jones et al. 2019; Henshaw and Van Vort 1990).

Caseloads of Abortion Providers

Specialized abortion clinics still account for most abortions in the United States (table 1.6). In 1992, specialized abortion clinics accounted for 69 percent of abortions (Henshaw and Van Vort 1994). By 2014, specialized abortion clinics still provided the majority of abortions (60 percent), even though they represented only 19 percent of the providers. By 2020, the percentage of abortions provided by specialized providers had declined to 54 percent, again reflecting the shift toward medication abortions.

Nonspecialized medical clinics, which offer a variety of medical services, now provide 35 percent of abortions, most of which are medication abortions. Together, hospitals and physicians' offices only provided 4 percent of abortions in the United States in 2020, down from 17 percent in 1985 (Jones et al. 2022a; Jones et al. 2019; NAS 2018).

Most abortion facilities offer both early medication and aspiration abortions. In 2014, 87 percent of nonhospital abortion providers offered medication abortions. Most "facilities offering only early medication abortions are located in metropolitan areas that are also served by facilities offering surgical abortion" (Jones and Jerman 2017a, 22). Across the coun-

TABLE 1.6
Percentage of Total Abortions Performed in Each Type of Facility, Various Years

Year	Specialized abortion clinic	Non-specialized medical clinic	Hospital	Physician's office
1985	60	23	13	4
1988	64	22	10	4
1992	69	20	7	4
1996	70	21	7	3
2000	71	22	5	2
2005	69	25	5	2
2008	70	24	4	1
2011	63	31	4	1
2014	59	36	4	1
2017	60	35	3	1
2020	54	43	3	1

Source: Data for 1985 from Henshaw et al. (1988), data for 1988 from Henshaw and Van Vort (1990), data for 1992 from Henshaw and Van Vort (1994); data for 1996 from Henshaw (1998), data for 2000 from Finer and Henshaw (2003), data for 2005 from Jones et al. (2008), data for 2011 from Jones and Jerman (2014), data for 2014 from Jones and Jerman (2017a), data for 2017 from Jones et al. (2019), and data for 2020 from Jones et al. (2022).

Note: Percentages may not add to 100 because of rounding in the original sources.

TABLE 1.7
Percentages of Medication Abortions by Type of Provider, Various Years

Year	Specialized abortion clinic	Non-specialized clinic	Physician's office
2005	57	40	3
2008	53	45	2
2011	52	46	2
2014	46	52	2
2017	53	45	2
2020	47	52	1

Sources: Data for 2000 from Finer and Henshaw (2003), data for 2005 from Jones et al. (2008), data for 2011 from Jones and Jerman (2014), data for 2014 from Jones and Jerman (2017a), data for 2017 from table 6 of Jones et al. (2019, 20), and data for 2020 from Jones et al. 2022a.

try, fewer facilities offer later-gestation procedures, and availability decreases with gestational age.[16]

Providers of Medication Abortion

Over time, nonspecialized providers have become more important in dispensing medication abortion (table 1.7). In 2005, most medication abortions were provided by specialized abortion clinics. By 2020, only 47 percent of medication abortions were provided by these clinics, and nonspecialized clinics provided the majority of clinic-based medication abortions. Doctors' offices played a minor and decreasing role.

Self-Managed Abortions and Telemedicine

This discussion of current abortion practice would be incomplete without mentioning self-managed abortion (SMA). SMA refers to the practice of a woman terminating her own pregnancy outside of a medical setting. SMA "encompasses a wide array of experiences—ingesting herbs, massage, drinking tisanes, using a combination of abortion medications (mifepristone and misoprostol), using misoprostol alone, inserting objects into the vagina, using a combination of these methods, and other methods" (Reed 2021, 232).

SMA is not a new practice, but its incidence is on the rise. A national survey conducted in 2017 estimated that 1.4 percent of reproductive aged women have attempted SMA, mostly with ineffective methods. The two most common reasons women gave for attempting self-managed abortion were (1) this method seemed faster or easier than other alternatives, and (2) a clinic-based abortion was too expensive (Ralph et al. 2020).

Although SMA and telemedicine abortion are separate concepts, in practice, they are increasingly convergent. Telemedicine abortion "refers to a medical abortion that is prescribed via a virtual abortion consultation and is supervised by an authorized health care professional" (Reed 2021, 233). Self-managed abortion refers to a person ending her "own pregnancy without a doctor's prescription or supervision" (Reed 2021, 233). As access to clinical abortion services has become more restricted in the US, more women have been turning to a hybrid of SMA and telemedical abortion.

This trend was in place even before the *Dobbs* decision. A study of US women requesting medication abortion through a telemedicine site in 2017 showed that women from states with more abortion restrictions (hostile) were more likely to request information about self-managed abortion than women from states with fewer abortion restrictions (supportive) (Aiken et al. 2020b). Data collected from 2019–2020 showed that this behavior intensified during the COVID-19 pandemic (Aiken et al. 2020a), with nearly 50,000 US residents requesting abortion medication from a single online provider, AID Access.[17] Similarly, after Texas' abortion ban went into effect in September 2021, the number of requests for abortion medication from the same provider increased dramatically (Aiken et al. 2022b).

Since the 2022 *Dobbs* decision, more research has documented an increase in requests for self-managed abortions, particularly from women in states that implemented total abortion bans. A recent study shows that the five states with the largest increases were Louisiana, Mississippi, Arkansas, Alabama, and Oklahoma (Aiken et al. 2022c). Another recent study demonstrated the safety of self-managed medication abortion in the US using online telemedicine, showing that it can be highly effective with low rates of serious adverse events (Aiken et al. 2022a).

For the most part, self-managed abortions are not included in estimates of the total number abortions or abortion rates, which reflect abortions that occur in clinical settings (Jones et al. 2022a). As the proportion of self-managed abortions increases, the undercount of total abortions will become larger if only pregnancy terminations occurring in clinical settings are enumerated.

Regulation and Abortion

Definition of Regulation

Regulation is any attempt by a government to control the behavior of individuals, organizations, or subgovernments[18] (Meier 1985). Regulations have the force of law; thus, governments can compel their implementation. Most regulatory policy is implemented by government agencies, which are charged with ensuring compliance with state or federal legislation. An example from abortion regulation is when states mandate their health departments or other administrative entities to inspect abortion clinics for compliance with state policies.

Regulations can target either the demand for or the supply of goods and services. In the case of abortion services, regulations can target patient behavior (demand side), or they can be aimed at modifying provider behavior (supply side) (Joyce 2011). For example, for patients, regulating the availability of contraception can cause demand for abortion to increase or decrease. For providers, licensing requirements for abortion clinics could cause the supply of abortion services to increase or decrease.

Scope of Abortion Regulation

Abortion regulations include both *restrictions,* policies that impede women's access to abortion, and *protections,* policies that safeguard abortion access.[19] This regulatory scope can be broadened to reproductive freedom, which also considers laws that restrict or promote access to contraception (NARAL Pro Choice America 2021; Petchansky 1980). Clearly, reproductive freedom and abortion are related; access to contraception lowers unintended pregnancy, which, in turn, decreases abortion demand.

The focus of this book is on abortion regulation. Therefore, the determinants and impacts of abortion restrictions and protections are central concerns. We are explicit when we broaden the analysis and discussion to include contraceptive access or reproductive freedom more broadly.

Forms of Government Regulation

Regulatory policies encompass many types of government interventions (Rice 2013, 9); six common regulatory forms are presented in the first column of table 1.8. The most prevalent regulatory strategy is **price regulation**, where a government entity or agent determines the price that can be charged for a good or service. A permutation of traditional price regulation is modified price regulation, which impacts the price consumers pay. **Franchising** or **licensing** is another form of regulation where public or quasi-public agencies "permit or deny an individual the right to do business in a specified occupation or industry" (Meier 1985, 1). **Standard setting** is when a government establishes regulatory standards for a product or production process. The **direct allocation of resources** is another regulatory strategy that governments can employ. A related strategy is **operating subsidies**; here, governments subsidize individuals or organizations for the purpose of changing behavior. Finally, regulations can promote **fair competition**, where a government agency monitors the market for fair practices (Meier 1985, 1–2).

Forms of Abortion Regulation

Five of the six types of government regulation are found in current abortion policies (table 1.8). If policies that address contraceptive access are included, then all six regulatory forms are represented.

TABLE 1.8
Forms of Regulation and Applications to Abortion Restrictions

Form of regulation	Application to abortion
Price regulation	Ban on Medicaid abortions (Hyde Amendment)
Franchising or licensing	Require physicians to have hospital privileges
Standard setting	Mandatory counseling with specific content
Direct allocation of resources	Applicable to contraceptive funding. The federal government gives grants to the states for contraceptive services
Operating subsidies	Funding CPCs to dissuade women from abortion
Fair competition	Protection of abortion clinics

Source: Adapted from Meier (1986).

Medicaid is a cost-sharing program funded by both the federal government and the states. The purpose of state Medicaid programs is to subsidize health care services for low-income persons. By prohibiting states from including abortion services in their Medicaid programs, the federal Hyde Amendment offers an example of **modified price regulation**. In traditional price regulation, the government regulator sets the price (or price range) that an individual can charge for a good or service. In the case of the Hyde Amendment, this regulation effectively raises the price of abortion for low-income individuals.[20] Low-income women, whose health care is subsidized by Medicaid for most services, have to pay the full price for abortion.[21] At upward of $500 for an early-gestation medication abortion (Knueven 2023),[22] this regulation makes the cost of abortion prohibitive for many women (Reed 2021, 236), especially because abortion is a time-sensitive service.[23]

Abortion regulation also employs **franchising** or **licensing**. Some states, such as Ohio (Chapter 5), license and inspect all facilities offering outpatient surgery, including abortion. Other states, such as Missouri, mandate that physicians performing these services must have hospital privileges within a certain distance of the clinic providing abortions. Many states require that only physicians provide surgical abortion or dispense medication abortion, despite the evidence that this service can be delivered safely by trained nurses, midwives, and physician assistants (Nippita and Paul 2018; Taylor et al. 2018; Paul and Stein 2011).[24]

In recent years, state abortion regulation through **standard setting** has become more common. Mandated counseling for abortion patients is one manifestation of this type of regulation. Here, states require abortion providers to use detailed counseling protocols, transmitting specific information, much of which is medically inaccurate (Daniels et al. 2016).

Neither the federal government nor the states **directly allocate funds or other resources** to clinics providing abortion services.[25] However, if the scope of regulation is broadened to include contraception, both the federal and state governments fund family planning services, albeit at different levels.[26]

Some states directly **subsidize** Crisis Pregnancy Centers (CPCs). Far more numerous than abortion providers, CPCs have the purpose of dissuading women from having abortions (Ehrlich and Doan 2019). States support CPCs directly with dedicated funding and indirectly by referring patients to them (NARAL Pro-Choice America 2014, 18).[27] This is discussed further in Chapter 3.

To a limited extent, some states and the federal government, issue regulations **to protect clinics from unfair practices.** These include regulations against blocking clinic entrances, harassing patients, and other actions designed to put abortion clinics out of business.

Politics of Regulation

Decisions about regulating specific activities are political. Politicians at both the state and federal levels have the authority to decide whether to limit or encourage specific activities. They can set penalties for violating regulations, and they can offer incentives for compliance. Because "the likelihood of coercion is more immediate and applicable to the individual," regulatory policies usually "result in more contentious politics than distributive policies[28] or redistributive policies"[29] (Smith and Larimer 2017, 34). High levels of bargaining and floor activity, along with numerous amendments, often accompany legislative deliberations about regulatory policies. In this highly charged arena, advocacy groups and politicians argue over the targets, conditions, and costs of government regulation. The result is "unstable, combative and divisive politics" (Smith and Larimer 201, 34).

Although generally contentious, regulatory politics also vary by the nature of the topic under consideration. Here, salience and complexity are the most important characteristics. Salience is the public prominence of an issue. Complexity refers to the degree of technical knowledge required to understand it (Gormley 1986, 597).

Most public issues have low salience, that is, they fly under the public radar. Exceptions occur when an issue affects a large number of people in a significant way. Highly salient issues include widely perceived threats to safety, economic security, and moral values (Gormley 1986, 601). COVID-19, for example, was highly salient throughout 2020 and 2021 and continued into 2022 because the pandemic threatened both people's lives and their economic security.

Technical complexity means that specialized knowledge and training are needed to address factual questions about an issue. In terms of public perception, an issue's technical complexity is not fixed. How advocates frame an issue can manipulate citizen perception (Haider-Markel 2020).

Participants in Regulatory Politics

Those who participate in regulatory politics can be divided into regular and irregular players. Regular players are nearly always present for regulatory politics; they include the public officials entrusted with the regulatory process and representatives of the regulated industry. Irregular (or sometimes) players are politicians, citizens, journalists, judges, and professionals (Gormley 1986).

Whether irregular (or sometimes) players become involved in regulatory politics depends on the issue at hand. Politicians are drawn to issues that are highly salient, but they are repelled by issues that are technically complex. Similarly, both citizens' groups and journalists are attracted to highly salient issues, but are less likely to become involved in technically complex issues. Judges are more likely to become involved in highly salient issues, regardless of their technical complexity. Business groups are more likely to become involved in issues that are both highly salient and technically complex. Bureaucrats[30] and professionals are both more likely to be involved in regulatory politics when the issues are technically complex, regardless of the salience of those issues (Gormley 1986).

Patterns of Regulatory Politics

Each combination of salience and complexity produces a distinct policy domain with a particular constellation of political players (table 1.9). In

TABLE 1.9
Typology of Issue Politics by Issue Salience and Complexity, with Dominant Participants

Salience	Complexity	
	Low	High
High	**Hearing room politics** Participants: politicians, citizens' groups, journalists (media), judges	**Operating room politics** Participants: upper-level bureaucrats, citizens' groups, journalists (media)
Low	**Street-level politics** Participants: lower-level bureaucrats	**Board room politics** Participants: business groups, bureaucrats, professionals

Source: Adapted from Gormley (1986).

the **hearing room domain** (high salience and low complexity), politicians, citizen groups, and journalists give the issue at hand an open airing. Politicians make the decisions here with input from citizen groups and with ample media coverage. Theoretically, at least, these decisions are subject to "gentle, judicial review" (Gormley 1986).

In **operating room** politics (high salience and high complexity), decisions are made largely by upper-level bureaucrats, with potential influence from politicians, citizen groups, and the media. Here, bureaucrats, most often highly trained professionals, must balance simultaneous pressures for accountability and expertise. Unless they have deep pockets, citizens' groups are disadvantaged by the issue's complexity. With enough resources, however, citizens' groups may challenge the factual claims of the regulated organizations, the bureaucrats, or both. Legal action may ensue. This policy domain is characterized by extensive low-quality media coverage, where the focus is on the human drama, rather than the facts.[31]

In **street-level politics** (low salience, low complexity), low-level bureaucrats make the decisions, however trivial. Lacking expertise, they tend to focus on regulatory minutia, not overall priorities. These patterns persist because there is little accountability.

In **board room politics** (low salience and high complexity), business groups dominate the decision-making about how industries are regulated. Bureaucrats and professionals also participate, but seldom make policy. Judicial review, however, is unusual (Gormley 1986).

Pathologies of Regulatory Politics

Pitfalls bedevil each of these regulatory policy domains. Hearing room politics are contentious, and even corrosive, as adversaries argue their positions. In this setting, politicians do respond to citizens, but rarely to underprivileged ones. Operating room politics often address crises, rushing upper-level bureaucrats to produce politically feasible and technically defensible regulations (e.g., COVID-19). Solutions are seldom cost-effective, and little planning occurs. Street-level politics foster ad hoc rules and uneven enforcement. There is little sense of overall goals, and even less progress. Private sector entities, usually those being regulated, make most of the decisions in board room politics. Government regulators tend to acquiesce and lend their support (Gormley 1986)

Regulatory Politics and Abortion

Most policies about regulating abortion are developed through hearing room politics. Abortion is a highly public salient issue, typically framed as having low technical complexity. Here, politicians dominate policy-making. The issue's high salience offers electoral rewards for acting, and its perceived low complexity means that messages about abortion regulation are easy to communicate to constituents (Meier 1988).

Citizens groups and journalists also participate in the hearing room. Because their pro-choice or anti-abortion messages are so understandable, citizens can easily mobilize and take part (Gormley 1986, 608). Picking up on citizen interest, the media often provides extensive coverage (Gormley 1986, 608).[32] In hearing room politics, each of these political players become involved at all levels of decision-making, including legislative committees, public hearings, press briefings, and legislative deliberations.

However, not all abortion regulations are decided in the hearing room. The range of possible abortion regulations is so extensive that, occasionally, regulatory decisions are made in operating room politics. In these cases, deliberations require technical expertise to understand the issue. Examples of this type of issue complexity are whether women suffer mental health, fertility, or economic problems because they had an abortion or were denied abortion (Foster 2020; Myers 2017). The fabricated link between abortion and breast cancer provides another example of where complex technical studies have been used to debunk this claim (NAS 2018, 148–149; Kulczycki 2015, 184).

Operating politics are the purview of upper-level bureaucrats who are charged with making technically and legally sound decisions. When these bureaucrats produce unacceptable results, advocacy or citizens groups may go to court. An example of this situation was the FDA requirement that women seeking medication abortion had to pick up their pills in person, even during the COVID-19 epidemic, as mentioned in the Introduction. The ACOG sued the FDA over this regulation. As regulatory politics theory would predict, at times, courts have been "willing to overturn important agency decisions in highly complex issue areas" (Gormley 1986, 614). That scenario certainly played out in this case, although the Supreme Court eventually stepped in, overruling the lower federal court and supporting the FDA regulation.[33]

Neither street-level nor board room politics are likely in abortion regulation. Abortion is too salient an issue for its politics to fly under the public radar. Even judicial bypasses permitting pregnant teens to obtain abortion without parental consent or minor abortion clinic violations (e.g., width of the clinic hall) are likely to be publicly reported and draw public attention.

Other Influences on Abortion Regulation

MORALITY POLITICS

State abortion policies are largely regulatory; they govern both access to and delivery of abortion services. The nature of the abortion issue also means that morality[34] politics come into play. These politics accompany issues where at least one set of participants "defines an issue in terms of morality–often based on religious principles" (Haider-Markel 2020, x). Opposing groups often frame morality issues in absolute terms, thus intensifying conflict and decreasing the likelihood of compromise (Weissert and Weissert 2019; Mooney 2001).

Morality politics intensify the hearing room dynamics found in regulatory politics. Religious groups often participate along with politicians and citizens' groups. In hearing room politics, messaging is easy to understand. However, discussions are likely to include declarations about morals and other core values. Whereas negotiation is common in most regulatory politics, the introduction of uncompromising positions precludes any negotiation.

In contemporary US society, abortion is a classic morality issue (Adam et al. 2020).[35] Often, both pro-choice and anti-abortion proponents frame their positions in stark moral terms, but not always. Recent evidence shows that both sides are strategic in how they frame issues during legislative debates (Candal 2020; Mucciaroni et al. 2019).[36] Although we would argue that the abortion issue embodies a great deal of profundity (Finer et al. 2005), this depth is usually missing from public discussions and public messaging. Most Americans think that they understand the issue, and they "have staked out a position. In a 1992 national survey, only five respondents, 0.3 percent of the sample had no opinion on the abortion question" (Weissert and Weissert 2018, 31). In a series of questions regarding the conditions under which abortion should be allowed and whether abortion should be funded (questions CC20_332a–g), the 2020 Cooperative Election Study (CES) revealed similar findings. Out of over 60,000 respondents, less than 0.05 percent failed to register an opinion in support or opposition to the abortion policy alternatives (Cooperative Election Study 2020).

MORALITY POLITICS AND THE US SUPREME COURT

Given its power of ultimate judicial review, the US Supreme Court frequently adjudicates disputes over morality policies. Consequently, "practically every piece of scholarship on morality policies includes a discussion of US Supreme Court decisions" (Patton 2007, 470). Within state legislatures, lawmakers are likely to be attentive to the Supreme Court when considering a particular policy based on the known or assumed future position of the Supreme Court (Patton 2007).

Among morality policies, abortion issues are emblematic. Since 1973, the US Supreme Court has heard over 40 abortion-related cases, most of which have come from the states. Empirical work on state abortion policies (1973–2005) showed that states were *most* likely to adopt abortion decisions prior to Court involvement and after the Court has deemed a policy constitutional. States were also more likely to adopt an abortion policy while it was under consideration by the Court than if it had been ruled unconstitutional (Patton 2007).[37]

GENDER POLITICS

In addition to being a morality issue, abortion is a gender or feminist issue, a manifestation of a polity's commitment to female autonomy and reproductive rights. Several scales have been developed to measure the ease with which women can access abortion services. Correlates of abortion policy include women's economic participation (e.g., women in the labor force), women's political power (e.g., women's political representation), and religion (e.g., degree of religiosity) (Forman-Rabinovici and Sommer 2018).

Religions differ widely in their perspectives on abortion (Forman-Rabinovici and Sommer 2018; Masci 2018); their abortion positions tend to be related to how they conceptualize the role of women. In the United States, the Roman Catholic Church, the Southern Baptist Convention, and the Lutheran Church–Missouri Synod are examples of denominations that oppose all abortion rights with rare exceptions. The United Church of Christ, the Presbyterian Church (U.S.A.), and Reform Judaism are representative of religions that support abortion rights with few exceptions. The Episcopal Church and the United Methodist Church support abortion rights with some limits (Masci 2018).

Recent work on global feminist policies has shown that the role of religion differs by type of abortion issue. Religion is a pivotal influence for legalizing abortion, but not for offering public funding for abortion. Leftist or progressive political strength and women's representation are associated with abortion funding (Htun and Weldon 2018)

In addition to religion, women's political representation influences abortion regulation. Critical mass theory posits that as the number of woman legislators grows, they are likely to become a coherent force in passing laws supporting women's rights (Childs and Krook 2008). Female legislators, however, are not always like-minded. Specifying the conditions under which a coalition of female legislators and their allies can lead to women's substantive representation in different policy areas, including abortion, is ongoing work (Lee and Jongkon 2020; Childs and Krook 2009).

Myths of Abortion Regulation

Several myths obfuscate the study of abortion regulation. These myths are widely accepted by politicians, advocacy groups, students and scholars of abortion regulation, and the general public. Because these myths are inaccurate or only partially accurate, they limit serious deliberations on abortion regulation reform. Consequently, lawmakers and advocates often respond to the myths rather than the true shortcomings of abortion regulation. Three prominent myths about abortion regulation (Meier 1985, 4) are highlighted in the next sections.[38]

ABORTION REGULATION MIRRORS PUBLIC OPINION

Most Americans favor legal abortion. Indeed, pro-choice public opinion has increased in recent years (Pew Research Center 2022). Yet the number of abortion restrictions has continued to mount. Moreover, the US Supreme Court recently vacated both *Roe v. Wade* (1973) and *Planned Parenthood of Southeastern Pennsylvania v. Casey* (1992), thus allowing states to ban abortion altogether.

One explanation for this contradiction is that abortion has not been a top priority for many voters. For example, Donald Trump campaigned on an anti-abortion platform in 2016, saying that he would appoint justices who would overturn *Roe*. Twenty-seven percent of those who voted for President Trump in 2016 said that abortion should be a matter of personal choice; 14 percent more thought that abortion should be permitted if need were established (ANES 2016). Clearly, these voters did not prioritize abortion. Public opinion polls since the *Dobbs* decision, however, show that abortion is becoming important to voters, especially Democrats (Tessler 2022).

Public opinion on abortion varies by how questions are framed (Cooperative Congressional Election Study 2016).[39] To some extent, the variance in state public opinion coincides with the variance in state abortion regulation. States with public opinion most opposed to abortion are among the states with the highest number of restrictions and fewest protections. Except for Rhode Island, states with the most pro-choice public opinion have among the fewest abortion restrictions.[40]

Lawmakers also misperceive public opinion. Recent work from political science showed that politicians from both parties dramatically overestimate their constituents' support for conservative policies on a range of issues, including abortion. Republican legislators drive much of this distortion, leading them to support policies far more conservative than public preferences (Broockman and Skovron 2018).

Other representational concerns with this myth remain. Low-income women, particularly low-income women of color, are less likely to participate in public opinion surveys, less likely to contact their legislators (Broockman and Skovron 2018), and less likely to vote. Consequently, the voices of the population most impacted by abortion regulation are muted.

ABORTION REGULATION IS ONLY SYMBOLIC

A second myth is that abortion regulation is only symbolic. Abortion restrictions may be on the books, but they can be overcome. In other words, any woman can get an abortion if she really wants or needs to terminate her pregnancy. Believing this myth may make it easier for a legislator to vote in support of a new abortion restriction pushed by a vociferous interest group.

But abortion restrictions matter. Before the *Dobbs* decision, women who lived in states with four or more abortion restrictions were much more likely to perceive that access to both procedural and medication abortions was difficult compared with women in states with fewer restrictions. These perceptions could discourage them from even seeking abortion (Perreira 2020), especially where there are gestational limits. So, if a woman lives in a state where abortion is heavily regulated or banned altogether, she may not even try to get one.

For those women who decide to seek abortion, this quest was aptly called an "obstacle course," well before the *Dobbs* decision (Cohen and Joffe 2020). Women in states with abortion restrictions, but not outright bans, face required waiting periods, state-mandated yet medically inaccurate counseling, unnecessary tests, state-supported fake clinics, high costs, and more. Moreover, these restrictions have real impacts. In Chapter 5, we demonstrate that abortion restrictions reduce state abortion rates, increase out-of-state travel for abortion, and disproportionately impact women of color.

ABORTION REGULATION PROTECTS WOMEN

This myth is the most long-lived. Over time, the canard has morphed somewhat, but its essence is the same: women need protection from their own decisions.

In the mid-nineteenth century, elite male physicians in the nascent American Medical Association noted that affluent women were increasingly turning to abortion to limit the size of their families. Drawing upon their purportedly learned beliefs, these doctors stressed that women's physiology rendered them "incapable of self-governance" (Ehrlich and Doan 2019, 9). In the political arena, they argued convincingly for replacing the flexible common law approach to abortion with a strict statutory regime. By 1900, abortion was a crime in every state (Mohr 1978, 229–230).

These criminal abortion laws were in place for much of the twentieth century. But they did not protect women. Instead, women faced back alleys, untrained operators, and often death. By the 1960s, even the American Medical Association was clamoring for changes in abortion law (Tribe 1992).

Similar justifications have been used to support abortion regulation in the late twentieth and early twenty-first centuries. Women need waiting periods to reconsider their abortion decisions. Certain types of abortion procedures and medications must be prohibited or heavily restricted because pregnant women do not really understand their ramifications (Erhlich and Doan 2019).

A recent exhaustive study revealed this myth's endgame. Women denied abortion because of state gestational limits fared far worse healthwise, economically, and psychologically than women who were able to access abortion. Over time, these differences persisted and even magnified (Foster 2020).

The Study of Abortion Regulation

There are many ways to study abortion regulation. Legal approaches focus on the law as well as legal concepts such as the right to privacy, criteria for informed consent, and what constitutes an undue burden (Goldman

2021; Ziegler 2020; Ehrlich 2018; Ziegler 2018; Tribe 1992). Historical approaches position abortion regulation within broader forces in society (Ziegler 2020; Ziegler 2015; Garrow 1998; Meier 1985; Mohr 1978). Economic approaches examine both the short-term and long-term impacts from abortion regulation (Myers 2017; Colman and Joyce 2011; Joyce 2011).

Abortion regulation has been fruitfully studied by scholars in a wide range of disciplines. Because the process of regulating abortion is complicated, it "contains facets amenable to study in different ways" (Meier 1985, 7). Evaluating the safety of a certain procedure or medication is a medical and epidemiological endeavor (NAS 2018). Assessing the constitutionality of a particular regulatory strategy is a legal question (e.g., Ziegler 2020; Tribe 1992). Determining the impact of an abortion regulation on the price of the procedure is an economic question (e.g., Gonzalez et al. 2020). Assessing the barriers for women seeking abortion is a sociological question (e.g., Cohen and Joffe 2020; Foster 2020).

This study borrows insights, concepts, and methods from each of these fields, but it relies most heavily on the perspectives of political science and public health. The book's approach, however, does deviate in some respects from both traditional political science and traditional public health.

Political science is an academic discipline devoted to the study of governments, public institutions, and political behavior at different levels, such as individuals, states, and countries. Political scientists describe and analyze how collective decisions are made and whom they impact. The traditional focus of political science is "on the broad picture and the search for general propositions about human behavior rather than on the specific levers that policymakers can manipulate in a particular situation" (Mazmanian and Sabatier 1989, 18). Most scholarly work in political science endeavors to understand political phenomena but takes a hands-off approach to the world of action.

Public health is an applied interdisciplinary field focused on population health at the local, state, national, and global levels. Public health has a preventive focus. Conducting applied research and developing policy recommendations are tools of public health (CDC Foundation 2023). Traditionally, public health has had an uneasy relationship with politics.

Public health endeavors to be scientific, which many public health professionals believe is antithetical to politics (Galea and Vaughan 2019; Institute of Medicine 1988). As a result, public health scholars seldom study how collective decisions are made.

This book merges the strengths of both political science and public health to analyze and understand abortion regulation and its impact. We use constructs from political science to understand how and why collective decisions are made. We use the population perspective from public health to assess how politics and political decisions influence the health status of women. We emulate both fields when we consider how Western European countries regulate abortion and what difference those regulations make. Then, at the end of our analysis, we offer policy prescriptions.

Our Approach to Studying Abortion Regulation

The purpose of this book is to explain state abortion regulation and assess its impact, not to test or advocate for a single theoretical approach. Accordingly, we rely on constructs from regulatory, morality, and feminist politics and more to study the development and implementation of state abortion policies. We use concepts, measures, and methods from public health, demography, economics, and more to examine the impact of abortion regulation. We draw liberally from other literature to understand the dynamics of specific trends in particular states and time periods (Sciubba 2011, 5).

Both regulatory and morality politics highlight the role of politicians. Gormley (1986)'s typology of regulatory politics does not separate these political principals into governors and legislators (Gerber and Teske 2020), but here, we examine both categories of state politicians. Because morality politics stresses politicians' adherence to partisanship (Doan and McFarlane 2012), we look at each category by political party. Borrowing from critical mass theory and more (Lee and Jongdon 2020), we examine how the presence of women legislators by party affects state abortion regulations. We note the dearth of racial and ethnic diversity among state politicians.

The hearing room scenario in Gormley's typology of regulatory politics stresses the role of citizens or advocacy groups. Although conceptually important, measuring the size and efforts of advocacy groups at the state level has proven to be a formidable task. State-level financial contributions for abortion-related issues are available, and we have used them as a proxy for citizens groups. We note that these data present challenges as well (further discussed in Chapter 4).

The morality politics literature stresses the role of religious groups (Haider-Markel 2020; Permoser 2019; Kreitzer et al. 2018; Kreitzer 2015). Drawing from an extensive database, we identify the denominations and congregants most likely to oppose abortion and examine their roles in the development of state abortion restrictions and protections.

By analyzing both policy development and implementation, this book implicitly incorporates sequential policy stages: policy development and policy impact.[41] This approach "is useful for its simplicity and direction" (Smith and Larimer 2017, 29). Although there is considerable discussion in political science about the merits of policy stages, this heuristic remains a useful way of organizing a policy narrative (Smith and Larimer 2017).

This book has two goals that sometimes come into conflict. One goal is to explain abortion regulation in the United States. The second goal is to suggest specific changes in how abortion is regulated. The positivist scientific tradition employed by both political science and public health scholarship suggests that empirical analysis should be separated from value judgments.

This separation seldom occurs with abortion policy. Most abortion research has policy objectives or was instigated by normative concerns. An example of a normative concern is what policy measures are most likely to improve women's health. We believe these kinds of concerns are entirely appropriate, and they are consistent with mores in both public health and political science. Public health is unabashedly dedicated to improving population health. Political science, particularly within the realm of public policy, does consider how to improve policy outcomes (Smith and Larimer 2017).

Accordingly, this book does not ignore normative issues, nor does it expect the reader to do so. Abortion regulation determines who will have access to pregnancy termination, a topic on which few people can claim neutrality. Rather than "disguise normative presentations as empirical arguments as much of the literature does," this book strives to make its normative contentions explicit (Meier 1985, 8). Although normative and empirical arguments cannot always be differentiated, we have made some effort to do so "by keeping the normative arguments in separate sections and labeling them as such" (Meier 1985, 8).

CHAPTER 2

Setting the Parameters for State Abortion Policies

Historical Background and US Supreme Court Decisions

States are key players in developing abortion regulations because the Tenth Amendment "reserves powers to the states, as long as those powers are not delegated to the federal government" (Cornell Law School 2022; Library of Congress 2022). The US Congress also enacts abortion policies. Of course, both state and federal laws are subject to judicial review (Ainsworth and Hall 2011), and abortion litigation at both levels is unceasing. The US Supreme Court alone has adjudicated more than 40 abortion cases[1] since the 1973 *Roe v. Wade* decision. During the first period (1973–1988), the Court struck down most state restrictions. After the *Webster* (1989) and *Casey* (1992) decisions, however, the Court allowed many more state restrictions to stand, ushering in a new period of upholding state restrictions. In vacating both *Roe* and *Casey*, the 2022 decision on *Dobbs v. Jackson Women's Health Organization* ushered in an entirely new epoch in abortion regulation.

This chapter begins with a brief history of abortion regulation and practice prior to the *Roe v. Wade* decision. Explaining this background is vital. American abortion politics "cannot be understood outside their historical context—past patterns illuminate present policies; and not just as 'background' but as explanations of why things happen" (Morone 1998, xii).

The historical section is followed by a chronology of myriad US Supreme Court decisions addressing abortion regulation. State and lower federal courts certainly issue opinions on abortion laws, but the Supreme Court has the ultimate authority. Well before 1973, the high court was ruling on abortion and reproductive rights at the state level;[2] this chronology, however, focuses on the cases following *Roe*, including the 2022 *Dobbs v. Jackson Women's Health Organization* decision.

No consensus exists among legal scholars, historians, or advocates about which US Supreme Court cases are pivotal for abortion regulation. To decide which cases to include, we consulted several authoritative sources and tallied which cases were cited most frequently in table A.1 of the Appendix. We used this tally as a guide along with our own knowledge and other references in the literature.

This section is divided into three chronological parts. Period One (1973–1989): Striking Down Most Restrictions presents cases following *Roe* up until, but not including, the 1989 *Webster* decision. Period Two (1989–2015): Upholding More State Restrictions begins with the *Webster* and *Casey* decisions, which provided the framework for upholding more, but not all, state restrictions. Period Three (2021–Forward): Undoing *Roe* begins after the death of Ruth Bader Ginsberg in September 2020 and leading up to the *Dobbs v. Jackson Women's Health Organization* decision. These delineations are not perfect, but they capture the overall trends in each period.

Brief History of Abortion (1800–1973)

As of 1800, none of the 16 American states and three territories (US Census Bureau 2021a) "had enacted any statutes whatsoever on the subject of abortion" (Mohr 1978, 3). The "legal status of the practice was governed by traditional British common law as interpreted by the local courts" (Mohr 1978, 3). US jurisprudence followed the tradition in English common law that abortions undertaken before quickening did not constitute homicide and were not considered criminal.[3] Quickening, a notion originating in thirteenth-century theological debates, is when a pregnant woman feels the first movement of the fetus, usually late in the fourth or early in the fifth month (Luker 1984; Mohr 1978). In the early nineteenth century, abortions in the United States performed before quickening were not punishable by law. For abortions occurring after quickening, the woman herself was immune from prosecution (Ehrlich and Doan 2019; Tribe 1992).

In the early nineteenth century, abortion information and services were widely available. Many home health manuals, including William Buchan's popular *Domestic Medicine*, prescribed abortifacient concoctions and other techniques. Folk remedies were also known; the most widely used was juniper extract. Midwives offered both services and abortifacient information, and "physicians sometimes used their knowledge to terminate unwanted pregnancies for their patients" (Mohr 1978, 14).

Abortion was not common, but nor was it rare. From 1820 to 1830, "an estimated one in every twenty-five to thirty pregnancies ended in induced abortion" (Sheeran 1987, 55). In order to hide illicit sexual behavior and avoid its social consequences, single women were more likely than married women to terminate pregnancies. Available evidence suggests that most Americans did not consider early abortion a serious moral issue.

Nevertheless, abortion, like childbirth, was risky in the early nineteenth century (Tribe 1992; Mohr 1978). The safety of pregnancy termination depended on the skill of the operator (e.g., midwife or doctor), the length of gestation, and the method employed (Mohr 1978). Based on the "dubious theory that a dosage sufficient to kill the fetus might spare the woman," a common method of the time was to administer poison to a pregnant woman to induce abortion (Tribe 1992, 29).

Politicians and physicians advocated for the first wave of anti-abortion legislation (1821–1841), ostensibly to protect women's health. Popular support, however, was nonexistent (McFarlane and Meier 2001; Sheeran 1987, 55). In 1821, Connecticut passed the first anti-abortion law, banning the administration of poisons to produce post-quickening abortions. In 1828, the state of New York went further, prohibiting all post-quickening abortions (Tribe 1992). Eventually, ten states and one territory restricted the practice of abortion to some extent (Sheeran 1987, 55), but these laws "were little noticed and rarely enforced" (Rosenblatt 1992, 86).

In 1846, "Massachusetts launched the second wave of anti-abortion legislation by enacting the most restrictive law in the nation" (McFarlane and Meier 2001, 35). Absent any public testimony, only physicians supported this law, which ignored the notion of quickening and included jail sentences for attempted abortions. That year, New York followed suit and passed another anti-abortion state law, disregarding quickening and requiring punishments for both pregnant women and abortionists (McFarlane and Meier 2001, 35; Sheeran 1987, 54–55).

Despite these regulations, the incidence of abortion was increasing. Abortion estimates for 1850–1860 range from one in four to one in six pregnancies. The patient profile was also changing. In 1840, most women seeking abortion were single, but by 1880, most women having abortions were wealthy or comfortably middle class, Protestant, married, and white (Ehrlich 2018; McFarlane and Meier 2001, 36; Sheeran 1987, 55). The practice of abortion was no longer confined to single women trying to hide illicit sexual activity. Prosperous married women were also using abortion to limit the size of their families.

In 1859, the American Medical Association (AMA), led by Dr. Horatio Storer, became the major proponent of anti-abortion legislation. The historical shorthand discussed in the *Roe v. Wade* decision attributes the AMA's efforts to criminalize abortion to protecting the unborn, but a deeper look reveals other motivations (Ehrlich 2018). The AMA's anti-abortion campaign coincided with the nascent organization's efforts to establish monopoly control by physicians over the practice of medicine. The abortion issue "proved the ideal vehicle for this task" (McFarlane and Meier 2001; Luker 1985, 31).

In mid-nineteenth-century America, midwives or other non-physician practitioners frequently provided abortion information and services. By attacking the laxity of abortion law, elite doctors, such as Horatio Storer, "could claim both *moral stature* (as a high-minded, self-regulating group of professionals) and *technical expertise* (derived from their superior training)" (Luker 1985, 31). By repressing abortion, these elite physicians could denigrate non-physicians and lower the demand for other health services that they delivered. Ironically, midwives, who attended childbirth, had better health outcomes during this period than did physicians (Reed 2020).

Storer and his colleagues drew "upon normative understandings of women's divinely ordained place in the domestic and social order, as shaped by racial, class, religious and ethnic considerations" (Ehrlich 2018, 183) to argue that the state should entrust the abortion decision not to women, but to their doctors. Physicians, after all, were "physical guardians" of their female patients, who were "too sure to be warped by personal considerations, and those of the moment" (Ehrlich 2018, 185). Storer warned of "the adverse consequences of trifling with the divine," when a married woman intentionally terminated a pregnancy (Ehrlich 2018, 191).

The AMA anti-abortion activists also fretted about the higher fertility of immigrants, particularly Catholics (e.g., Italian and Irish women), compared with native-born American women (Ehrlich 2018, 183). On this point, Storer was blunt, noting that abortions were "infinitely more frequent among Protestant women than among Catholic" (Mohr 1978, 90). He worried about the future composition of American settlements in the west and south, wondering if "these regions would be peopled by our own children or those of aliens? This is a question our women must answer; upon their loins depends the future destiny of the nation" (Reagan 1997, 11).

Given their demographic aspirations—to people the growing country with native-born white Protestants—it is not surprising that the AMA's anti-abortion campaign ignored non-white women. Although offensive, the racial views of many doctors in that period are noteworthy (Erlich 2018). Some physicians believed the "negro pelvis" had specific characteristics and that whereas "savage women of the dark races gave birth painlessly, civilized white women suffered greatly in childbearing" (Rich 2016, 64).

Religious faiths did not participate in the anti-abortion campaigns occurring before 1850 and did so only sporadically thereafter. Eventually, a few conservative Protestant clergy and an occasional Catholic bishop supported the AMA position. Despite the overblown nativist fears of the AMA physicians, Catholics accounted for only about 10 percent of the country's population in 1860 (Mohr 1978).

The Catholic Church altered its 300-year-old abortion doctrine in 1869, when Pope Pius IX decreed that there was no distinction between an animated and an unanimated fetus. Although this doctrinal change laid the groundwork for "the theological position that all abortion is homicide" (Tribe 1992, 32), the decree was hardly noticed in the United States. No American diocesan papers even reported the Pope's anti-abortion stance (Mohr 1978, 187). The implications of this silence are unclear, however, because nineteenth-century clergy, both Catholic and Protestant, were reticent to address sexual matters (Sheeran 1987, 56).

Organized religion's faltering support did not quell the AMA's anti-abortion momentum. After the Civil War, the anti-obscenity or social purity crusaders, spearheaded by Anthony Comstock, joined forces with the anti-abortion movement. Between 1860 and 1880, 40 state anti-abortion laws were passed. The common element in these laws was that the interruption of gestation at any time during pregnancy was a crime. In large part, this legal situation persisted until the 1960s (Sheeran 1987, 56–57).

Separate from the AMA, Comstock and his social purity movement pushed to restrict contraception as well as abortion. These efforts culminated in 1873, when the US Congress passed the Act for the Suppression of Trade in and Articles of Immoral Use, more commonly known as the Comstock Act. This law prohibited interstate trade in obscene literature and materials, "including any article whatever for the prevention of conception or for causing unlawful abortion" (Brodie 1994, 255–56). Passage of this act marked the federal government's first foray into contraception, abortion, and censorship (Mohr 1978, 197). During the next 15 years, 22 states passed similar legislation. Known as "little Comstock laws," many of these state regulations were more stringent than the federal Comstock law (McFarlane and Meier 2001; Brodie 1994, 257).[4]

By 1900, all but one state[5] had outlawed induced abortion at any stage and made it a criminal offense (Mohr 1978). "Therapeutic abortion," performed to save the life of the woman, was usually the only exception (Rosenblatt 1992, 88). Despite these regulations, an estimated one in three pregnancies ended in abortion during the first half of the twentieth century (Luker 1985).

Over time, the rationale for therapeutic abortions expanded. During the Great Depression, poverty was a widely accepted reason for performing therapeutic abortions. In the 1940s and 1950s, doctors increasingly performed "therapeutic" abortions for psychiatric reasons, especially for women of means. Most abortions in the early twentieth century were not "therapeutic," but illegal and unregulated, resulting in especially high morbidity and mortality rates for poor and rural women. Across the country, however, there were few indictments for performing illegal abortions and even fewer convictions (Tribe 1992, 35).

During the 1950s, local hospital boards increasingly reviewed physicians' decisions to perform therapeutic abortions. Responding to the added scrutiny, the American Law Institute (ALI) revised its Model Penal Code in 1959 to include three defenses against the charge of criminal abortion. The first was that continuation of the pregnancy would gravely impair the physical or mental health of the mother. The second was that the child was likely to be born with grave physical or mental defects. The third defense was that the pregnancy was the result of rape or incest. This widely copied code required certification by two physicians describing the circumstances that justified an abortion (Tribe 1992, 37). At the time the ALI was being drafted, the only opposition came from a Catholic attorney and a priest (Reagan 1997, 221).

Two events in the 1960s attracted more public attention to the abortion issue. One was the large number of babies born with missing or undeveloped limbs because their mothers had taken the sedative thalidomide during pregnancy. The most publicized case was that of Sherri Finkbine, an Arizona mother of four and a television personality. In 1962, Mrs. Finkbine was unable to obtain a legal abortion in the United States despite having taken thalidomide early in pregnancy. The second event was the rubella outbreak of 1962–1965, causing severe birth defects in an estimated 15,000 infants (Tribe 1992, 37).

Ironically, the medical profession, which had successfully lobbied for making abortion a crime a century earlier, became a principal advocate for changing the abortion laws. In 1967, the AMA issued a statement favoring liberalization of these laws. By this time, abortion had become a relatively safe procedure. In 1955, 100 of every 100,000 abortions resulted in the woman's death. By 1972, this number was three in 100,000 (Tribe 1992, 36, 38). Women of color, however, suffered far higher abortion mortality rates, mirroring inequities in the health system and overall health (Reagan 1997, 211–214).

During this period, the last vestiges of the state Comstock laws were coming to an end. In 1965, in *Griswold v. Connecticut*, the US Supreme

Court overturned Connecticut's little Comstock law, which banned the use of birth control by anyone, married or single. In 1972, in the *Eisenstadt v. Baird* decision, the Court struck down a Massachusetts law prohibiting unmarried persons from obtaining contraception (McFarlane and Meier 2001; Brodie 1994; Craig and O'Brien 1993).

From 1967 to 1970, most state legislatures considered changes in their abortion laws. Nineteen states passed new abortion laws. Although more liberal than in the past, most of these new abortion codes were based on the ALI's modest Model Penal Code (Tribe 1992). In 1970, Hawaii became the first state to repeal its criminal abortion law and to legalize abortion performed before the twentieth week of pregnancy. In the same year, New York enacted the most liberal of these laws, allowing abortion to be performed up until 24 weeks of gestation. As a result of these changes, women from more restrictive states flocked to less restrictive states to obtain abortions (Sheeran 1987, 57).

In 1971, the US Supreme Court issued a 5–4 decision in *United States v. Vuitch*, the first abortion case to reach the high court. In this case, a physician, Dr. Milan Vuitch, challenged the constitutionality of a District of Columbia abortion law that permitted abortion only to preserve a woman's life or health (ACLU 2003; Garrow 1994). The Court disagreed, rejecting the claim that the statute was unconstitutionally vague and concluding that health included both psychological and physical well-being.

Roe v. Wade (401 U.S. 113)

No state repealed any criminal abortion law during 1971 and 1972, but on January 22, 1973, the US Supreme Court struck down every abortion law in the land. In handing down *Roe v. Wade* (41 U.S. 113), the Court held 7 to 2 that a woman's right to choose was constitutionally protected as part of her right to privacy (table 2.1).[6] Only Justices William Rehnquist and Byron White dissented.

Justice Harry Blackmun, appointed by President Nixon in 1970 (table 2.2) and a former general counsel for the Mayo Clinic, wrote the majority opinion. That opinion was based in part on research that he conducted in the Mayo Clinic library during the Court's 1972 summer recess. In that process, he "reviewed social, religious, medical and legal approaches to abortion going back to ancient times" (Greenhouse 1999). Justice Blackmun "concluded that abortion, at least in early pregnancy, was widely tolerated both under English common law and at the time of the adoption of the United States Constitution, with legal prohibitions becoming widespread only late in the 19th century" (Greenhouse 1999).

Writing for the majority, Justice Blackmun laid out a trimester framework for restrictions that would follow. In the first trimester of pregnancy, *Roe* prohibited any level of government from interfering "with a woman's right to terminate a pregnancy in any way, except to insist that it be performed by a licensed physician" (Tribe 1992, 11). During the second trimester, states only had the power to regulate abortion to preserve and protect women's health. By the third trimester, *Roe* permitted states to restrict the right to choose to protect fetal life (McFarlane and Meier 2001; Tribe 1992).

First Period (1973–1989): Striking Down Most, but Not All, Restrictions

On the same day that the Court issued the *Roe* decision, it also ruled on a companion case, *Doe v. Bolton*, which had specific ramifications for state abortion laws. This decision articulated some of the implications of *Roe*. It struck down state residency requirements for abortion patients along with state laws mandating "that all abortions had to be performed in specifically accredited hospitals." States were disallowed from requiring hospital committees or other doctors to oversee the performing physician's judgment (McFarlane and Meier 2001, 62; Tribe 1992, 42, 140; Alan Guttmacher Institute 1983a).

Following *Roe v. Wade*, some states moved quickly to regulate abortion access and practice. By 1975, two state restrictions were on the Supreme Court docket. The *Bigelow v. Virginia* decision (41 U.S. 809) struck down a state law prohibiting advertisements for legal abortion. *Connecticut v. Menillo* (423 U.S. 9) upheld a state law requiring physicians to perform abortions.[7] In the same year, "the Supreme Court dealt access to abortion a blow when it refused to review—and therefore let stand—a decision by a U.S. circuit court (*Greco v. Orange Memorial Hospital Corporation)* that permitted a private hospital financed largely by private funds, to refuse to perform 'elective abortions'" (McFarlane and Meier 2001, 65).

In 1976, the Court disallowed three Missouri abortion restrictions in *Planned Parenthood v. Danforth* (428 U.S. 52): granting an abortion veto to the man that shared responsibility for the pregnancy, prohibiting saline abortions after 12 weeks of gestation, and allowing an absolute parental veto for a minor daughter's abortion. The *Danforth* case also upheld two restrictions. The state could require written informed consent from the pregnant woman that she was not coerced to have an abortion. Missouri was also allowed to require health facilities and physicians to report all abortions to the health department and keep those records for seven years (McFarlane and Meier 2001; Tribe 1992; Alan Guttmacher Institute 1976).

That year, the Court also issued an opinion in *Singleton v. Wulff* (428 U.S. 106), another Missouri case. This case was brought by two doctors challenging the exclusion of abortion in Missouri's Medicaid program. The issue was whether the physicians had standing to litigate on behalf of their patients. Writing for the Court, Justice Blackmun stated unequivocally, "Aside from the woman herself, the physician is uniquely qualified, by virtue of his confidential, professional relationship with her, to litigate the constitutionality of the State's interference with, or discrimination against, the abortion decision." The question of Medicaid funding was remanded to a lower court, but this case established third-party standing for abortion doctors on behalf of their patients (Sobel et al. 2020). Forty-five years later, the question of third-party standing in an abortion case was raised again by the state of Mississippi in *Dobbs v. Jackson Women's Health Organization*.[8]

In 1977, the Court upheld state restrictions on the use of public funds for abortion. Here the Court decided three companion cases: *Beal v. Doe* (432 U.S. 438), *Maher v. Roe* (432 U.S. 464), and *Poelker v. Doe* (432 U.S. 519). In *Beal* and *Maher*, the Court found that refusals by Pennsylvania and Connecticut to use Medicaid funds for non-therapeutic[9] abortions did not violate the federal Medicaid law. In *Poelker*, the Court held that a St. Louis public hospital was not constitutionally compelled to provide non-therapeutic abortions even if it funded childbirth services (Mezey 2011; McFarlane and Meier 2001; Tribe 1992; Alan Guttmacher Institute 1977).

In the 1979 *Bellotti v. Baird* decision (443 U.S. 622), the Court struck down a Massachusetts law requiring the consent of both parents. Eight justices agreed that a state could not require parental consent for a minor's abortion unless it offered a confidential alternative. The Court insisted that states provide minors a judicial bypass, rejecting the constitutionality of any absolute requirement of parental consent or notification for minors of any age (Drucker 1990; Alan Guttmacher Institute 1980, 1979;).

In the same year, the Court issued a 7–2 ruling in *Colautti v. Franklin* (49 U.S. 379) concerning the Pennsylvania Abortion Control Act. At issue was the requirement that a physician performing an abortion had to first "make a determination of viability and then use only those abortion procedures that gave the fetus the best chance of a live birth" (Goldman 2021, 83; Drucker 1990; Alan Guttmacher Institute 1983). The law was struck down because the Court considered it too vague to implement.

A Major Ruling: The Hyde Amendment Upheld

Congress entered the policymaking fray in Medicaid funding for abortions in 1976 when it passed the Hyde Amendment prohibiting "the use of federal monies to fund abortions except in cases where the life of the pregnant woman would be endangered if the fetus were carried to term" (Alan Guttmacher Institute 1980, 1). Appended to the 1977 Appropriations bill, the Hyde Amendment applied to all federal funds. Its major effect was to curtail federal funding for poor women (Alan Guttmacher Institute 1978). Until this rider, the federal government alone had been paying for about 300,000 abortions a year (Rose 2007, 72).

Due to judicial injunctions, the Hyde Amendment was not immediately implemented throughout the country.[10] In 1980, a federal judge held that the Hyde Amendment "violated a woman's First and Fifth Amendment rights" (Mezey 2011, 214). The US Supreme Court, however, was not persuaded by this reasoning.

Later that year, in a 5–4 ruling, the Court upheld the Hyde Amendment in *Harris v. McRae* (448 U.S. 917). Supporting the contention of the Carter administration, which argued the case, the Court noted that the Hyde Amendment placed "no government obstacle in the path of a woman choosing to terminate her pregnancy, but . . . encourages an alternative" (Ziegler 2020, 54; Mezey 2011, 214). Notwithstanding the meaning of poverty, the majority opinion explained, "the Hyde Amendment leaves an indigent woman with at least the same range of choice in deciding whether to obtain a medically necessary abortion as she would have had if Congress had chosen to subsidize no health costs at all" (Garrow 1994, 635).

In reaching its decision in *Harris*, the majority used the rational basis review, also known as minimum scrutiny, the lowest legal standard[11] to determine the constitutionality of the Hyde Amendment. Only "seven years after *Roe v. Wade* had been decided, the Court in *Harris* departed from its holding in *Roe* that abortion regulations be subject to strict scrutiny. . . . Under the strict scrutiny standard of review, the government must show that any abortion restriction is narrowly tailored to further a compelling governmental interest" (Adams and Arons 2014, 28) Writing for the majority, however, Justice Potter Stewart stated that *Roe* merely " 'protects the woman from *unduly burdensome interference* with her freedom to decide whether to terminate her pregnancy' and does not prevent the state from making a value judgment favoring childbirth over abortion, and . . . implement[ing] that judgment by the allocation of public funds" (Adams and Arons 2014, 28).

The dissent saw this issue differently; all four filed dissenting opinions, concurring that *Harris* was a departure from precedent. Joined by Justices Blackmun and Marshall, Justice William Brennan asserted that Congress's "deliberate effort to discourage the exercise of a constitutionally protected right" burdened and intruded upon "a pregnant woman's freedom to choose" (Garrow 1994, 635).[12] Justice Thurgood Marshall "predicted that women seeking abortions would be forced to resort to dangerous methods to secure them. He contended that the majority opinion was a 'retreat' from *Roe* and 'a cruel blow to the most powerless members of our society' " (Mezey 2011, 215). Justice John Paul Stevens's dissent pointed out that *Roe* allowed for no burden whatsoever on the right to an abortion before viability (Adams and Arons 2014, 29). Justice Harry Blackmun stated that the consequence of this decision "is a devastating impact on the lives and health of poor women" (48 U.S. 297). Nonetheless, the Hyde Amendment, with some variation—namely, the addition of rape and incest to the allowed exemptions (McFarlane and Meier 2001, 73)—has been in effect for more than four decades.

In *Williams v. Zbaraz* (448 U.S. 917), also a 5-4 decision, the Court found that a state did not have to provide reimbursement for medically necessary abortions for Medicaid-eligible women (Alan Guttmacher Institute 1983). This and other decisions concerning funding for low-income women were especially important. Funding restrictions have been shown to be especially consequential for abortion access in the states (Meier et al. 1996) and they disproportionately impact women of color (Ziegler 2020).

In 1981, the Court ruled on *H.L. v. Matheson* (445 U.S. 959), a case that addressed a Utah law requiring a physician to notify a minor's parents before performing an abortion. The Court held that a state may require parental notification when an immature and unemancipated minor seeks an abortion. In this context, emancipation refers to "the partial or complete extinguishment of parental rights and duties," which was most commonly through marriage at the time (Alan Guttmacher Institute 1978, 102). Unlike *Bellotti* and *Danforth*, the *Matheson* decision did not address whether a state may require parental notification for mature and emancipated minors (McFarlane and Meier 2001).

City of Akron v. Akron Center for Reproductive Health (462 U.S. 416) was decided in 1983. In this 6–3 ruling, the Court struck down a variety of state and local restrictions, "including a 24-hour waiting period, elaborate 'informed consent rules,' parental or judicial consent for all minors, and hospitalization for all second trimester abortions" (Alan Guttmacher Institute 1983b, 1–4). In this case, the Court reaffirmed that any statutory requirements must provide for an alternative method of approval for a minor who (1) is sufficiently mature to make the decision herself, or (2) has good reason for not seeking parental consent and can demonstrate that abortion would be in her best interests. In addition, the Court ruled that any parental consent rule must be accompanied by procedures ensuring that the judicial bypass would be accomplished quickly and confidentially (McFarlane and Meier 2001, 67; Tribe 1992, 14).

Justice Sandra Day O'Connor's dissent in the Akron case is noteworthy. Here, she adapted the undue burden standard championed by antiabortion groups (Ziegler 2020, 8).[13] Under "this approach, abortion restrictions would be constitutional unless the law created 'an absolute obstacle . . . or severe limitation on the abortion decision.'" The articulation of this new standard foreshadowed upholding many more state abortion restrictions (Ziegler 2020, 72). O'Connor also criticized Roe's trimester framework, writing that it was "clearly on a collision course with itself" because "it is certainly reasonable to believe that fetal viability in the first trimester of pregnancy may be possible in the not-too-distant future" (Garrow 1994, 643).

The Supreme Court issued two other abortion-related opinions on the same day it ruled on *Akron*. In *Planned Parenthood of Kansas, Missouri Inc. v. Ashcroft* (462 U.S. 476), the Court struck down a requirement in the Missouri abortion law that second-trimester abortions be performed in hospitals. However, in *Simopoulos v. Virginia* (462 U.S. 506), the Court upheld a similar Virginia requirement because Virginia's hospital law included licensed outpatient clinics in the definition of hospital (McFarlane and Meier 2001; Drucker 1990; Alan Guttmacher Institute 1983a).

In June 1986, the Court handed down *Thornburgh v. American College of Obstetricians and Gynecologists* (476 U.S. 747). This 5–4 ruling struck down informed consent and reporting requirements for abortions as well as standards of care for post-viability abortions (i.e., abortions performed after a fetus has become viable, or able to survive outside the womb). The Court found the elaborate requirements for informed consent mandated by the Commonwealth of Pennsylvania were designed to persuade the woman to withhold consent; moreover, they intruded on the discretion of the physician. The Court also struck down the Pennsylvania abortion reporting requirements, stating that they went well beyond the patient's health-related interests and showed no tolerance for extreme reporting requirements that might be made public.[14] The post-viability standards of the law were struck down because they failed to make maternal health the physician's "paramount" consideration (Tribe 1992, 14–15; Drucker 1990, 128; Alan Guttmacher Institute 1986).

Second Period (1989–2015): Upholding More State Restrictions

The 1989 *Webster v. Reproductive Health Services* decision was a milestone for state abortion restrictions. By this time, three justices appointed by President Ronald Reagan sat on the Court (table 2.2). Writing for the majority, O'Connor stated *Roe* had struck the wrong balance between women's rights and the government interest in fetal life, instead putting

TABLE 2.1
Supreme Court Cases Pertinent to State Abortion Regulations, 1973–2022

Year	Ruling	Case	Major points for state laws
1973	7–2	*Roe v. Wade*	Legalized abortion. Articulated trimester framework.
1973	7–2	*Doe v. Bolton*	Struck laws requiring state residence and specifically accredited hospitals for abortion.
1975	7–2	*Bigelow v. Virginia*	Upheld advertisements for legal abortion.
1975	9–0	*Connecticut v. Menillo*	Upheld requiring physicians to perform abortions.
1975	N/A	*Greco v. Orange Memorial Hospital Corporation*	Allowed private hospitals financed by public funds not to perform elective abortions.
1976	6–3	*Planned Parenthood v. Danforth*	Struck down partner veto, saline abortion ban (>12 weeks), absolute parental veto. Upheld written informed consent and state of Missouri reporting requirements.
1976	5–4	*Singleton v. Wulf*	Established third-party standing for doctors who perform abortions on behalf of their patients.
1977	6–3	*Beal v. Doe*	Upheld Pennsylvania's refusal to use Medicaid funds for non-therapeutic abortions.
1977	6–3	*Maher v. Roe*	Upheld Connecticut's refusal to use Medicaid funds for non-therapeutic abortions.
1977	6–3	*Poelker v. Doe*	Upheld St. Louis public hospital funding childbirth services, but not non-therapeutic abortions.
1979	8–1	*Bellotti v. Baird*	Struck down Massachusetts law requiring consent of both parents. Insists on judicial bypass.
1979	7–2	*Colautti v. Franklin*	Struck down Pennsylvania law requiring doctor save the life of a fetus that may be viable.
1980	5–4	*Harris v. McRae*	Upheld Hyde Amendment prohibiting use of federal funds for abortion (Medicaid), unless pregnant woman's life endangered.
1981	5–4	*Williams v. Zbaraz*	Upheld Illinois in not paying for medically necessary abortions through Medicaid program.
1981	6–3	*H.L. v. Matheson*	Upheld Utah law requiring parental notification for unemancipated minors.
1983	6–3	*City of Akron v. Akron Center for Reproductive Health*	Struck down Ohio law requiring 24-hour waiting period and elaborate reporting requirements.
1983	6–3	*Planned Parenthood of Kansas City v. Ashcroft*	Struck down hospital requirement after 12 weeks, but upheld other restrictions.
1983	8–1	*Simopoulos v. Virginia*	Upheld Virginia hospitalization requirement because outpatient clinics included.
1986	5–4	*Thornburgh v. ACOG*	Struck down Pennsylvania restrictions, including informed consent and post-viability requirements.
1989	5–4	*Webster v. Reproductive Health Services*	Upheld Missouri prohibition on state-employed physicians, state facilities ban, requirement for fetal viability determination ≥ 20 weeks gestation.
1990	5–4	*Hodgson v. Minnesota*	Upheld notification of two biological parents if judicial bypass is provided and 48-hour waiting period between notification and abortion procedure.

(continued)

TABLE 2.1
Continued

Year	Ruling	Case	Major points for state laws
1990	6–3	*Ohio v. Akron Center for Reproductive Health*	Upheld one-parent notification with judicial bypass without requiring anonymity for minor, a more stringent standard for minor bypass.
1991	5–4	*Rust v. Sullivan*	Upheld gag rule prohibiting abortion counseling in federally funded family planning clinics.
1992	5–4	*Planned Parenthood of Southeastern Pennsylvania v. Casey*	Upheld *Roe v. Wade* in principle, but replaced trimester framework with undue burden standard. Upheld 24-hour waiting period, informed consent, reporting to state, and parental or judicial consent. Struck down spousal consent.
1993	6–3	*Bray v. Alexandria Women's Health Clinic*	Struck down the use of a federal civil rights law to protect abortion patients from protestors.
1994	9–0	*National Organization of Women v. Scheidler*	Upheld use of federal anti-racketeering law in lawsuits against violent anti-abortion protestors.
1994	6–3	*Madsen v. Women's Health Center*	Upheld some court-ordered restrictions on abortion clinic protests.
1995	N/A	*Cheffer v. Reno*	Supreme Court let stand lower court ruling upholding constitutionality of FACE.
1997	8–1	*Schenck v. Pro-Choice Network, W. New York*	Struck down floating bubble zone for protection of abortion clinic and patients.
2000	5–4	*Steinberg v. Carhart*	Struck down Nebraska law banning partial birth abortion, with no health-of-mother exception.
2000	6–3	*Hill v. Colorado* 120 S. Ct. 2480	Upheld Colorado law for "a no-approach zone to protect patients and clinics from violence, harassment, and intimidation" (NARAL 2001, v).
2006	8–0	*Scheidler v. NOW*	RICO laws could not be invoked to challenge abortion clinic protests, which were protected by the First Amendment.
2006	9–0	*Ayotte v. Planned Parenthood of Northern New England*	Remanded New Hampshire's 48-hour notification with no health exception to lower court.
2007	5–4	*Gonzales v. Carhart*	Upheld partial birth abortion with life endangerment clause, but no health exception.
2014	5–4	*Burwell v. Hobby Lobby*	Upheld a closely held corporation to block its employees' access to no-copay birth control coverage as guaranteed by the Affordable Care Act (ACA) on the basis of religious objection (NARAL 2021).
2016	5–3	*Whole Women's Health v. Hellerstedt*	Struck down two Texas abortion restrictions.
2018	5–4	*National Institute of Family & Life Advocates v. Becerra*, 138 S. Ct. 2361	Struck down two sections of California's Reproductive Freedom Act: (1) requiring medical facilities to post notices informing patients of California's free and low-cost family planning, prenatal, and abortion services, and (2) notifying patients if clinic not medically supervised.

(continued)

TABLE 2.1
Continued

Year	Ruling	Case	Major points for state laws
2019	7–2	*Box v. Planned Parenthood of Indiana and Kentucky, Inc.*	Upheld Indiana's fetal cremation and burial law. Did not consider undue burden.
2020	5–4	*June Medical Services v. Russo*	Struck down Louisiana TRAP law requiring that physicians performing abortions must have admitting privileges at local hospital.
2020	7–2	*Little Sisters of the Poor Saints Peter and Paul v. Pennsylvania* *Trump v. Pennsylvania*	Upheld the Trump administration's authority to issue rules that allow an employer or a university to deny no-copay birth control coverage as guaranteed by the ACA on the basis of a religious or moral objection (NARAL 2021).
2021	6–3	*FDA, et al. v. ACOG, et al.*	Allowed in-person requirement for medication abortion during COVID-19 pandemic.
2022	6–3	*Dobbs v. Jackson Women's Health Organization*	Upheld pre-viability abortion ban in Mississippi. Vacated *Roe v. Wade* and *Planned Parenthood of Southeastern Pennsylvania v. Casey*.

forward the undue burden standard that was to replace *Roe's* trimester framework.

Webster is also pivotal because after years of striking down state abortion restrictions, the Court finally upheld three. A state's right to prohibit state-employed physicians from performing elective abortions was allowed to stand. States were also permitted to ban abortions in state facilities, regardless of how loosely public facility was defined.[15] This decision also upheld Missouri's law that required physicians to determine fetal viability at or after 20 weeks gestation, a mandate that absolutely contradicted best medical practices (McFarlane and Meier 2001, Tribe 1992).

In his dissent from the majority opinion, Justice Blackmun warned that "a plurality of this Court invites every state legislature to enact more and more test cases" (Drucker 1990; Greenhouse 1990). Blackmun predicted dire consequences in the future:

> Hundreds of thousands of women, in desperation, would defy the law, and place their health and safety in the unclean and unsympathetic hands of back-alley abortionists, or they would attempt to perform abortions on themselves, with disastrous results. Every year, many women, especially poor and minority women, would die or suffer debilitating physical trauma, all in the name of enforced morality or religious dictates or lack of compassion, as it may be. (Mezey 2011, 225)

TABLE 2.2
Supreme Court Justices

Supreme Court justice	Nominator	Party	Start date	End date	Chief	Roe	Webster	Casey	Dobbs
William Douglas	Franklin D. Roosevelt	Democrat	1939	1975		1	0	0	0
William Brennan	Dwight Eisenhower	Republican	1956	1990		1	1	0	0
Potter Stewart	Dwight Eisenhower	Republican	1958	1981		1	0	0	0
Byron White	John F. Kennedy	Democrat	1962	1993		1	1	1	0
Thurgood Marshall	Lyndon B. Johnson	Democrat	1967	1991		1	1	0	0
Warren Burger	Richard Nixon	Republican	1969	1986	1969–1986	1	0	0	0
Harry Blackmun	Richard Nixon	Republican	1970	1994		1	1	1	0
Lewis Powell	Richard Nixon	Republican	1972	1987		1	0	0	0
William Rehnquist	Richard Nixon	Republican	1972	2005	1986–2005	1	1	1	0
John Paul Stevens	Gerald Ford	Republican	1975	2010		0	1	1	0
Sandra Day O'Connor	Ronald Reagan	Republican	1981	2006		0	1	1	0
Antonin Scalia	Ronald Reagan	Republican	1986	2016		0	1	1	0
Anthony Kennedy	Ronald Reagan	Republican	1988	2018		0	1	1	0
David Souter	George H.W. Bush	Republican	1990	2009		0	0	1	0
Clarence Thomas	George H.W. Bush	Republican	1991	Present		0	0	1	1
Ruth Bader Ginsburg	William Clinton	Democrat	1993	2020		0	0	1	0
Stephen Breyer	William Clinton	Democrat	1994	Present		0	0	0	1
John Roberts	George W. Bush	Republican	2005	Present	2005–present	0	0	0	1
Samuel Alito	George W. Bush	Republican	2006	Present		0	0	0	1
Sonia Sotomayor	Barack Obama	Democrat	2009	Present		0	0	0	1
Elena Kagan	Barack Obama	Democrat	2010	Present		0	0	0	1
Neil Gorsuch	Donald Trump	Republican	2017	Present		0	0	0	1
Brett Kavanaugh	Donald Trump	Republican	2018	Present		0	0	0	1
Amy Coney Barrett	Donald Trump	Republican	2020	Present		0	0	0	1
Ketanji Brown Jackson	Joseph Biden	Democrat	2022	Present		0	0	0	0

Note: 1 = participated in the case, 0 = did not participate in the case.

Blackmun concluded, "For today, at least, the law of abortion remains undisturbed. For today, the women of this Nation still retain the liberty to control their own destinies. But the signs are evident and very ominous, and a chill wind blows" (Mezey 2011, 225).

The Court allowed further restrictions in 1990 in *Hodgson v. Minnesota* (497 U.S. 417) and *Ohio v. Akron* (497 U.S. 502). Both cases dealt with parental notification for minors seeking abortions. In *Hodgson*, the Court ruled that although states could not impose a blanket two-parent notification on minors seeking abortions, they could require notification of both biological parents as long as they provided a judicial bypass for minors who did not want to inform their parents about their plans. The Court also upheld a state requirement that minors wait 48 hours between the notification of parents and the abortion procedure (McFarlane and Meier 2001, 68; Alan Guttmacher Institute 1991a; Alan Guttmacher Institute 1990).

In *Ohio*, the state's policy to require notification of one parent and provide a judicial bypass was upheld. Here, the Court explicitly refused to decide whether a state had to provide a bypass when there was a one-parent notification requirement. This decision weakened the judicial bypass option in two ways: first, by ruling that a state was not required to guarantee anonymity to minors seeking abortion and second, by requiring that minors meet a difficult standard of proof: to show that they were sufficiently mature to consent to abortion on their own or that parental notice was not in their best interest (McFarlane and Meier 2001, 68; Alan Guttmacher Institute 1991a; Alan Guttmacher Institute 1990).

In May 1991, the Court ruled 5–4 on *Rust v. Sullivan* (500 U.S. 173). The majority upheld the federal regulation, popularly known as the "gag rule," barring employees of federally financed family planning clinics from all discussion of abortion with their patients. The dissenting justices expressed great concern about an abrogation of First Amendment rights (McFarlane and Meier 2001, 68; Alan Guttmacher Institute 1991b).

In June 1992, the Court handed down *Planned Parenthood of Southeastern Pennsylvania v. Casey* (510 U.S. 1309). The Court reaffirmed 5–4 "'the essential holding of *Roe v. Wade*' that prior to fetal viability, a woman has a constitutional right to obtain an abortion" (Alan Guttmacher Institute 1992, 1). At "the same time, however, the Court discarded *Roe's* trimester framework that severely restricted a state's power to regulate abortion in the early stages of pregnancy. The trimester framework 'undervalues' a state's interest in potential life,' which exists throughout pregnancy, the Court explained" (Alan Guttmacher Institute 1992, 1). The four dissenting justices, including the then-recently-appointed Justice Clarence Thomas, called for an outright reversal of *Roe* (McFarlane and Meier 2001; Alan Guttmacher Institute 1992).

Applying the undue burden standard, the *Casey* decision upheld four sections of Pennsylvania's Abortion Control Act and struck down one. The Court found that requiring teenagers to have the consent of one parent or judge did not constitute an undue burden, nor did the requirement that a 24-hour waiting period follow a state-mandated "informed consent" presentation intended to persuade the woman not to have an abortion. Also upheld was the section of the act requiring the doctor or clinic performing the abortion to make statistical reports to the state, as well as a related section specifying the medical emergencies under which other state requirements would be waived. The Court did overturn the section that required a married woman to inform her husband of her intent to have an abortion (McFarlane and Meier 2001, 69; Alan Guttmacher Institute 1992).

The undue burden standard set no guidelines. As a result, each new state law had to be considered anew in order to ascertain "if a majority of the Court feels it creates an undue burden for a pregnant woman" (Goldman 2021, 86). In the end, *Casey* retained a woman's right to choose, yet it allowed states greater latitude in regulating abortions, gratifying neither side of the abortion debate (Mezey 2011, 243).

In 1993, the Supreme Court decided *Bray v. Alexandria Women's Health Clinic* (506 U.S. 263). It ruled that a Reconstruction-era federal civil rights statute could not be invoked to protect abortion patients in the Washington, DC, metropolitan area from protestors who blocked access to abortion clinics. Writing for the majority, Justice Antonin Scalia said that women seeking abortions do not qualify for this class-based protection because anti-abortion protesters are not targeting them because of their gender.

A major consequence of this ruling was to make abortion providers more dependent on state and local law enforcement, considered less reliable and less effective than federal intervention. Before this decision, abortion providers "had used the law to obtain federal court injunctions barring blockades of clinics" (McFarlane and Meier 2001; Alan Guttmacher Institute 1993; *CQ Weekly* 1993). Dissenting from the majority in *Bray* were Justices Stevens, Blackmun, and O'Connor. Stevens said applying the 1871 law to the clinic blockades was wholly consistent with its Congressional purpose "to protect this Nation's citizens from what amounts to the theft of their constitutional rights by organized and violent mobs across the country" (*Congressional Quarterly* 1993, 130).

In January 1994, "the Supreme Court again ruled on anti-abortion protests, this time in *National Organization for Women v. Scheidler* (510 U.S. 249), a case brought on behalf of abortion clinics in Delaware and Wisconsin. "In this unanimous ruling, the Court allowed the Racketeering Influenced and Corrupt Organizations Act (RICO), a federal anti-racketeering statute, to be invoked in lawsuits brought against protestors who engage in violent activities intended to put abortion clinics out of business" (McFarlane and Meier 2001, 69; Alan Guttmacher Institute 1994).

This decision did not determine whether anti-abortion protesters had engaged in activities prohibited by RICO. Instead, the Court determined that RICO was an appropriate vehicle for pressing litigation against certain anti-abortion activities (Idelson 1994). Those found guilty of violating RICO's civil provisions would be liable for triple monetary damages, and criminal defendants would face up to 20 years in prison for each violation of the law. The use of RICO also allowed abortion providers "to target the masterminds of anti-abortion activity, rather than just the protesters at the scene" (McFarlane and Meier 2001, 70; Alan Guttmacher Institute 1994b).

Legislation (Freedom of Access to Clinics Entrances Act)

In May 1994, President Bill Clinton signed the Freedom of Access to Clinics Entrances Act (FACE). This Act was a Congressional response to the increasingly vociferous abortion demonstrations and the violence that was perpetrated against abortion providers during this period (discussed in Chapter 3). FACE amended the federal criminal code to prohibit the use of physical force, the threat of physical force, and the physical obstruction or destruction of property intended to interfere with access to reproductive health services (Mezey 2009a; McFarlane and Meier 2001, Alan Guttmacher Institute 1994a). Although FACE was challenged by a conservative activist group in 1995, the Supreme Court let a lower court ruling stand, upholding its constitutionality in *Cheffer v. Reno* (McFarlane and Meier 2001).

In June 1994, the Court ruled on another case concerning anti-abortion protests, *Madsen v. Women's Health Center* (512 U.S. 1277). This case addressed an injunction by a Florida judge, which placed buffer zones and noise restrictions around an abortion clinic and the private residences of clinic employees. The Court upheld a 36-foot buffer zone around the clinic's entrances and driveway, as well as noise restrictions on clinic protestors, but it struck down a 300-foot buffer zone around the residences of the clinic's staff. The decision emphasized that "'more narrowly targeted noise, time and/or place restrictions would be permissible'" (McFarlane and Meier 2001, 70).

1994 Midterm Election and Abortion

The midterm elections of 1994 gave Republicans control of both the US House and Senate for the first time in 40 years. Their majority status and the party's anti-choice platform changed federal abortion-related policies in important ways during President Clinton's second term. Congress reinstated a ban on induced abortions in US military hospitals overseas, even if with private funds,[16] excluded abortion coverage from health insurance plans offered to federal employees, banned the use of fetal tissue in federally funded research; achieved an 85 percent reduction in international assistance for family planning, and passed the partial birth abortion ban, which President Clinton vetoed (Ziegler 2020).

In the February 1997 *Schenck v. Pro-Choice Network of Western New York* (519 U.S. 357) decision, the Supreme Court upheld a New York law establishing a "15-foot fence around facilities providing abortion services" (Alan Guttmacher Institute 1997). However, the Court struck down a floating bubble zone, which would have established a protected zone around patients and vehicles entering and leaving the clinic. The Court explained that a floating bubble zone would be an undue burden on protesters' right to free speech because such a zone would be difficult to des-

ignate, measure, and enforce (McFarlane and Meier 2001; Alan Guttmacher Institute 1997).

In 2000, the Court decided *Stenberg v. Carhart* (530 U.S. 914), another
5–4 decision. This case addressed a Nebraska law banning a particular
abortion procedure, known politically, but not medically, as partial birth
abortion. The Court ruled the law unconstitutional because it lacked any
exception for preservation of health of the mother. Moreover, "the language defining the procedure was too broad," thereby imposing an undue
burden on a woman's ability to choose abortion (Palmer 2000, 1612).

The Court issued another abortion decision in 2000, *Hill v. Colorado*,
upholding the constitutionality of the zone-of-separation provision in
Colorado's 1993 clinic-protection statute, enacted before the federal FACE
law. This state law prohibited a person from knowingly approaching
within eight feet of another person without consent for the purpose of
passing a leaflet or handbill, displaying a sign, or engaging in oral pro-
test, education, or counseling, and it applied within a 100-foot radius
from clinic entrances. Responding to a First Amendment challenge from
three anti-abortion activists, the Court ruled that states have a legitimate
interest in protecting the health and safety of their citizens, especially at
medical care facilities. The opinion stressed the difference between states
restrictions on a speaker's right to address a willing audience and those
that protect listeners from unwanted communication, saying that the
Colorado statute only dealt with the latter (Mezey 2011, 250–251).

In *Scheidler v. National Organization for Women* (547 U.S. 9), the Supreme Court ruled that RICO laws could not be invoked to challenge
abortion clinic protests, which were otherwise protected by the First
Amendment freedom of speech. The case "had been in the courts for
almost two decades" (Mezey 2009b). The ruling precluded the ability of
abortion clinics to obtain injunctions to stop protesters from blocking
clinic entrances and more.[17] This decision ended the National Organization of Women's (NOW's) use of civil law provisions in RICO "to halt
the actions of protestors whose aim was to stop women from obtaining
abortions" (Mezey 2011, 247).

The Supreme Court returned to parental involvement in the 2006
Ayotte v. Planned Parenthood of Northern New England (546 U.S. 320)
decision. At issue was New Hampshire's Parental Notification Prior to

Abortion Act (PNPAA), prohibiting a physician from performing an abortion on a pregnant minor until 48 hours after written notice of the pending abortion had been delivered to her parent or guardian. The Supreme Court unanimously remanded the case back to a lower court, ruling that the lower courts should not have completely invalidated a New Hampshire parental notification law just because it lacked a health exception. In doing so, the Court upheld the plaintiffs' ability to challenge the law's constitutionality pre-enforcement, and it affirmed that states could not enact abortion restrictions that failed to protect women's health and safety. The New Hampshire legislature repealed the PNPAA in 2007, before further action occurred (Center for Reproductive Rights 2019; ACLU 2006; Perrine 2006).

The Supreme Court addressed partial birth abortion again in 2007 in a 5–4 decision, *Gonzales v. Carhart*. Although several lower courts had invalidated the constitutionality of the Partial Birth Abortion Ban Act (PBABA) passed by Congress in 2003 (Congress.Gov. 2004), the Supreme Court overruled them. By this time, President George W. Bush's two appointees sat on the Court: Chief Justice Roberts and Justice Samuel Alito (table 2.2). The Court upheld the state of Nebraska in banning a specific late-term abortion procedure except when the pregnant woman's life was endangered.

This decision was important for several reasons. *Gonzales v. Carhart* marked the first time since *Roe* that the Court had upheld a ban on a specific type of abortion. In addition, the explanation for this decision was written in political, not medical terms.[18] Also, for the first time since *Roe*, the Court upheld an abortion restriction that lacked an exception for preserving a woman's health (Goldman 2021; Ahmed 2020; Perrine 2007).

Writing for the majority, Justice Anthony Kennedy (appointed by President Reagan in 1988) relied on the notion that women require protection from the harms of abortion, including the regret that some women face because of that choice. Acknowledging "the lack of 'reliable data'" (Ehrlich and Doan 2019, 124) to measure this phenomenon, the majority decision, nonetheless, pivoted on abortion regret.[19] This decision propagated the myth that abortion regulation protects women, and its subtext: women need to be protected from their own decisions (Ehrlich and Doan 2019).

Justice Ginsberg (appointed by President Clinton in 1993) wrote a scathing dissent, which she read aloud to the Court for emphasis (Gutgold 2010; Greenhouse 2007). The majority opinion's decision to protect women from their own choices, she said, relied on "ancient notions about a woman's place in the family and under the Constitution that have long been discredited" (Ehrlich and Doan 2019, 124–125).

In June 2014, the US Supreme Court issued another 5–4 reproductive health decision, *Burwell v. Hobby Lobby Stores, Inc.* At issue were regulations promulgated by the Department of Health and Human Services (HHS) under the Patient Protection and Affordable Care Act of 2010 (ACA), requiring health insurance policies to cover all FDA-approved contraception. The majority sided with two family-held corporations, which enjoyed corporate tax advantages but claimed religious objections to birth control methods. The majority agreed that these businesses did not have to offer contraceptive coverage through their health insurance programs even if their employees did not share their beliefs. This far-reaching decision had the potential to affect more than half of all US workers.

Again, Justice Ginsberg dissented, this time with a 35-page tome, joined by Justice Stephen Breyer and Justice Kagan. She noted the "startling breadth of the decision," a ruling that opened the door to denial of other kinds of health care and employment policies based on the beliefs of their employers. Justice Ginsberg pointed out that women already spent far more money on preventive health care than men did.

She noted that in previous cases, the Court had already clarified that "accommodations to religious beliefs or observances . . . must not significantly impinge on the interests of third parties." Clearly, this decision would disadvantage those employees "who do not share their employer's religious beliefs." The dissent continued:

> Religious organizations exist to foster the interests of persons subscribing to the same religious faith. Not so of for-profit corporations. Workers who sustain the operations of those corporations commonly are not drawn from one religious community. (Cornell Law 2014, Ginsberg dissent in *Burwell v. Hobby Lobby*)

The Court has "ventured into a minefield," she asserted (Cornell Law 2014; Henderson 2014).

In 2018, the Court addressed a California law that protected a woman's right to choose in *National Institute of Family and Life Advocates (NIFLA) v. Becerra* (138 S. Ct. 2361). At issue was a state law that required clinics serving pregnant women (1) to reveal if they were unlicensed with no medical providers onsite, and (2) to notify patients about the health services, including abortion, funded by the state of California. At the time, there were over 200 crisis pregnancy centers (CPCs) in the state dedicated to dissuading pregnant women from seeking abortion, but posing as medical clinics, which they were not. Nevertheless, the CPCs, under the umbrella of NIFLA, sued, stating that these state requirements violated their first amendment rights. The Court agreed. Justice Thomas (appointed by President George H. W. Bush) wrote the majority opinion in this 5–4 decision, "holding that the law constituted a content-based regulation of speech prohibited by the First Amendment" (NARAL Pro-Choice America 2018).

Justice Breyer (appointed by President Clinton in 1994) dissented, pointing out that under the majority's reasoning many ordinary disclosure laws" including "numerous commonly found disclosure requirements relating to the medical profession" could be struck down (138 S. Ct. 2361, 2381 (2018)). He also highlighted that the "marketplace of ideas," as mentioned in the majority opinion, "is fostered, not hindered, by providing information to patients to enable them to make fully informed medical decisions in respect to their pregnancies."

The verdict in this case continues to be of great concern to those who practice public health, medicine, and law. For years, public health practitioners have worked to control deceptive advertising that affects human health (Parasidis 2019; Pomerantz 2019). For physicians, this case challenged medical ethics (Bryant and Swartz 2018). For legal scholars, "the rationales underlying the decision seem intended to justify differential treatment of abortion opponents and reproductive rights supporters" (*Harvard Law Review* 2018, 355).

Two Cases Striking Down State Restrictions—An Interval, but Not a Trend

In June 2016, the Court issued the *Whole Woman's Health v. Hellerstedt* (136 S. Ct. 2292) decision. At this point, only eight justices were on the

Court due to the February 2016 death of Justice Scalia. The Court voted 5–3 to strike down two provisions of a 2013 Texas law regulating abortion (Vaida 2016). The first restriction required doctors who provided abortion services to obtain admitting privileges at local hospitals no farther than 30 miles away from the clinic. The second restriction struck down by the Court was a mandate that every health care facility offering abortion care had to meet the building specifications of ambulatory surgical centers.[20] The majority stated

> We have found nothing in Texas' record evidence that shows that, compared to prior law (which required a "working arrangement" with a doctor with admitting privileges), the new law advanced Texas' legitimate interest in protecting women's health. (Cornell Law School 2016)

In her concurrence with the decision, Justice Ginsberg commented that "it is beyond rational belief that H. B. 2 could genuinely protect the health of women, and certain that the law would simply make it more difficult for them to obtain abortions." Justices Alito, Roberts, and Thomas dissented from the majority opinion.

In the 2020 *June Medical Services v. Russo* (140 S. Ct. 2103) decision, the Court issued another 5–4 decision striking down a Louisiana law almost identical with the Texas law that was addressed in the 2016 *Whole Woman* case, requiring physicians who perform abortions to have hospital admitting privileges. Noting the similarity of the case with *Whole Woman's Health v. Hellerstedt,* this time Chief Justice Roberts concurred with the majority based on the principle of *stare decisis.* Justices Alito, Neil Gorsuch, Brett Kavanaugh, and Thomas dissented.

Both the *Whole Woman* and *June Medical Services* decisions addressed state laws that regulate only abortion providers far in excess of standard medical protocols (NAS 2018; Nippita and Paul 2018). Dubbed Targeted Regulation of Abortion Providers or TRAP laws, this constellation of laws is discussed at length in Chapter 3.

In 2019 the US Supreme Court issued another 7–2 decision, *Box v. Planned Parenthood of Indiana and Kentucky, Inc.* (39 S.Ct. 1780). Here, in a *per curiam* decision,[21] the Court upheld an Indiana law signed by the anti-abortion then-Governor Mike Pence that required abortion providers to bury or cremate fetal remains (Williams 2019). The Court left intact lower court rulings "that invalidated a broader measure that would prevent a woman from having an abortion based on a fetus's gender, race or genetic disorder." The majority opinion dodged the undue burden standard, stating

> Respondents have never argued that Indiana's law imposes an undue burden on a woman's right to obtain an abortion. This case, as litigated, therefore does not implicate our cases applying the undue burden test to abortion regulations. (Cornell Law School 2019; Wolf and Rudavsky 2019)

Justice Ginsberg dissented from the decision to uphold the disposal of fetal remains and concurred with invalidating the second restriction. Justice Sotomayor also dissented.

In 2020, the Court returned to religious exemptions from the contraceptive and women's preventive health services mandates of the Affordable Care Act in the companion cases *Little Sisters of the Poor Saints Peter and Paul v. Pennsylvania, et al.* (140 S. Ct. 2367) and *Donald J. Trump, President of the United States, et al., Petitioners v. Pennsylvania, et al.* (930 F. 3d). In a 7–2 decision, the Court sided with the Trump administration and allowed "employers and universities to opt out of the Affordable Care Act requirement to provide contraceptive care because of religious or moral objections" (Barnes 2020). This decision greatly expanded the ability of employers to claim the exception, resulting in the loss of access to contraceptive coverage for an estimated 70,000 to 126,000 women (Barnes 2020; Liptak 2020; SCOTUSblog 2020).

In her final dissent, which was joined by Justice Sotomayor, Justice Ginsberg stated, "Today, for the first time, the Court casts totally aside countervailing rights and interests in its zeal to secure religious rights to the *n*th degree." Congress, she said, meant to provide "gainfully employed women comprehensive, seamless, no-cost insurance coverage for preventive care protective of their health and wellbeing." However, this ruling, "leaves women workers to fend for themselves, to seek contraceptive coverage from sources other than their employer's insurer, and, absent another available source of funding, to pay for contraceptive services out of their own pockets" (Barnes 2020).

A New Period Begins

Justice Ginsberg died on September 18, 2020, less than two months before the presidential election. Senate Republicans reversed their rhetoric from 2016, when they had refused to hold hearings for Judge Merrick Garland nominated by President Obama in March 2016 because it was too close to a presidential election.

Trump nominated Amy Coney Barrett to replace Justice Ginsberg in record-breaking speed, and the Republican majority in the US Senate confirmed her just a week before the November 2020 presidential election. Judge Coney Barrett had already made her anti-abortion views public. In 2006, for example, Barrett signed her name to an ad declaring that it was "time to put an end to the barbaric legacy of *Roe v. Wade*" (Talbot 2022).[22] As a member of the Notre Dame Faculty for Life, she voted to condemn Notre Dame University's decision to award then Vice-President Joe Biden a medal for "service to Church and society" because Biden supports the right to abortion. In less than two months, the Court had changed profoundly, a fact that was not lost on Mississippi Attorney General Lynn Fitch, who had filed a petition to the Supreme Court in June 2020 to hear *Dobbs v. Jackson Women's Health Organization.*

In January 2021, in *Food and Drug Administration, et al. v. American College of Obstetricians and Gynecologists, et al.*, the Court reinstated (6–3) a federal requirement issued by the Trump administration that women seeking to end their pregnancies using medication abortion must pick up the pills in person from a hospital or medical office. The ACOG, whose 60,000 members deliver much of women's reproductive health services in the country, had sued the FDA. The ACOG noted that "of the over 20,000 FDA-approved drugs, mifepristone [for medication abortion] is the only one that the FDA requires to be picked up in person for patients to take at home" (Supreme Court 2021; ACOG 2020). By issuing an injunction, a federal district court had blocked the in-person requirement considering the coronavirus pandemic. The district court noted that "a needless trip to a medical facility during a health crisis very likely imposed an undue burden on the constitutional right to abortion" (Liptak 2021b).

But just eight days before President Biden was to take office, the Supreme Court tossed out the injunction issued by a federal district court judge. Women now had to obtain medication abortion pills in person. In her dissent, Justice Sotomayor noted that the inevitable delays, exacerbated by the COVID-19 pandemic, would cause some women to miss the 10-week gestation limit for medication abortion.

Dobbs v. Jackson Women's Health Organization

In June 2021, the US Supreme Court agreed to hear *Dobbs v. Jackson Women's Health Organization*. At issue was Mississippi's abortion law passed on March 19, 2018, that prohibited abortion after 15 weeks of gestation, with only narrow exceptions "for medical emergency or severe fetal abnormality" (Howe 2021). There were no exceptions for rape and incest.

Within hours, Jackson Women's Health Organization, the only remaining abortion provider in Mississippi, filed a complaint and a request for a temporary restraining order to block the ban. On March 20, the US District Court for the Southern District of Mississippi granted emergency relief, blocking enforcement of the ban. On November 20, 2018, the same federal district court that had ruled the ban unconstitutional issued a permanent injunction, thus striking down the ban. The ruling cited the Supreme Court precedent, *Roe v. Wade*, pointing out that abortions are not allowed to be banned before a fetus becomes viable, occurring at approximately 24 weeks gestation.

The State of Mississippi appealed to the US Court of Appeals. On December 14, 2019, a three-judge panel of the US Court of Appeals for the Fifth Circuit unanimously affirmed the lower court's decision to strike down the 15-week ban. In doing so, the Court of Appeals affirmed another section of *Roe*:

> In an unbroken line dating to *Roe v. Wade*, the Supreme Court's abortion cases have established (and affirmed, and re-affirmed) a woman's right to choose an abortion before viability. States may regulate abortion procedures prior to viability so long as they do not impose an undue burden on the woman's right, but they may not ban abortions. The law at issue is a ban. (Center for Reproductive Rights 2022a)

On June 15, 2020, the State of Mississippi filed a certiorari petition[23] with the US Supreme Court asking the court to reverse the decision of the US Court of Appeals. Mississippi argued that, as a third party, Jackson Women's Health Organization had no standing to challenge the state restriction.[24] In this document, Mississippi noted that "the questions presented in this petition do not require the Court to overturn *Roe* or *Casey*" (Marcus 2021). On May 17, 2021, 11 months after the writ of certiorari was filed, the US Supreme Court announced that it would hear Mississippi's petition.

The interval between the cert petition and the Supreme Court's decision to take up the case was unusually long. During that period, Justice Ginsberg died and Justice Barrett was appointed to the high court. On average, it takes the US Supreme Court six weeks from an appeal to act once a petition has been filed (Supreme Court Public Information Office 2021). After the case was accepted by the Supreme Court, the State of Mississippi submitted a second writ of certiorari on July 22, 2021. In this petition, Mississippi argued that *Roe* and *Casey* should both be overruled.

Over 140 amicus briefs were filed in the *Dobbs v. Jackson* case. Among them was an amicus brief initiated by the American College of Obstetricians and Gynecologists that argued that implementation of the Mississippi law would be harmful to women's health. Scores of medical, nursing, and public health organizations, including the American Medical Association, the American Academy of Nursing, and the American Academy of Family Physicians, signed on to this brief (Center for Reproductive Rights 2021).

Oral arguments for *Dobbs v. Jackson Women's Health Organization* took place on December 1, 2021. In a nearly-two-hour session, both sides presented their arguments (Supreme Court of the United States 2021). Given the questioning from the justices, most analysts thought that Mississippi would prevail.

The Leak

On May 2, 2022, *Politico* leaked a draft *Dobbs* opinion from the Court. This draft, written by Justice Alito in February 2022, was "a full-throated, unflinching repudiation of the 1973 decision which guaranteed federal con-

stitutional protections of abortion rights and a subsequent 1992 decision—
Planned Parenthood v. Casey—that largely maintained the right" (Gerstein and Ward 2022). Alito wrote that "*Roe* was egregiously wrong from
the start. . . . We hold that *Roe* and *Casey* must be overruled. . . . It is time
to heed the Constitution and return the issue of abortion to the people's
elected representatives." The draft also discounted the history of abortion in the United States, saying that "a right to abortion is not deeply
rooted in the Nation's history and traditions" (Gerstein and Ward 2022).

Although a Supreme Court leak is rare, this draft opinion was surprising in its stridency. Given the composition of the Court and the questions asked by the justices during oral arguments, most analysts thought
the case would tilt toward the anti-abortion side.[25] Overturning both *Roe*
and *Casey* was not as widely anticipated. The draft showed that four justices, namely, Barrett, Gorsuch, Kavanaugh, and Thomas, had signed onto
the opinion. At this point, Chief Justice Roberts had not signed on to the
draft, so his position was unclear (Gerstein and Ward 2022).

The Opinion

On June 24, 2022, the Court announced its opinion for *Dobbs v. Jackson
Women's Health Organization*. Written by Justice Alito, the decision did
not deviate substantially from the leaked draft. Justices Thomas, Gorsuch, Kavanaugh, and Barrett joined the majority opinion. Both Thomas
and Kavanaugh filed concurring opinions. Chief Justice Roberts filed
an opinion concurring in the judgment. Justices Breyer, Sotomayor, and
Kagan filed a joint dissenting opinion.

The majority opinion stated

> We hold that *Roe* and *Casey* must be overruled. The Constitution
> makes no reference to abortion, and no such right is implicitly pro-
> tected by any constitutional provision, including the one on which the
> defenders of *Roe* and *Casey* now chiefly rely—the Due Process Clause
> of the Fourteenth Amendment. That provision has been held to guar-
> antee some rights that are not mentioned in the Constitution, but any
> such right must be "deeply rooted in this Nation's history and tradi-
> tion" and "implicit in the concept of ordered liberty" . . . The right to
> abortion does not fall within this category. (*Dobbs v. Jackson*, 5)

Moreover, *Roe* and *Casey* have "enflamed debate and deepened division" because they have not brought about a "national settlement" of the abortion issue (*Dobbs v. Jackson*, 6).

The majority engaged in a five-factor test[26] to overturn legal precedents and "justify its failure to adhere to stare decisis" (Lindgren 2022, 240). The result was the removal of "the constitutional floor that has protected the abortion right for fifty years. States are now free to "regulate, restrict, criminalize, or protect abortion at the state level" (Lindgren 2022, 236). The Court did not rule on the issue of standing for Jackson Women's Health Organization, but the majority signaled their willingness to entertain future challenges that abortion providers and doctors "lack standing to enjoin enforcement of a state's restrictive abortion laws" (Lindgren 2022, 241—note 40). In his concurrence, Chief Justice Roberts sought "a measured course" that would "leave for another day whether to reject any right to abortion at all." Instead, he would have preferred to uphold the Mississippi 15-week pre-viability ban, but not overturn *Roe* and *Casey* at that time. He "argued for revising the legal standard applied in abortion cases from the previous 'undue burden' test with a 'reasonable opportunity test' that provides that states can ban abortion so long as a woman has had a reasonable opportunity to obtain an abortion" (Lindgren 2022, 245).

In his concurrence, Justice Kavanaugh acknowledged that this decision returned abortion regulation to state legislatures. Beyond that, he wrote blithely, "other abortion-related questions raised by today's decision are not especially difficult as a constitutional matter" (*Dobbs v. Jackson Women's Health Organization*, 10). One of his examples was whether a state "could bar a resident of that State from traveling to another State to obtain an abortion? In my view, the answer is no based on the constitutional right to interstate travel" (*Dobbs v. Jackson Women's Health Organization*, 10). Other legal scholars have argued that this question is much more unsettled than Justice Kavanaugh suggested (Lindgren 2022, 256). Justice Kavanaugh also reiterated that the Dobbs decision would not impact other cases or "cast doubt on those precedents" (*Dobbs v. Jackson Women's Health Organization*, 10).

Justice Thomas' concurrence, however, called Kavanaugh's reassurance into question. Dismissing substantive due process as an oxymoron, he argued that future cases should revisit this precedent. In the future, the Court should reconsider *Griswold* (right to use contraception), *Lawrence* (right to same-sex sexual activity), and *Obergefell* (right to same-sex marriage).

In their powerful joint dissent,[27] Justices Breyer, Kagan, and Sotomayor noted that "just as the majority wrote about how abortion is not deeply rooted in the nation's history or tradition, the same could be said about other rights" (Lindgren 2022, 244). They took aim at the majority's "originalist interpretation of the Constitution in striking down the abortion right" (Lindgren 2022, 258). At the time the Fourteenth Amendment passed, "the period to which the majority looks to determine if a right is deeply rooted in the nations' history—women were not viewed as equals and did not have rights to vote, own property, or control their bodies" (Lindgren 2022, 258), so if they are considering this period, they are consigning women to second-class citizenship (Cruickhank 2022). The dissent argued "that the Framers drafted the Constitution in broad language so that it would endure the ages and respond to changing times" (Lindgren 2022, 258). The dissent also included different sources to show that abortion was indeed deeply rooted in the nation's history (e.g., Mohr 1978).

The dissent closed "with sorrow for this Court, but more for the many millions of women who have today lost a fundamental constitutional protection" (Lindgren 2022, 258).

Court Composition Changes Again

The split decisions on abortion show the importance of the composition of the Court for substantive abortion cases (table 2.2) (Chotiner 2019). The April 2022 appointment to the US Supreme Court of Ketanji Brown Jackson, nominated by President Biden, did not change either the vote or the outcome in *Dobbs v. Jackson*. She was not involved in the deliberations, as she replaced Justice Breyer, who retired at the end of the Supreme Court's Summer 2022 term.

Conclusion

Neither abortion practice nor abortion politics have been short-lived in America. Despite the assertions of the *Dobbs* majority, history shows that women terminated pregnancies before and after the American Revolution (Mohr 1978). At various junctures, banning abortion by the state has not quashed its practice.

The judicial branch, especially the US Supreme Court, plays a pivotal role in deciding the parameters of how the states regulate abortion. In the years since the 7–2 *Roe v. Wade* decision, most Supreme Court rulings on topics related to abortion have been close split decisions, showing the importance of the composition of the Court. For that reason, appointments to the high court have become even more politicized over time.

This chapter explained that the 2022 *Dobbs* decision vacated nearly a half-century of precedent in abortion law. The ramifications of *Dobbs* will be felt for many years. As the dissent stated, "young women will come of age with fewer rights than their mothers and grandmothers had" (*Dobbs* 42, 2326). The legality of abortion has been returned to the states, and already, most abortions are banned in 14 states (*New York Times* 2023). More state bans are likely to follow, even as other states scramble to protect the right to choose.

The impact of *Dobbs* extends beyond abortion. Given its originalist philosophy, the Court is likely to revisit other issues for which there is judicial precedent. Moreover, this case has affected public perception of the Court itself, which was already at a historic low just before the decision (Pew Research Center 2022b; Pew Research Center 2022c; Jones 2021; Weschler 2018). More recent polls have shown that 58–62 percent of Americans disapproved of the *Dobbs* decision (ANES 2022; Pew Research Center 2022a).

CHAPTER 3

Weakening *Roe*

The Proliferation of Abortion Regulations in US States

State abortion regulation began long before the 1973 *Roe v. Wade* decision, but *Roe* reset its parameters. At the time, many Americans, particularly pro-choice activists, thought the abortion issue was settled (Ziegler 2020, 30; NARAL 1989). Nothing could have been further from the truth.

Roe v. Wade catalyzed the anti-abortion movement, which quickly became more active in the federal and state legislative arenas (Madden 1973). By March 1973, two different types of federal constitutional amendments had been introduced in the US House of Representatives (Rosoff 1973). Eventually, these constitutional amendment efforts stalled, but Congress did pass the Church Amendment in 1973 "allowing any medical facility or provider receiving federal funds to refuse for reasons of conscience to perform abortion or sterilization" (Simon 2021; US Department of Health and Human Services 2021; Ziegler 2020, 34).

Other restrictive national abortion legislation followed. At the end of 1974, Congress had enacted two more funding exclusions. First, lawmakers prohibited the Legal Services Corporation, the federally funded legal aid program for those on low incomes, from assisting low-income women to obtain legal abortions. Second, Congress banned the inclusion of abortion in the US Foreign Assistance Act, which authorized monies for overseas family planning programs (Rosoff 1975, 2).[1] In 1976, Congress passed the Hyde Amendment, excluding abortion from the federal Medicaid program.[2] Although its proponents disingenuously pitched it as a way to shrink government, the Hyde Amendment directly targeted low-income women's access to abortion.

In addition to federal legislative actions, national interest groups, which proliferated after the *Roe* decision, also promulgated state abortion regulations. Over the years, these groups have become instrumental in developing model legislation as well as pushing for and defending abortion restrictions. Americans United for Life (AUL), for example, publishes a lengthy report each year, called *Defending Life*, which they send to state legislators and now post on their website. Each year, this document includes model bills for abortion restrictions, easy for state legislators to introduce. The Alliance Defending Freedom (ADF) is another anti-abortion group[3] whose model legislation was used to craft the 15-week viability law in Mississippi that was challenged in the *Dobbs* case. The Federalist Society has promoted anti-abortion litigation for many years as well (Gerstein 2022).

On the pro-choice side, both NARAL Pro-Choice America, formerly the National Abortion Rights League, and the Guttmacher Institute monitor state developments. Thus far, these pro-choice groups have not developed strategies for model legislation to counteract the effects of abortion restrictions. However, the Reproductive Freedom Project of the American Civil Liberties Union (ACLU) has challenged state restrictions over the years, particularly the Medicaid funding for abortion (ACLU 2022). Over the last three decades, the Center for Reproductive Rights (CRR) has participated in every abortion case argued before the US Supreme Court, but CRR does not develop model legislation for the states.

Much of the control, particularly by the end of the 1980s, would be at the state level, regulations would vary greatly among the states, and many state abortion regulations would emanate from national strategies. Both state and federal courts would be involved in their implementation. Additionally, because of their limited resources and dependence on public programs, low income women—disproportionately women of color—would feel the impact of those restrictions far more than affluent women.[4]

This chapter focuses on state abortion regulations since 1973, emphasizing the period from 1988 to 2022. Although states did enact abortion regulations between 1973 and 1988, the variety and velocity of regulations accelerated after the *Webster* (1989) and *Casey* (1992) decisions. Moreover, systematic information about state abortion regulation became more readily available after 1987.

For the most part, information about individual regulations is presented chronologically. First, we discuss the status of state regulations prior to *Webster*, between *Webster* and *Casey*, and after *Casey*. Second, we describe state restrictions and protections by decade as they appeared or as they proliferated. Third, we consider the role of the US Supreme Court in state abortion regulation. Fourth, we examine the role of partisanship in state abortion regulation. Finally, we compare the intensity and velocity of abortion regulation in individual states.

After *Roe*

Prior to 1989, after the legalization of abortion in *Roe v. Wade,* the US Supreme Court had upheld three major types of abortion restrictions: limits on abortion after fetal viability, parental involvement in minors' abortion decisions, and curtailing public funding (table 3.1).[5] The authority for restricting post-viability abortions emanated from *Roe*. States were permitted to prohibit abortion after viability, occurring roughly at the twenty-fourth week of pregnancy. By 1988, 27 states had enacted regulations prohibiting all or most post-viability abortions (NARAL 1989).[6] Post-viability abortion laws can be classified as standard setting regulations (table 1.8).

By 1988, 33 states had parental involvement laws on the books, including parental consent and/or parental notification mandates.[7] Parental consent laws require written permission from one or more parents before a minor can access abortion services. Parental notification laws require that one or more parents must be informed before a minor can obtain abortion services. At the time, only 11 states (Alabama, Indiana, Louisiana, Maryland, Massachusetts, Missouri, Rhode Island, South Carolina, Tennessee, West Virginia, and Wyoming) could enforce their parental involvement laws; various judicial decisions had deemed the rest unconstitutional.[8] Parental involvement laws can be considered standard-setting regulations (table 1.8).

TABLE 3.1

State Abortion Restrictions Impacted by Supreme Court Rulings:
After Roe, *after* Webster, *and after* Casey

After *Roe* (1973–1988)	After *Webster* (1989–1991)	After *Casey* (1992–2020)
Post-viability bans on abortions	Public facility prohibitions	Informed consent/mandatory counseling requirements
Parental involvement requirements	Public employee bans	Waiting period requirements
Medicaid funding prohibitions	Viability testing requirements	State abortion reporting requirements
	Conscience exemption requirements	

In 1988, only 12 states were funding abortions through their Medicaid programs; five of these states funded abortions for low-income women only because of a court order.[9] The impact of the Hyde Amendment was obvious: more than three-quarters of states did not fund abortion services for Medicaid-eligible women. In those 38 states, low-income women had to pay full price for abortion, even if Medicaid subsidized their other medical services. The Hyde Amendment is an example of regulation that impacts price (table 1.8).[10]

Initiation of Annual State Abortion Reports

In January 1989, the National Abortion Rights League (NARAL)[11] published a comprehensive report,[12] *Who Decides? A State by State Review of Abortion Rights in America.* This report detailed specific abortion legislation in every state for 1988, including laws on the books and laws that could not be enforced because of a court injunction or another reason. It also included political information about whether governors and legislative bodies supported the right to choose.[13] In 1988, both houses in 24 states favored making abortion illegal; in 15 of those states, the governor also did not favor abortion rights (NARAL 1989, vi).

The timing of this NARAL publication was not serendipitous. A pending case at the US Supreme Court, *Webster v. Reproductive Health Services,* had the potential to change the landscape for state abortion regulation and allow more restrictions to stand. This inaugural *Who Decides?* report served as a blueprint for the annual volumes that NARAL has issued since that time.[14] These reports continue to provide detailed information about the development and enforcement of each state's abortion regulations.

After *Webster* (before *Casey*), 1989–1991

After 15 years of striking down most state abortion regulations, the Supreme Court upheld three in *Webster v. Reproductive Health Services* (1989). Missouri's ban on the provision of abortion in public facilities, its prohibition against the participation of public employees in pregnancy terminations, and its requirement for viability testing prior to abortion after 20 weeks gestation were each found to be constitutional (table 3.1).

This ruling encouraged other states to pass similar restrictions, especially banning public facilities from being used for abortions. Because *Webster* was litigated on a very broad definition of "public facility," upholding this restriction implied that many types of hospitals and clinics could be categorized as public facilities.[15] By 1991, five more states (Arizona, Kentucky, Louisiana, North Dakota, and Pennsylvania) had enacted public facility bans[16] (NARAL 1993, vii). By 2000, nine states had passed this kind of restriction, adding Iowa, Kansas, Mississippi and Missouri to the list.

The other two newly constitutional restrictions were not as popular. No other state passed a prohibition on the participation of public employees in pregnancy terminations.[17] Few states adopted regulations similar to the Missouri requirement for viability testing for pregnancies at or above 20 weeks. By 1992, only two more states (Alabama and Louisiana) had similar regulations.[18]

Conscience-Based Exemptions or Refusal-of-Care Restrictions

Between *Webster* and *Casey*, states passed more and different types of restrictions. Conscience-based exemptions are an example of an abortion restriction that multiplied during this interval between major judicial decisions. These types of regulations are also called refusal-of-care restrictions; in many communities they are "a significant barrier to care" (NARAL Pro-Choice America 2021, 21). These state laws permitted "medical personnel, health facilities, or both to refuse to participate in abortion on the basis of 'conscience'" (NARAL 1999, xiv).

In 1988, 15 states had employed refusal-of-care restrictions for abortion services.[19] That number increased to 17 in 1989, 19 in 1990, 28 in 1991, and 45 states by 1992. By 2005, three more states, Kentucky, Mississippi, and West Virginia, as well as the District of Columbia, had enacted this type of abortion restriction. Alabama followed in 2017, leaving only two states, New Hampshire and Vermont, that had not passed refusal-of-care restrictions for abortion care.

Casey and Beyond, 1992 to Present

For state abortion regulations, the *Casey* decision was even more significant than *Webster*. *Casey* abandoned the strict scrutiny *Roe v. Wade* had applied to the abortion right.[20] In their attempt to reconcile the state of Pennsylvania's interest in procreation with "the woman's constitutionally protected liberty" (Ziegler 2020, 117), the *Casey* decision replaced *Roe*'s trimester framework with a more lenient undue burden standard of review. Instead of minimal regulation in the first trimester, for example, restrictions were now presumed to be constitutional unless they posed an "undue burden"[21] to abortion. The result was the Court began to uphold some abortion restrictions that it had only recently struck down.

At issue was Pennsylvania's 1989 Abortion Control Act (Garrow 1994). The Court upheld provisions of the Pennsylvania abortion law requiring parental consent for a minor before an abortion, informed consent from any patient before an abortion, a 24-hour waiting period between the informed consent and the procedure, and a detailed report from the abortion provider to the state following the procedure (NARAL 1991–93, iv). The only disputed provision of Pennsylvania's abortion law struck down by the Court was spousal consent (table 3.1).

Here, *Casey* presented extensive evidence about domestic violence, pointing out that women who feared for their safety and that of their children should not be subject to a husband's veto (Ziegler 2020).[22] The Court explicitly rejected the view of marriage written into Pennsylvania's spousal consent requirement.[23] Nonetheless, state laws requiring a married woman to notify her husband or get his consent for her pending abortion stayed on the books in 10 other states (Colorado, Florida, Illinois, Kentucky, Louisiana, Montana,[24] North Dakota, Rhode Island, South Carolina, and Utah). However, *Casey* did render these laws unenforceable. No state enacted a spousal consent law after 1992, and Florida repealed its unconstitutional spousal consent law in 1997 (NARAL 1998, vii).

Informed Consent

Informed consent laws, also called mandatory counseling (Ziegler 2020, 145) or even biased counseling laws (NARAL 2014), began to proliferate in the period between *Webster* and *Casey*. In 1989, only 13 states (Delaware, Florida, Idaho, Louisiana, Maine, Massachusetts, Michigan,[25] Missouri, Nebraska, Pennsylvania, Rhode Island, South Dakota, and Wisconsin) mandated informed consent for abortion (ICAs) before an abortion could be performed. By 1991, 25 states required this type of consent; by 1992, 30 states had adopted this abortion law. However, by 1992, ICAs had been judicially enjoined in all 30 states, so they were not able to be enforced.[26] *Casey* changed that. By 1993, 30 state laws were again in effect. By 2020, 30 states still had ICAs, with only one state law (Iowa) enjoined.[27]

On the surface, ICAs may not appear to be abortion restrictions. After all, informed consent (IC) for medical treatment is fundamental in both medical ethics and health law (American Medical Association 2021). The standard process for informed consent is that a physician or another health care provider gives the patient information about the diagnosis (when known), the nature and purpose of recommended treatments or interventions, and "the burdens, risks, and expected benefits of all options, including forgoing treatment" (American Medical Association 2021). Ideally, informed consent is an interactive communication process between a patient and health care provider (American Cancer Society 2021) that results in a patient legally authorizing or not authorizing to undergo a specific medical intervention (American Medical Association 2021).

Shared decision-making is a vital part of the informed consent process, allowing patients to play an active role in making decisions that affect their health. For abortion patients, this process is especially important (Joffe 2013). In shared decision-making, the health care provider and patient work together to choose tests, procedures, and treatments, and then to develop a plan of care (American Cancer Society 2021). Essential to informed consent is the provision of medically accurate and unbiased information (table 3.2).

State laws requiring specific informed consent for abortion did not and

TABLE 3.2

Comparison of Standard Informed Consent and
State-Mandated Informed Consent for Abortion

Types of informed consent	Unbiased toward a particular treatment	Medically accurate	Shared decision making
Standard informed consent (IC)	Yes	Yes	Yes
Informed consent abortion laws (ICA)	No	No	No

do not adhere to standard informed consent protocols (Paul and Stein 2011). The *Casey* decision permitted states to provide patient information biased toward childbirth and against abortion. In many states, abortion providers are required to read a state-mandated script to prospective abortion patients.

Recent evidence showed that at least one-third of the information in these scripts is medically inaccurate (Daniels et al. 2016). These erroneous facts are concentrated in descriptions of fetal development in the first trimester, when the vast majority of abortions occur (Daniels et al. 2016). However, misrepresentations are not limited to fetal development. State-mandated counseling may associate abortion with suicidal ideation, psychological trauma, and infertility—all of which are untrue (Ziegler 2020; Daniels et al. 2016). South Dakota's 2005 law, for example, required the attending physician to discuss all of the above and more (Lazzarini 2008).

Waiting Periods

State regulations requiring ICAs for prospective abortion patients and those mandating a waiting period following the informed consent are frequently conjoined, as they were in Pennsylvania's 1989 Abortion Control Act. Waiting period regulations began to grow after the *Casey* decision, doubling from 13 in 1993 to 26 a decade later. Anti-abortion advocates lobbied for both regulations so that women would receive state-mandated abortion counseling and then have a waiting period during which they could reconsider their abortion decisions. Both types of restrictions purport to protect women from making abortion decisions that they would later regret—a widely touted, but largely unsupported concern (Ehrlich and Doan 2019).

TABLE 3.3

Relationship between Waiting Period Laws and Mandated Counseling

State mandates counseling before abortion	State mandates waiting period before abortion		
	No	Yes	Total
No	709	11	720
Percentage	73.5	1.5	42.8
Yes	256	707	963
Percentage	26.5	98.5	57.2
Total	965	718	1,683
Total percentage	100	100	100

Note: Pearson chi-squared = 870.39. Probability = 0.00. First row has frequencies and second row has column percentages. Total = 50 states plus the District of Columbia from 1988–2020.

By 1996, about two-thirds of states with ICAs also required waiting periods. Since that time, waiting periods and informed consent have become even more intertwined. As shown in table 3.3, over 98 percent of the years when American states have had a waiting period, these states have also had another regulation requiring abortion counseling.

In 2020, 28 of the 30 states (as discussed in endnote 27) with ICAs also have waiting periods (the exceptions are Alaska and Rhode Island), ranging from one to 72 hours. In 2020, the average waiting period was 35.4 hours, with the majority of state waiting periods being longer than 24 hours. No "other common medical procedure has a legally mandated waiting period of this kind" (Joyce et al. 2009, 3).[28]

Abortion Reporting

Casey upheld this section of the Pennsylvania abortion law, requiring the abortion provider to submit two different reports to the state regarding the pregnancy termination. The first report was to be confidential, collecting such data as the gestational age of the aborted fetus, the number of third-trimester abortions performed by the provider, and the number of abortions performed as a result of a medical emergency. These data, if made public, were to appear only in summary statistical form.

The second report to the state was quarterly, showing the number of abortions performed, the trimester of pregnancy in which the abortion occurred, and age of the woman having the abortion as well as her county of residence. These reports were to be publicly available if the facility had received state funds during the preceding 12 months (Richardson 1992, 298). Pennsylvania justified this regulation by claiming that this report provided accountability for tax dollars spent (Richardson 1992).[29]

Now, as in 1992, the balance between public health surveillance and patient confidentiality is a fundamental concern for any state abortion reporting requirement (Dreweke 2015). At the time of *Casey*, abortion providers and women's health advocates worried that the level of detail publicly reported about the abortion procedure, as well as the residence of the woman, could compromise patient confidentiality, particularly for women residing in sparsely populated counties. Those concerns about the Pennsylvania Department of Health's abortion reporting system persist to this day (Pennsylvania Department of Health 2020).

Annual data on the characteristics of state abortion reporting systems are unavailable. NARAL Pro-Choice America has not collected annual data on state abortion reporting systems, and the Guttmacher Institute only reports on characteristics of current systems, such as reasons for procedure, method of payment, and adherence to select state requirements (Guttmacher Institute 2023a). Consequently, this type of state abortion regulation was not included in our analysis.[30] Nevertheless, the disparate state abortion reporting systems merit scrutiny. Some important considerations are whether state monitoring systems treat abortion like other health services, whether state reports might inadvertently identify individuals if detailed information is publicly released, and whether abortion providers are scrutinized more than other health providers.

Parental Involvement

The *Casey* decision upheld the parental control provision in the Pennsylvania Control Act of 1989. Any pregnant woman under the age of 18 had to obtain the consent of a parent or guardian, but the law did provide a judicial bypass, "a process by which a minor could go to court and ask a court to allow an abortion without parental permission" (Goldman 2021, 83). Interestingly, the Pennsylvania parental control provision required that the minor's parent or guardian be given the same information as an adult seeking an abortion (Richardson 1992, 298).

As discussed in Chapter 2, states began to regulate minors' rights to abortion shortly after the *Roe* decision, "usually by requiring one or both parents to consent to the procedure" (Mezey 2011, 209). In addition to parental consent, state parental involvement laws also include regulations that require notifying one or both parents before a minor's abortion. In 1979, the US Supreme Court ruled that states requiring parental consent for minors must also offer a judicial bypass.[31] A 1981 decision, however, upheld parental notification without a judicial bypass.[32]

In 1988, 24 states already had laws on the books requiring a minor to have parental consent before an abortion. Seventeen states required one parent to consent, and seven states required the consent of two parents. However, two-thirds of those laws were enjoined. By 1993, after *Casey*, only one-third of those laws were still enjoined. In the same period, parental notification laws followed a similar pattern. In 1988, there were 15 parental notification laws, only three of which were being enforced. By 1993, 10 state parental notification laws were being enforced. Since that time, the number of both parental consent and parental notification laws has increased. In 2020, 31 states had parental consent laws, with 26 enforced, and 20 states had parental notification laws, with 16 enforced.

The Decades Following *Casey*: State Abortion Regulations in the 1990s, 2000s, and 2010s

Beyond the direct impact of the *Webster* and *Casey* decisions on the proliferation of state abortion regulations, new restrictions have continued to appear in the decades since *Casey*. In the two decades following *Roe*, only a few states had any regulations protecting women's rights to abortion. Beginning in the 1990s, some states enacted abortion protections to protect the right to choose. This section documents the emergence of new state abortion restrictions and protections in each decade since the *Casey* decision (table 3.4).

New Restrictions in the 1990s

Gestational Viability Restrictions for Abortion. The probability of survival increases with gestational age (Allen et al. 1993), but "there is no clear bright line denoting the point at which an extremely premature baby can be deemed to have reached the point of viability" (British Pregnancy Advisory Service 2015). Survival outside of the womb is related to the maturity of fetal organs, which varies greatly (Kelly and Welch 2018).

TABLE 3.4
New State Abortion Restrictions and Protections Introduced over the Decades

State abortion restrictions	State abortion protections
1990s	
• Ban abortion after viability • Gag rules for state employees • Ban on abortion coverage for state employees • Prohibit specific abortion procedures • Sponsor "Choose Life" license plates	• State funds abortions for low-income women • Security for abortion providers • State constitutional protection
2000–2009	
• Targeted Regulation of Abortion Providers (TRAP) laws • Prohibit abortion coverage in private market • Prohibit specific abortion procedure (partial birth abortion)	• State Freedom of Choice Act (FOCA) • Require emergency contraception for rape victims (contraceptive access, not abortion) • Access to prescription birth control (contraceptive access, not abortion)
2010–2022	
• Ban based on weeks of gestation • Prohibit abortion in state health insurance exchanges • State funds Crisis Pregnancy Centers • Reason-based bans • Require physician administration of medication abortion • Ban on telemedicine medication abortion • Mandate discussion of reversal • COVID-19 bans on abortion	• State Supreme Court has affirmed right to abortion • Increasing number of abortion clinicians • Mandate abortion coverage in private insurance market • COVID-19 protections for abortion

Nonetheless, the longer the gestation, the greater the likelihood of viability.[33]

Despite this uncertainty, the *Roe* decision permitted states to ban abortion beyond the second trimester, approximately 26–27 weeks, and *Webster* upheld viability testing for abortion beyond 20 weeks gestation, considerably earlier than viability occurs. In 1988, 27 states had banned abortion beyond viability. Between 1988 and 1993, 14 more states banned abortion beyond viability, bringing the total to 41. The number of states with viability restrictions has remained between 41 and 42 since that time. Although the number of these bans has remained steady, many of these laws were not enforced—the number of injunctions had reached 16 by 2020.

By 2021, five states (Alabama, Kansas, Louisiana, Missouri, and Ohio) required viability testing for abortions beyond 20 weeks gestation. At this point, early gestational limits for abortion, bans based on the number of weeks a woman had been pregnant, had mostly superseded viability test-ing. These restrictions included "heartbeat laws," which banned abortion after approximately six weeks gestation (Smythe 2022). Eight of these were in place, but enjoined, by 2021 (Georgia, Iowa, Kentucky, Louisiana, Mississippi, North Dakota, Ohio, and Tennessee) (NARAL Pro-Choice America 2021). After the *Dobbs* decision, each of these states, except for Georgia, banned abortion altogether (Guttmacher Institute 2023d).

Gag Rules for State Employees. Intended to curtail referrals to abor-tion providers, this type of restriction began with three states in 1991. Louisiana, Missouri, and North Dakota each prohibited state workers from discussing abortion, including referrals, with their patients. Penn-sylvania enacted similar legislation in 1995. Michigan followed in 1996, and the following year, Wisconsin and Ohio banned state employees from discussing abortion with clients.

By 1999, 15 states prohibited health care providers employed by the state as well as organizations receiving state funds from counseling about or referring women for abortion services (NARAL 2000, xiii). By 2010, 21 states forbad state workers as well as employees in state-supported orga-nizations from discussing abortion with their patients. As of 2021, this restriction was still enforced by 21 states.

Ban on Abortion Coverage for State Workers' Health Insurance. In 1995, Massachusetts became the sixth state to forbid abortion coverage in the health insurance plans offered to public employees (NARAL 1996). By the end of the decade, 11 states had followed suit. By 2004, 17 states banned abortion coverage for public employees' health insurance, regu-lations that have persisted through 2021.

Prohibit Specific Abortion Procedures. In 1995, Ohio became the first state to outlaw a specific abortion procedure, dilation and extraction, which is used rarely and only in abortion later in pregnancy (ACOG 2021; NAS 2018; Nippita and Paul 2018). Ohio made it a felony for physicians to use dilation and extraction for abortions and offered no exceptions for a woman's health or even her life (NARAL 1996).

By 1996, 19 states had adopted legislation forbidding specific abortion procedures. Dilation and extraction (D&X) and sometimes dilation and evacuation (D&E) were dubbed "partial birth abortion" by anti-abortion forces. By 2000, 31 states banned partial birth abortion, an imprecise political term that is not used in medicine. In 18 of those states, court injunctions were issued to prohibit the enforcement of these bans (NARAL 2000, 238). By the following year, 29 of the 31 states' partial birth abortion bans were enjoined by a court order.

Choose Life License Plates. In 1999, Florida became the first state to officially offer license plates featuring the phrase "Choose Life." Not only did the license plates advertise a particular point of view, but public revenues also realized from the sale of these plates were designated for non-governmental, not-for-profit agencies that limit their services to counseling and meeting the physical needs of pregnant women who are committed to placing their children up for adoption.

In 2001, Louisiana and South Carolina enacted similar laws. Oklahoma and Mississippi followed suit in 2002; Arkansas, Connecticut, Maryland, and Tennessee started offering Choose Life plates in 2003. The number of states offering Choose Life license plates as an option grew virtually every year after 2003, with 34 states allowing the official production of Choose Life license plates by 2022 (Guttmacher Institute 2022b).

State Protections Emerge in the 1990s

State Funding for Abortions for Low-Income Women. In 1993, 12 states funded abortions for low-income women.[34] That number jumped to 18 in 1994. The District of Columbia, New Mexico, Idaho, Illinois, Maryland, and Minnesota funded abortion with their own funds for Medicaid-eligible women. In 1997, the District of Columbia stopped funding abortions. In 1998, Alaska, Idaho, and Illinois no longer funded most abortions for low-income women.

Because of court challenges, there was some fluctuation during the early 2000s. Abortion funding became somewhat stable, with 17 states supporting abortion for low-income women from 2002 to 2017. Arizona stopped abortion funding in 2018. By 2023, 17 states funded abortion for Medicaid-eligible women.

Security for Abortion Providers. By the end of 1991, five states (California, Maryland, Nevada, Oregon, and Washington) had laws on the books criminalizing clinic harassment and violence. By 1994, this number had more than doubled; 11 states banned intimidation and violence against abortion clinics and providers. Six of these state laws followed the enactment of federal legislation. In 1994, the Freedom of Access to Clinic Entrances Act (FACE) was passed, prohibiting "the use of force, threats, or physical obstruction to block access to abortion clinics" (NARAL 1995, iv).

FACE and the growth in this protective regulation stemmed, in no small part, from the grim events of 1993 and 1994. In 1993, Dr. David Gunn, who performed abortions, was murdered in Pensacola, Florida. In 1994, two more physicians and a clinic escort were shot and killed by an anti-abortion activist. Two abortion clinic receptionists in Boston were murdered the same year. These killings were in addition to the death threats, bombings, blockades, chemical attacks, and other violent acts perpetrated against abortion providers and their families (Hern 2021; NARAL 1995; Stack 2015; Feminist Majority 1993).

State bans against abortion provider violence and harassment grew to 15 in 1999, following the 1998 assassination of Dr. Bernard Slepian in Buffalo, New York. In 2009, Dr. George Tiller, an abortion provider, was murdered while he served as an usher for church services in Topeka, Kansas. By 2021, 19 states had laws protecting abortion clinics, providers, and patients from blockades, harassment, and/or other anti-choice violence (NARAL Pro-Choice America 2021, 20).

State Constitutional Protection. By 1994, courts in 13 states[35] had decreed that their constitutions provided more protection for choosing abortion than did the US Constitution. Over half of these decisions were issued after the *Casey* decision. These state judicial rulings were not just pro-forma. Two states, California and Florida, invalidated both ICAs and mandatory waiting periods under their state constitutions (NARAL 1995, x). Over the years, few fluctuations have occurred; the number of states with state constitutional protections was 15 in 2021.

State Abortion Regulations 2000–2009

The new millennium ushered in new and more restrictions along with a new anti-abortion president, former Texas governor George W. Bush. The FDA finally approved medication abortion, which had been used in Europe since 1988. In December 2000, the US Equal Employment Opportunity Commission found that two employers that denied coverage for prescription contraceptives violated Title VII of the Civil Rights Act of

1964, as amended by the Pregnancy Discrimination Act (Kaiser Family Foundation 2023b; Paul and Stein 2011; NARAL 2001, v).

RESTRICTIONS 2000–2009

Targeted Regulation of Abortion Providers (TRAP). These laws place more onerous regulations on abortion providers than necessary for patient safety; they are a form of franchising or licensing (Chapter 1) determining the conditions under which a clinic or a private practice can operate if they offer abortion services. Using this regulatory mechanism as a political strategy instead of a quality control measure, state TRAP laws aim to "drive doctors out of practice and make abortion care more expensive and difficult to obtain" (Goldman 2021, 108). All state abortion regulations apply to abortion clinics, but in some states, TRAP laws apply to "physicians' offices where abortions are performed or even to sites where medication abortion is administered" (Guttmacher Institute 2022j, 1).

TRAP laws cover a constellation of abortion restrictions. Most "requirements apply states' standards for ambulatory surgical centers to abortion clinics, even though surgical centers tend to provide more invasive and risky procedures and use higher levels of sedation" (Guttmacher Institute 2022j, 1). Common TRAP regulations include limiting the provision of care to physicians only, forcing abortion clinics to convert into mini-hospitals,[36] requiring abortion providers to get hospital admitting privileges, and mandating that facilities have a transfer agreement with a local hospital. Because no state requires or even encourages hospitals to grant such privileges, local hospitals in states with this type of regulation have a de facto veto over "qualified and willing abortion providers" (Goldman 2021).

These types of restrictions are not new. In the years immediately following *Roe*, several states imposed unnecessarily strict regulations on abortion clinics. In the 1980s, lower federal courts struck down many of these requirements, but TRAP laws resurfaced in the 1990s and grew rapidly after 2000.

NARAL began reporting TRAP laws in 2001. At that time, 35 states had some type of TRAP law (NARAL 2002). By 2007, that number had climbed to 45.[37] Of those 45 states, 25 restricted the provision of abortion to a hospital or another specialized facility. These states impose far more stringent regulations on abortion clinics than are necessary for patient safety (NAS 2018).

TRAP Admitting Privileges. Proponents of this type of TRAP law claim that it promotes patient safety. In fact, TRAP laws that require admitting privileges for physicians offering abortion services aim to make pregnancy terminations less available. However, in states with this kind of TRAP law, providers that offer abortion services cannot be licensed unless they adhere to this regulation. Complications from abortion are rare, and if they do occur, hospitals must admit emergency patients (Mukpo 2020). Admitting privileges usually require a minimum number of annual hospital visits. Many physicians providing abortion services simply do not have the requisite number of cases with complications to qualify, precisely because they are competently delivering a safe service (Joffe 2019).

After the 2016 Supreme Court *Whole Woman* decision struck down the hospital privileges mandate in Texas,[38] only a few states were able to enforce laws requiring that doctors working in clinics performing abortions have admitting privileges at local hospitals. To circumvent the unconstitutionality of this type of regulation, nine states required that a doctor performing abortions must have hospital admitting privileges or alternative agreements. Indiana, for example, required "an abortion provider to either have admitting privileges or an agreement with another physician who has admitting privileges at a local hospital" (Guttmacher Institute 2022j).[39]

Ban on Abortion Coverage in Private Markets. In 2001, six states (Idaho, Kentucky, Missouri, North Dakota, Rhode Island, and Wisconsin) prohibited private coverage for abortion unless the woman paid an extra premium for insurance for an unplanned pregnancy. The Rhode Island law was ruled unconstitutional. Pennsylvania required insurers to offer a policy alternative excluding abortion, and a Massachusetts law specifically stated that health maintenance organizations (HMOs) were not required to pay or refer for abortion (NARAL 2002). Oklahoma banned the private coverage of abortion in 2004; Nebraska and Utah followed suit in 2011. Indiana and Michigan enacted similar bans in 2014. Texas joined this group in 2017.

Ban Specific Abortion Procedures. The crusade against partial birth abortion—a political term, not a medical procedure—continued into the 2000s. In 2001, following the 2000 *Stenberg v. Carhart* decision, 31 states had laws on the books banning partial birth abortion. Twenty-nine of those state laws were enjoined largely because they did not provide an exception for a woman's health. The 2000 *Stenberg* ruling "temporarily took the steam out of state legislative efforts to ban abortion procedures" (NARAL 2001, x).

Stenberg, however, was followed by the federal Partial Birth Abortion Ban of 2003, similar to the Nebraska law struck down in 2000. The Supreme Court upheld this federal law in *Carhart v. Gonzales* in 2007, despite that fact that the federal law had no exception for a woman's health.[40] In doing so, the Court overturned its *Stenberg* ruling decided only seven years earlier (Goldman 2021, 89–90).

PROTECTIONS

State Freedom of Choice Acts. A state's Freedom of Choice Act (FOCA) helps to ensure that a woman's right to choose is protected, by making essential provisions of *Roe* a permanent part of state law. In 1990, Connecticut became the first state to codify a woman's right to choose abortion before viability. Maryland and Washington followed with similar legislative affirmations in 1991. The following year, Maryland voters supported the right to choose by approving the pro-choice legislative affirmation through referendum, thus overturning the state's pre-*Roe* criminal abortion law.[41] Hawaii and Nevada each codified *Roe v. Wade* in 2006, the latter by referendum.

From 2006 to 2017, no other states passed FOCA legislation. In 2018, however, two more states, Delaware and Oregon, passed FOCA laws. California, New York, Rhode Island, and Vermont added the right to choose in state laws in 2019. The following year, the District of Columbia and Massachusetts enacted measures to improve abortion access.

CONTRACEPTIVE PROTECTIONS

Although not abortion protections per se, state contraceptive mandates do protect women's reproductive health choices. They aim to reduce unintended pregnancy, and thus the need for abortion. Two of these are discussed below.[42]

Emergency Contraception. This is any method "that women can use after unprotected sexual intercourse to prevent pregnancy" (Trussell and Schwarz 2011, 113). Emergency contraception, most commonly in the form of pills (ECPs), "does not cause abortion or harm an established pregnancy" (Trussell and Schwarz 2011, 121).[43] Estimates show that "increased use of ECPs could reduce the number of unintended pregnancies and abortions by half" (NARAL 2000, ix). They could also prevent the more than 22,000 pregnancies each year resulting from rape (Stewart and Trussell 2000).

In 2002, California and Washington became the first states to enact laws requiring hospitals to inform rape survivors about emergency contraception. At the time, 82 percent of Catholic hospitals did not provide emergency contraception, even to women who had been raped (NARAL 2000, x). The following year, New Mexico and New York passed similar legislation, and in 2005, eight states mandated that emergency contraception be offered to rape survivors. The Commonwealth of Massachusetts was one of those states. Not only did Massachusetts require that victims of sexual assault receive information about and access to emergency contraception, but that year, the state also passed a law allowing pharmacists to dispense emergency contraception to women without a prescription (NARAL 2006, 5).

By 2014, 17 states and the District of Columbia had laws that improved sexual-assault survivors' access to emergency contraception or required information about emergency contraception in hospitals (NARAL Pro-Choice America 2014). By 2023, 21 states and the District of Columbia required hospital emergency rooms to provide emergency contraception–related services to sexual assault victims (Guttmacher Institute 2023b).

States have also expanded access to emergency contraception by allowing pharmacists "to dispense emergency contraception without a physician's prescription under certain conditions" (Guttmacher Institute 2023b). Five states allow pharmacists to distribute ECP "when acting under a collaborative-practice agreement with a physician" (Guttmacher Institute 2023b). Three states "allow pharmacists to distribute emergency contraception in accordance with a state-approved protocol" (Guttmacher Institute 2023b).

Access to Prescription Birth Control. In 2005, two states, California and Illinois, passed laws mandating access to contraceptive prescriptions. California "enacted a guaranteed access to prescriptions law, prohibiting pharmacists from refusing to fill women's prescriptions based on their personal beliefs."[44] Illinois required pharmacies selling contraceptives to dispense prescription birth control without delays (NARAL Pro-Choice America 2006, 4).[45] Maine, Nevada, and New Jersey passed similar legislation in 2005, with Washington State doing so the following year. Wisconsin joined this group of seven states in 2010, which has not increased since that time.

State Abortion Laws 2010–2021

RESTRICTIONS

Abortion Bans by Week of Gestation. In 2010, only two states had bans on abortion based on the weeks of gestation. By 2018, 22 states had unenforceable bans on abortion at or below 20 weeks gestation. Two states (Iowa and North Dakota) had an unenforceable ban at six weeks, before many women know they are pregnant. By 2022, at least 12 states had six-week bans (Nash 2021).

Abortion Bans in State Health Exchanges or Marketplaces. In 2010, Congress passed and President Obama signed the Affordable Care Act (ACA) extending health insurance coverage to millions of Americans. A cornerstone of this program was health insurance exchanges (also called marketplaces), where citizens and small employers in each state could shop (online) for health insurance (Kaiser Family Foundation 2013).

By the end of 2010, five states (Arizona, Louisiana, Mississippi, Missouri, and Tennessee) had banned abortion from any plan included in its state health insurance marketplace. This ban was in addition to the complex federal rules for abortion coverage.[46] Since that time, more states passed this abortion restriction; this number reached 24 states in 2017 (NARAL Pro-Choice America 2018).

State Funding for Crisis Pregnancy Centers. Crisis Pregnancy Centers (CPCs)[47] are facilities set up to discourage women from having abortions.

CPCs advertise as if they were abortion providers, but their purpose is to dissuade women from having abortions (Goldman 2021, 93). They often provide free pregnancy tests, and some offer sonograms (Ehrlich and Doan 2019). Across the United States, there are far more CPCs than abortion providers.[48]

In 1996, the first states, Missouri and Pennsylvania, began to fund CPCs. In its first year of funding CPCs, Pennsylvania appropriated $2 million for this purpose. Both states only gave funding to organizations that did not refer for abortions. More than a decade later, only a handful of other states had followed Missouri and Pennsylvania's lead in funding CPCs. By 2011, however, 10 states had followed suit. As of 2021, 16 states financially supported CPCs. Funding CPCs is an abortion restriction because the purpose of CPCs is to talk women out of having abortions.

Reason-Based Bans. In 2013, North Dakota became the first state to prohibit abortions in cases of fetal abnormality, even in cases where the fetus had a condition that is incompatible with life and would die before or soon after birth (Guttmacher Institute 2021a). By 2016, 10 states enacted reason-based restrictions, laws holding physicians liable for performing abortions for specific reasons. Three states (Indiana, Louisiana, and North Dakota) would hold the physician liable if the abortion were performed because of a fetal anomaly. Two states (Arizona and Indiana) banned abortion if it were being sought because of the race or sex of the pregnancy. Nine states (Arizona, Illinois, Indiana, Kansas, North Carolina, North Dakota, Oklahoma, Pennsylvania, and South Dakota) banned abortion if sought because of the sex of the pregnancy (NARAL Pro-Choice America 2017). By 2020, the number of states with reason-based bans had increased to 16.

Mandate That Only Physicians Can Prescribe Medication Abortion. As of 2021, 32 states insisted that only physicians can prescribe medication abortions. These state regulations contradict recommendations from the World Health Organization, the National Academies of Science, Engineering, and Medicine, and the National Abortion Federation that mid-level providers or advanced practitioners, such as physician assistants and nurse practitioners, can safely provide medication abortion (Guttmacher Institute 2023c).

Ban on Telemedicine Medication Abortion. Nineteen states require the clinician, usually a physician, to be in the same room as the patient when dispensing abortion-inducing drugs (Kaiser Family Foundation 2022b). These regulations effectively ban "telemedicine provision of medication abortion despite clinical evidence that this practice is appropriate and safe" (Guttmacher Institute 2023c, 1). For patients in rural areas and other regions with few abortion providers, this type of restriction greatly limits access to medication abortion. (Guttmacher Institute 2023c).

Informed Consent and Reversing Medical Abortion. In 2019, five states (Arkansas, Kentucky, Nebraska, North Dakota, and Oklahoma) enacted legislation requiring abortion providers "to counsel pregnant patients about unproven claims about 'reversing' a medication abortion" (NARAL 2020, 4). This information is incorrect and has no support in the medical literature (Grossman et al. 2015). Nonetheless, abortion providers had to provide unsubstantiated information to their patients in these states, a violation of the patient–physician relationship.

COVID-19 Restrictions. During the COVID-19 pandemic, anti-abortion officials in 13 states[49] attempted to restrict access to abortion care (Webber 2020). In these states, the governor or the state health director issued executive orders "that limited access to or resulted in a complete ban on abortion services" (Rebouche 2021, 117). In Alabama, for example, the state health director issued an order postponing surgical procedures not necessary to treat an "emergency medical condition" or "avoid serious harm from an underlying condition" (Rebouche 2021, 117). In Ohio, the director of the state health department prohibited all nonessential surgeries and procedures that used personal protective equipment (PPE). This order included abortion services, and it was enforced by the state attorney general, who sent cease and desist letters to abortion providers. In Texas and Tennessee, governors issued these orders.

These bans did not remain in force for long. Several of these orders were enjoined by state and federal courts or they expired (e.g., Alaska). Arkansas had the longest lasting ban on abortion services, roughly two months. Eight weeks of pregnancy, of course, is not trivial and could easily put a woman beyond the gestational limits for an abortion in many states (Jones et al. 2020). Reports from these states indicate that while these bans were in place, patients seeking abortion experienced abruptly cancelled appointments and more. Once clinics reopened, there were long waiting lists for appointments (Rebouche 2021).

PROTECTIONS

State Supreme Courts and the Right to Abortion. By 2018, nine states (Alaska, California, Florida, Iowa, Massachusetts, Minnesota, Montana, New Jersey, and New Mexico) had rulings from their states' highest courts affirming that the state constitution protects the right to abortion, separate from the federal Constitution. The following year, the Kansas Supreme Court affirmed that the state constitution protects the right to abortion (NARAL Pro-Choice America 2020; NARAL Pro-Choice America 2019).

Increasing Abortion Clinicians. By 2015, 10 states and the District of Columbia had expanded the scope of practice for advanced-practice clinicians so that they could prescribe or dispense medication abortion or perform early aspiration abortions (California, Connecticut, Illinois, Montana, New Hampshire, New York, Oregon, Rhode Island, Vermont, and Washington). Six of these states (California, Montana, New Hampshire, New York, Oregon, and Vermont) permitted both.

By 2020, that number had increased to 13 states, with Maryland, Massachusetts, and Virginia expanding the scope of practice for advanced practice clinicians so that they could provide abortion care. Both Massachusetts and Maryland allowed advanced practice clinicians to provide surgical abortion care (NARAL Pro-Choice America 2021, 18).

Requiring Abortion Coverage in the Private Insurance Market. In 2014, California became the first state to require that all health insurance plans in the state cover abortion. This policy was a stark contrast to the 26 states that banned abortion coverage in either their private insurance or health exchange markets (NARAL Pro-Choice America 2015, 2). New York and Oregon passed similar protections in 2017. They were joined by Washington State in 2018, and Maine in 2019.

COVID-19 Protections. During the COVID-19 crisis, governors in 12 states[50] issued executive orders stating that essential medical services included abortion. Many of these states also recognized family planning and other reproductive health services as essential. As Chapter 6 explains, these orders stopped short of some of the Western European provisions implemented during the pandemic (Jones et al. 2020).

PERIPHERAL PROTECTIONS FOR REPRODUCTIVE HEALTH

States also passed peripheral protections aimed at reducing unintended pregnancy and improving maternal outcomes. California, Connecticut, Illinois, Maryland, Rhode Island, and Washington all enacted policies to improve sex education in the state (NARAL Pro-Choice America 2021; NARAL Pro-Choice America 2019). Multiple states, including Connecticut, Indiana, Louisiana, Maryland, Oregon, and the District of Columbia, enacted measures to improve maternal mortality—or at least begin to evaluate the care and support that pregnant women can receive (NARAL Pro-Choice America 2019, 2). Other states began to offer services and protections for pregnant women who are incarcerated.

THE SUPREME COURT AND THE STATES

Starting in 2017, states were passing more abortion protections than restrictions. Of course, the existing restrictions were still on the books, and the number of aggregate restrictions greatly exceeded the number of abortion protections. There was much pro-choice legislation at the state level, but also more extreme abortion restrictions.[51]

After the Trump appointment of Justice Gorsuch in 2017 to the seat that President Obama had been unable to fill, anti-abortion states seemed to be baiting the US Supreme Court. These states were enacting laws that had previously been ruled unconstitutional. This trend continued with two more conservative Trump appointments: Justice Kavanaugh (2018) and Justice Coney Barrett (2020).

The acceleration of state abortion regulation continued: more state protections passed, but more restrictions as well (Wilson 2020). In 2020, Colorado voters turned down a proposed ban on abortion later in pregnancy that would have forced someone to carry a pregnancy to term (with no exceptions for risks to health, a lethal fetal diagnosis, or rape). At the same time, Louisiana voters approved an amendment to the state constitution to make clear that it did not protect the right to abortion or require public coverage of abortion care (NARAL Pro-Choice America 2021). In 2021, New Mexico overturned its pre-*Roe* criminal abortion law from 1969, which is explained in Chapter 4. States seemed to be poised for a Supreme Court decision that would overturn *Roe v. Wade* or considerably weaken a woman's right to choose abortion.

In abortion politics, the process of states gauging the likely position of the Supreme Court is nothing new (Patton 2007). The 1989 *Webster* decision, as well as the 1992 *Casey* decision, precipitated an increasing number of state abortion bills and enactments. New state laws included informed consent before an abortion, spousal and parental consent requirements, conscience clauses for abortion providers, mandatory waiting periods, hospital board approval requirements, and stringent licensing requirements for abortion providers (NARAL 1991, iii). More recently, anticipation of the Supreme Court's *Dobbs* decision incentivized states to enact more and new restrictions (Bouie 2022; Collins 2022).

State Party Control and Abortion Regulation

Partisanship plays an important role in abortion regulation. The rapid rise in the overall number of abortion restrictions in the latter half of the 1990s and again between 2010 and 2014 (figure 1.1) coincided with a shift in state political party control from the Democrats to the Republicans. The number of Republican governors hovered around 20 from 1988 to 1994, but that number jumped to 32 in 1995. In 2007, the number of Republican governors was back down to 22, only to increase again in 2010 to 24, then to 30 in 2011.

A similar shift occurred in state legislatures. Republican control of state houses shifted from 15 to 24 states between 1994 and 1995. Republican control rose again from 16 to 29 states between 2010 and 2011. On the Senate side, 18 state senates were under Republican control in 1994, rising to 25 in 1995. Similarly, the number of state senates under Republican control increased from 19 in 2010, to 27 in 2011, and to 30 in 2012.

Trifecta Control

The likelihood of policy adoption increases when the same party controls a state's executive and legislative branches. Over time, Republican trifecta control at the state level has increased. In 1994, the Republican Party controlled all three bodies of government in six states. This number jumped to 15 states in 1995. In 2010, 10 states were governed by Republican trifectas. This number jumped to 21 states in 2011 and 24 states in 2012. These shifts in Republican control of state governments contributed to the rise in state abortion restrictions over time. This phenomenon is examined in more detail in Chapter 4.

Average Change in Restrictions

State party control (Republican, Democratic, or divided) also affects the average change in abortion restrictions and protections. Over the time period 1989–2020,[52] the Republican Party controlled state government for a total of 463 state/years, just over 28 percent of the cases. Under Republican control, the average change in the number of restrictions is a 2.2 increase; the average change in the number of restrictions for the remaining state/years not under Republican control is a 0.7 decrease. This represents a 2.9 difference in means, statistically significant at better than a $p = 0.0001$ level.

For state abortion protections, the average number under Republican control is a 0.8 decrease compared with an average 0.3 increase in the number of protections under divided government or Democrat control. This represents a 1.1 difference in means, statistically significant at better than a $p = 0.0001$ level.

The results are similar when comparing states and years under Republican trifecta control versus Democrat trifecta control. The average number of restrictions increases by 2.2 under a Republican trifecta versus a 1.1 decrease in the average number of restrictions under a Democratic trifecta. This represents a 3.3 difference in means, statistically significant at better than a $p = 0.0001$ level. The average number of protections under a Republican trifecta decreased by 0.8 compared with a 0.8 increase under a Democratic trifecta, a difference in means of 1.6, again significant at better than a $p = 0.0001$ level.

Overall, partisanship in state government clearly has an impact on the adoption of state restrictions and protections.[53] Under Republican party control, on average, restrictions increase and protections decrease. Conversely, under Democratic party control, on average, restrictions decrease and protections increase. The impact of partisanship is addressed in more depth in the multivariate models in Chapter 4.

State Abortion Regulations over Time

State Abortion Restrictions

Over time, the number of abortion restrictions[54] in individual states has risen. In 1988, the average number of state restrictions was 2.55 per state. Between the *Webster* and *Casey* decisions, the yearly state average increased to 3.08. In the post-*Casey* period (1993–2020),[55] the average number of state restrictions rose to 7.64. The average number of state restrictions rose each decade from 4.55 in the period from 1990–99 to 6.98 between 2000 and 2009 and to 9.82 in the period from 2010 to 2019. By 2020, the last year for which we have comprehensive data, the average number of state restrictions reached 11.39.

Figure 3.1 shows the average number of state restrictions (and protections) over time. In Appendix table A.2, we separate the restrictions into the individual regulations to give us the total number of abortion restrictions; here we report the number of years that each regulation was in existence for each state. The number of years varies from zero for states that never enacted a regulation during our period of study, 1988 to 2020, to 33 for states that had regulations throughout our time period. As we can see, Vermont, Oregon, and New Hampshire are among the states with the fewest enacted regulations (the most zeros), and Missouri and Pennsylvania are among the states with the most long-standing regulations that extended through the entire time period of 33 years.

States passed a record number of abortion restrictions in 2021 (Nash and Ephross 2022; Nash and Naide 2021). New 2021 restrictions included near-total abortion bans (Arkansas and Oklahoma), bans on abortions after six weeks of pregnancy (Idaho, Oklahoma, South Carolina, and Texas), trigger bans (Oklahoma and Texas) that would ban all abortions if *Roe v. Wade* were overturned, gestational bans (Montana) starting at 20 weeks of pregnancy, reason-based bans (South Dakota and Arizona) for Down syndrome and fetal abnormalities, medication abortion restrictions (Arizona, Arkansas, Indiana, Montana, Ohio, Oklahoma, South Dakota, and West Virginia), regulations prohibiting or restricting telehealth for medication abortion, counseling requirements (Arkansas, Indiana, South Dakota, and West Virginia), and additional TRAP restrictions

(Arizona, Arkansas, Indiana, Kentucky, Ohio, Oklahoma, and Tennessee) on abortion providers (Sobel et al. 2022a).

State Abortion Protections

State abortion protections have also risen over the years, but much more slowly than restrictions. In 1988, no state laws protected a woman's right to choose or access abortion services. Twelve states had enacted a single abortion protection, allowing state funds to be used to fund abortion for low-income women. Between the *Webster* and *Casey* decisions, the yearly state average number of protections was only 0.37. After 1992, the average climbed to only 1.44.

Looking at the state abortion protections by decade, the yearly state average was only 0.71 in the 1990s, 1.26 in the 2000s, and 1.89 in the 2010s. There was a significant uptick in 2020, when the average number of state protections rose to 2.82. More state abortion protections passed in 2021 and 2022 than in previous years, but most protections are only from a few states (Nash and Ephross 2022; Sobel et al. 2022b). Overall, the average number of state protections lags far behind the average number of state abortion restrictions (figure 3.1).

Similar to Appendix table A.2, Appendix table A.3 shows each protection used in the study along with the number of years each type of protection was in existence in each state. A number of states have no enacted protections throughout our period of study; these include Alabama, Georgia, Kentucky, Louisiana, Mississippi, Missouri, Nebraska, North Dakota, Ohio, and Wyoming. States with the among the most long-standing protections include California, Massachusetts, Minnesota, Oregon, Vermont, and Washington.

Abortion Regulations by State

With few exceptions, state abortion regulations have been cumulative. For example, if a state enacted an abortion restriction in 1988, that abortion restriction will be on the books in subsequent years. As a result, the number of abortion restrictions for each state mounts over time. The number of restrictions, however, varies dramatically by state. By 2020, states that had enacted the greatest number of abortion regulations included Kansas, Kentucky, Louisiana, Mississippi, Missouri, North Da-

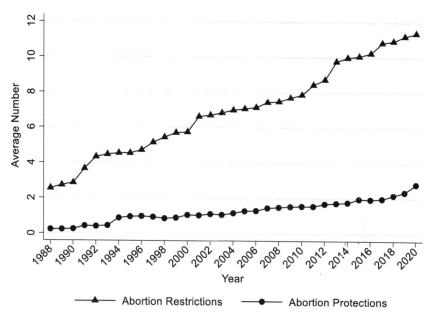

FIGURE 3.1. Average Number of Abortion Regulations per State, 1988–2020

kota, Ohio, and Oklahoma, each with 20 or more restrictions, followed by Arizona, Arkansas, and Texas, each with 19. At the other extreme are Vermont and Oregon, each with no more than one restriction in the entire period from 1988 through 2020. Only a few states—such as Virginia, Delaware, Illinois, and Massachusetts—have reduced the number of restrictions in recent years (figure 3.2).

Protections also vary dramatically by state, with many states—Alabama, Georgia, Kentucky, Louisiana, Mississippi, Missouri, Nebraska, North Dakota, Ohio, South Dakota, and Wyoming—enacting no protections from 1988 to 2020. In most states, the enactment of protections occurred far later than did restrictions. Nonetheless, abortion protections, like restrictions, increased over time. California has enacted the most protections of any state, reaching 10 by 2015, followed by Illinois, Massachusetts, and Washington, each with nine protections by 2020 (figure 3.3).

Abortion Regulations by Region

Figure 3.4 reveals regional differences in abortion restrictions. Southern states have far more abortion restrictions than any other region, and these have been growing at a steeper rate in recent years. The Midwest is next

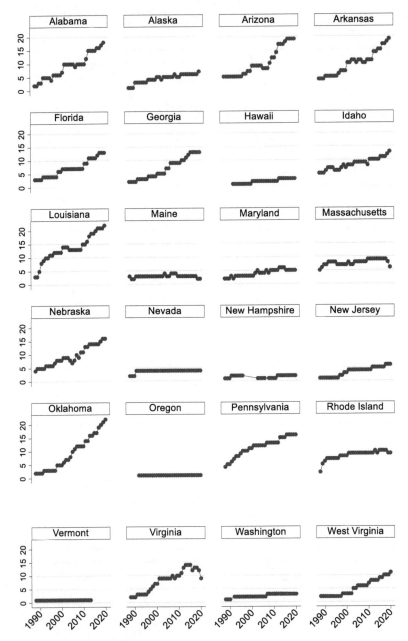

FIGURE 3.2. Number of Abortion Restrictions by State, 1988–2020

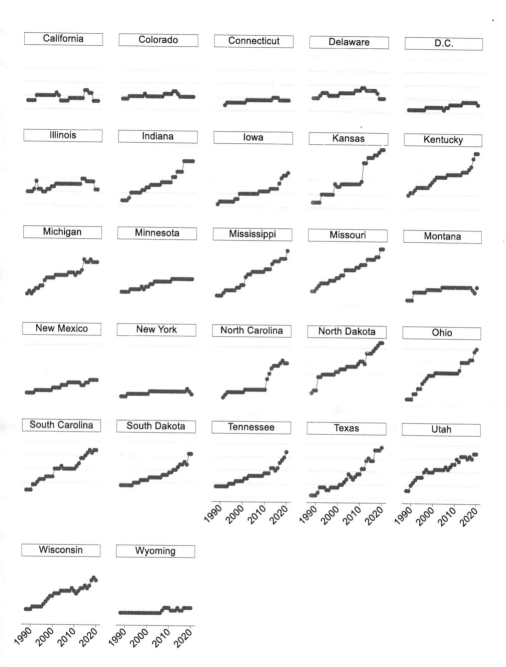

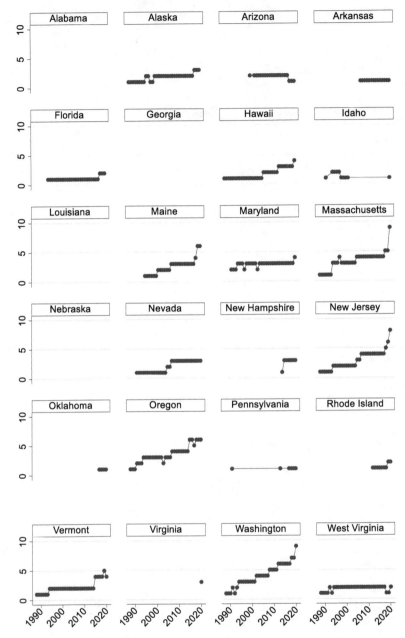

FIGURE 3.3. Number of Abortion Protections by State, 1988–2020

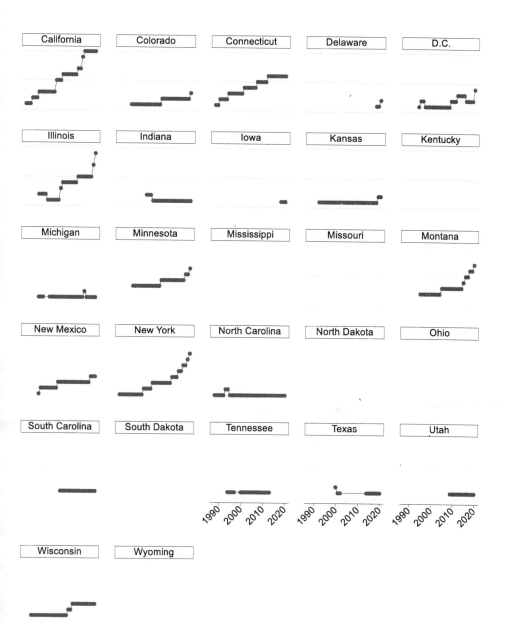

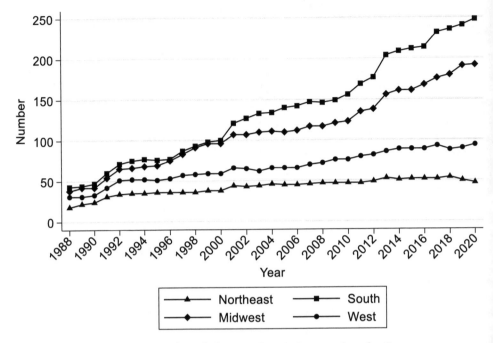

FIGURE 3.4. Average Number of Abortion Restrictions per State by Census Region, 1988–2020

in terms of restrictions, with a significant gap between the Midwest and the West, which is third. Northeastern states have the fewest restrictions, and these have been declining in recent years.

Not surprising, there is nearly an opposite relationship with the number of regional abortion protections (figure 3.5). The West has the most protections, followed in recent years very closely by the Northeast. In most years of the study period, the Midwest is third in the number of abortion protections, and the South is last.

Demand-Side versus Supply-Side Abortion Regulations

State abortion restrictions and protections can be aimed at abortion patients or abortion providers, or both. In other words, some regulations specifically target the women seeking abortion (demand-side), whereas others specifically target providers of abortion (supply-side). An example of a demand-side restriction is requiring parental involvement in a minor's decision to seek abortion services. An example of a supply-side restriction

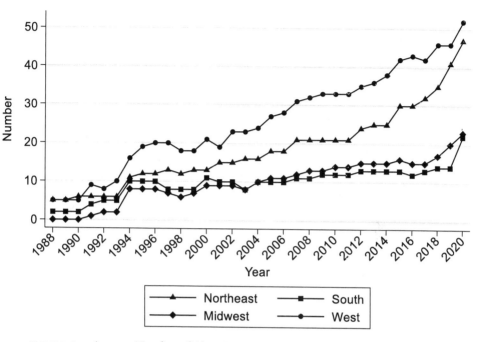

FIGURE 3.5. Average Number of Abortion Protections per State by Census Region, 1988–2020

is state TRAP laws requiring abortion providers to comply with facility specifications of ambulatory surgical centers.

Since 1988, most states have enacted more demand restrictions that target women seeking abortion than supply restrictions that target providers. The average number of state demand-side restrictions rose from 2.6 in 1988 to 6.8 in 2020, whereas the average number of state-supply restrictions increased from 0.3 to 4.2. The overall averages for the entire period are 4.6 (demand) and 2.3 (supply). Only a handful of states (Alaska, Connecticut, Hawaii, New Jersey, Oregon, and Washington) enacted more supply than demand restrictions, but these are also the states with among the lowest number of restrictions overall.

States that have the highest average number of demand-side restrictions across the whole time period (1988 to 2020) are North Dakota (9.1), Utah (8.5), Kentucky (7.9), Pennsylvania (7.8), Louisiana (7.3), Nebraska (7.3), and Missouri (7.2), followed by Idaho, Kansas, Rhode Island, South Carolina, Ohio, Wisconsin, Michigan, Arkansas, and Mississippi, all with an average of more than six demand-side restrictions. Hawaii, Oregon, and Vermont have no demand-side restrictions, and New Jersey, New York, and Washington State all have an average of less than one restriction over the period.

Supply-side restrictions are far fewer and have less variance. The state with the largest average number of supply-side restrictions is Utah with 3.6, followed by Missouri, Arizona, Ohio, Michigan, South Dakota, South Carolina, Oklahoma, Louisiana, Indiana, Arkansas, and North Dakota, all with more than three supply-side restrictions on average. Vermont is the only state with no supply-side restrictions, followed by New Hampshire, Oregon, and Washington, DC, all with fewer than one restriction on average over the period.

Protections that specifically target patients or providers (consumers or suppliers) are far fewer in number. Examples of a demand-side protections are when states guarantee that birth control prescriptions will be filled or when the state requires private health insurance companies to cover abortion services. An example of a supply-side protection is when a state expands the scope of practice for nurse practitioners to include medical or surgical abortion.

The first demand-side protections appeared in 2005 in California and Illinois. By 2007, in addition to these, Maine, Nevada, and New Jersey had enacted one demand-side protection. By 2020, only 16 states had any demand-side protections, the most in Illinois and Washington at three each. The first supply-side protections appeared in 1991 in California, Maryland, Nevada, Oregon, and Wisconsin, with one protection each. Kansas joined these states in 1992, followed by Colorado, North Carolina, and Wisconsin in 1993. By 2020, 26 states had enacted between one and three supply-side protections, the most in California, Massachusetts, Montana, New Hampshire, New York, and Washington.

State-level protections were adopted much later than restrictions, and thus the averages over the study period are much smaller. California stands out as the state with the highest average number of both demand- and supply-side protections. On the demand side, California is followed by Illinois and Washington. On the supply side, beyond California, the states with the next highest averages are New York, Oregon, and Washington State. Most states (35) have no demand-side protections, and half (25) have no supply-side protections. Many of the states with no protections are also among the states with the highest average number of restrictions.

Not All Abortion Restrictions Are Enforced

Abortion restrictions are frequently challenged in both state and federal courts. At any point in time, some restrictions are likely to be enjoined (or not enforced). For some types of abortion restrictions, this difference is not trivial. For example, in 2019, courts enjoined one-fifth of the 30 enacted waiting period state laws, meaning that six states with waiting period laws could not enforce them, either permanently or temporarily (NARAL 2020).

Women's Perceptions and Abortion Restrictions

To comply with state laws, abortion providers must know the difference between enacted and enforced abortion restrictions. Women seeking abortion may not understand this distinction. Moreover, at any point in time, many women are unlikely to know if a particular abortion restriction is enforced or enjoined.

A woman's perception of her state's abortion regulations, even if incorrect, can affect her decision to seek abortion services. Findings from a recent study showed that women in states with four or more enacted abortion restrictions think that access to both medical and surgical abortion is difficult (Perreira et al. 2020). Over time, more states have reached this four-restriction threshold. In 1988, 15 states had enacted four or more restrictions, although only three states enforced that many. By 1992, 30 states had enacted four or more restrictions, with only 11 enforcing four or more. By 2010, the number of states with four or more enforced restrictions (40) almost equaled the number of states with four or more enacted restrictions (43). By 2020, the comparable number of states was 42 (enacted) and 41 (enforced).

After Dobbs

By overturning *Roe v. Wade*, the US Supreme Court's *Dobbs* decision reset the parameters of state abortion regulation. By November 2023, abortion was banned in 14 states (Arkansas, Alabama, Idaho, Indiana, Kentucky, Louisiana, Mississippi, Missouri, North Dakota, Oklahoma, South

Dakota, Tennessee, Texas, and West Virginia). Georgia and South Carolina also prohibit abortion after six weeks of pregnancy, "before many women know they are pregnant" (*New York Times* 2023). Courts have temporarily blocked enforcement of bans in six other states (Arizona, Iowa, Montana, Utah, Wisconsin, and Wyoming). In states where abortion is available, "the influx of patients from states with severe restrictions has created lengthy waiting times" for abortion services (Nash and Ephross 2022).

Legislatures and governors in other states reacted to the *Dobbs* decision by implementing pro-choice abortion laws, policies, and programs. Eighteen states (California, Colorado, Connecticut, Delaware, Hawaii, Illinois, Maine, Maryland, Massachusetts, Michigan, New Mexico, Nevada, New Jersey, New York, Oregon, Rhode Island Vermont, and Washington) adopted a total of 77 protective provisions[56] through the legislative process or executive orders that focused on abortion funding, clinic access and safety, and "shield laws" to protect providers from out-of-state lawsuits for providing abortions. In sum, more abortion protections were passed in 2022 than in 2021, but most of these measures came from only a few states.

In an August primary vote and the November midterm elections, voters in six states (California, Kansas, Kentucky, Michigan, Montana, and Vermont) confirmed via ballot initiatives that they support abortion rights. California, Michigan, and Vermont explicitly added protections for reproductive health and rights, including abortion, to their constitutions. Kansas voters "rejected language that would have explicitly excluded abortion rights from the state constitution" (Nash and Ephross 2022). Kentucky voters "rejected a similar amendment in November to the one rejected in Kansas" (Nash and Ephross 2022). Montana voters turned down another anti-abortion measure (Nash and Ephross 2022).[57]

Undoing the right to abortion and sending the issue back to the states means that more changes in state abortion policies are inevitable over the next few years. Readers wishing to be current on this issue are directed to data sources that have been useful for us:

Guttmacher Institute (2023d)
https://www.guttmacher.org/state-policy/explore/overview-abortion
  -laws

Kaiser Family Foundation (2022)
https://www.kff.org/womens-health-policy/dashboard/abortion-in
-the-u-s-dashboard/
New York Times (2023)
https://www.nytimes.com/interactive/2022/us/abortion-laws-roe-v
-wade.html
Washington Post (Kitchener et al. 2023)
https://www.washingtonpost.com/politics/2022/06/24/abortion-state
-laws-criminalization-roe/
Center for Reproductive Rights
https://reproductiverights.org/maps/abortion-laws-by-state/

CHAPTER 4

Politics across the States

Explaining State Differences in Abortion Regulation

I-40 is a major interstate highway traversing the southern American states. Its most eastern point is Wilmington, North Carolina; its most western is Barstow, California. Between those points, I-40 connects eight states, including New Mexico and Tennessee. Their state capitals of Santa Fe and Nashville are only about 1,200 miles apart, roughly a 16-hour drive.

Besides I-40, New Mexico and Tennessee share other connections. Both states have lower average incomes and are more religious than the rest of the country. Tennessee ranks forty-third among the 50 states in median household income, and New Mexico ranks forty-sixth (Kaiser Family Foundation 2021). Tennessee ranks third among the states in its percentage of highly religious adults, and New Mexico ranks eighteenth (Lipka and Wormald 2016). The citizen legislatures of both states are ranked among the least professionalized[1] in the country with few staff, low pay, and limited sessions (Weissert and Weissert 2019; Squire 2017). Despite these similarities, New Mexico and Tennessee are light years apart in how they regulate abortion.

A Tale of Two States

New Mexico

On February 26, 2021, Democratic governor Michelle Lujan Grisham signed N.M. Senate Bill 10, repealing New Mexico's 1969 criminal abortion ban (Associated Press 2021; Bodkin 2021). That law, invalidated by *Roe v. Wade*, had classified all pregnancy terminations as criminal unless a highly regulated local hospital board deemed otherwise.[2] Shortly after *Roe*, a state court also ruled New Mexico's abortion code unconstitutional.[3] Nearly a half-century later, however, New Mexico women's rights advocates and others worried that the increasingly conservative US Supreme Court could overturn or weaken *Roe v. Wade*, thus allowing for the enforcement of the 1969 abortion law (Chacon 2021; Murguia 2018).

Upon signing the repeal, Governor Lujan Grisham stated:

> A woman has the right to make decisions about her own body. Anyone who seeks to violate bodily integrity, or to criminalize womanhood, is in the business of dehumanization. New Mexico is not in that business—not anymore. Our state statutes now reflect this inviolable recognition of humanity and dignity. I am incredibly grateful to the tireless advocates and legislators who fought through relentless misinformation and fearmongering to make this day a reality. Equality for all, equal justice and equal treatment—that's the standard. And I'm proud to lead a state that today moved one step closer to that standard. (Lujan Grisham 2021)

The path to revoking New Mexico's criminal abortion law was not straightforward. Pro-choice advocates had to wait for a governor who would sign such a repeal as well as a legislature that would pass it. In 2018, Democrat Michelle Lujan Grisham was elected governor. She succeeded Republican governor Susanna Martinez, who certainly would not have supported repealing the 1969 law.

Senate Bill 10 (SB 10), Repeal Abortion Ban, was introduced on the opening day of the 2019 legislative session. The bill made it all the way to the New Mexico Senate floor during that session. Despite the Democratic trifecta[4] in New Mexico's government that year, SB 10 "failed when eight moderate and conservative-leaning Democrats joined all 16 Republican senators in voting to keep the anti-abortion law on the books" (Chacon 2021).

By the 2021 session, six of the Democrats who voted against SB 10 were no longer in office. One Democratic state senator died later in 2019. Five others lost their June 2020 primary races to more progressive candidates, who had made repealing the criminal abortion code a major campaign issue. The November 2020 general election yielded a slightly widened Democratic majority in the senate (Ballotpedia 2020), making it easier to pass the repeal in the 2021 legislative session (Chacon 2021).

As neighboring states, particularly Texas with SB 8, enacted more restrictive abortion laws, women from out of state increasingly sought abortion services in New Mexico. When Oklahoma banned abortions in May 2022, this trend accelerated. After the *Dobbs* ruling, New Mexico abortion clinics stretched even further to accommodate the increased demand. One clinic reported scheduling about four weeks out, noting that 75 percent of the patients were from Texas (McCullough 2022).

After Dobbs

Three days after the US Supreme Court overturned *Roe v. Wade*, Democratic governor Michelle Lujan Grisham signed an executive order to protect both abortion patients and providers in New Mexico. This order shielded "health care providers targeted by lawsuits from losing their licenses or being disciplined for providing abortion services." It also asserted that the state would not comply with abortion-related arrest warrants or extradition requests from other states (Boyd 2022c). "We will not further imperil the rights and access points of anyone in New Mexico," Governor Lujan Grisham stated, adding that "abortion is and will continue to be legal, safe and accessible, period" (Boyd 2022c).

Given the vastly different state regulatory situation, Whole Women's Health, one of the largest abortion providers in Texas, announced its intention to relocate to New Mexico (Associated Press 2022c). In making her July 2022 announcement, the CEO of Whole Woman's Health had said that community support would be required because the organization did not have sufficient resources to set up a new facility. As of mid-

2023, Whole Woman's Health's plan to open a clinic near the Texas border had not yet materialized.

Abortion became a major issue in the 2022 New Mexico gubernatorial race (Boyd 2022b). Reflecting his party's position, Republican candidate Mark Ronchetti commented that the *Dobbs* decision "paves the way for measured dialogue on the issue of abortion that will save lives and should result in politics that are more mainstream" (Candelaria 2022). If elected, Ronchetti promised to pursue a 15-week limit on abortion.

Incumbent governor Lujan Grisham, however, took another tack. In September 2022, she issued another executive order for the construction of a $10 million state-funded reproductive health clinic that would provide abortion services (Boyd 2022a). Not surprisingly, this race drew national attention; both candidates received media support from their respective parties[5] (Boyd 2022b).

Executive orders, such as those issued by Governor Lujan Grisham to protect abortion access, can be repealed by future governors. But Governor Lujan Grisham defeated Mark Ronchetti by more than 6 percentage points in the November 2022 election (Ballotpedia 2022). Her victory meant that abortion rights were secure in New Mexico, at least for her second four-year term, despite an unsuccessful lawsuit and two counties and two cities near the Texas border trying to outlaw abortion (McKay 2022a; McKay 2022b).

In January 2023, Raul Torrez, New Mexico's Attorney General (Democrat), filed an emergency petition "challenging a series of anti-abortion ordinances passed by communities in eastern New Mexico" (McKay 2023). During the state legislature's biennial 60-day session in early 2023, the Democratic-controlled state legislature passed two measures addressing abortion. The first aimed to "block cities, counties, or other government bodies from barring access to abortions, reproductive health care, or gender affirming treatment" (Boyd 2023, A3–A4). The second was to enshrine into law Governor Lujan Grisham's executive order from June 2022 that protected both abortion patients and providers (Boyd 2023).

Figure 4.1 depicts New Mexico's approach to abortion regulation, and figure 4.2 shows the number of New Mexican abortion restrictions and protections over more than three decades. Both the number of restric-

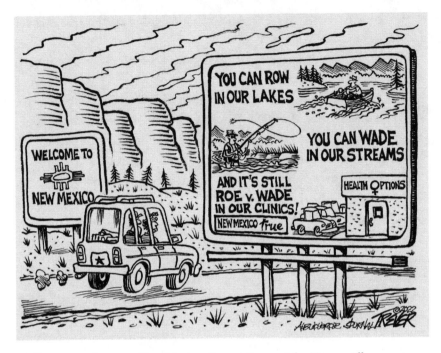

FIGURE 4.1. Welcome to New Mexico. *Source:* © 2022 John Trever, *Albuquerque Journal*. Reprinted with permission of the artist.

tions and protections have grown modestly over time, with slightly more restrictions than protections.

Tennessee

Tennessee's trajectory for abortion regulation could not have been more different. In 2019, the Tennessee legislature passed the Human Life Protection Act, making it a felony to provide abortion services throughout the state. Signed by Republican governor Bill Lee, this legislation was a trigger law: it could not be enforced unless specific circumstances were met or changed. Those conditions were anticipated in the body of the statue: either the Supreme Court of the United States (SCOTUS) would issue a judgment that "in whole or in part" would overrule *Roe v. Wade* as modified by *Planned Parenthood of Southeastern Pennsylvania v. Casey*, or an amendment to the US Constitution that "in whole or in part" would restore the authority to ban abortions to the states is enacted (Tennessee Advocates for Planned Parenthood 2022).

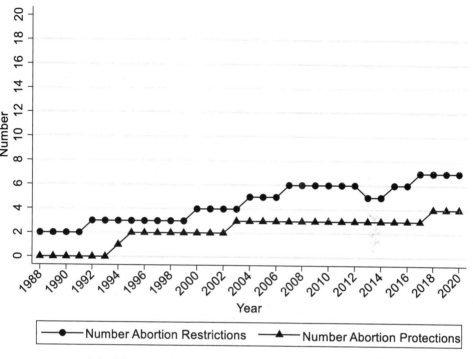

FIGURE 4.2. New Mexico's Abortion Restrictions and Protections, 1988–2020

The following year, on July 13, 2020, just eight months before New Mexico repealed its criminal abortion law, Governor Lee signed one of the country's most restrictive abortion laws (Stracqualursi and Kelly 2020). Included in this legislation was a ladder provision—a cascading prohibition of abortion at multiple points in pregnancy. This law forbid abortion at 24, 23, 22, 21, 20, 18, 15, 12, 10, eight, and six weeks of pregnancy, ensuring that an abortion ban would be in effect no matter what gestational limits the courts might strike down (Timms 2020).

In addition to multiple gestational limits, the 2020 Tennessee abortion law had other mandates. The state required ultrasounds for all women seeking abortion services, regardless of medical necessity.[6] Abortion was prohibited if the attending doctor knew that a patient was seeking abortion because of the sex, race, or a Down syndrome diagnosis of the fetus (Guttmacher Institute 2022i; NARAL Pro-Choice America 2020; Timms 2020). Physicians offering abortion services were subject to criminal penalties if they did not adhere to the law. All abortion providers were required to display information about and counsel pregnant patients about "unproven claims that it is possible to 'reverse' a medication abortion" (NARAL Pro-Choice America 2020, 4).

Less than one hour after Governor Lee signed the 2020 abortion law, a federal court enjoined this statute (Timms 2020). As a result, Tennessee was unable to enforce the law it just enacted. Subsequent state judicial appeals were unsuccessful (Timms 2021). After the *Dobbs* ruling, this law was superseded by the 2019 trigger ban.

On May 5, 2022, Governor Lee signed another bill intended to counteract the FDA decision to allow medication abortion at home. This law was set up to take effect if *Roe* were overturned. It outlawed mail-order medication abortion and stiffened the penalties for abortion providers. If caught, they "would be charged with a felony, fined up to $50,000, and sentenced to up to 20 years in prison" (Naftulin 2022).

Tennessee's 2019, 2020, and 2022 anti-abortion laws are consistent with earlier state efforts to thwart the right to choose. In 2014, Tennessee voters amended their state constitution to remove access to abortion as a fundamental right in the state.

After Dobbs

The Tennessee trigger ban went into effect on August 25, 2022, because the 2019 law explicitly stated that if *Roe v. Wade* were overturned "in whole or in part," then the statute would become effective 30 days later. Added to the final version of the law, this provision required the Tennessee Attorney General to determine if the Supreme Court's decision was indeed a reversal. The Supreme Court issued its *Dobbs* opinion on June 24 but released its Dobbs judgment on July 24. Therefore, Tennessee Attorney General Herbert Slattery (Republican) announced the effective date of the law as August 25 (El-Bawab 2022).

This now implemented Tennessee law has few exceptions—only to save the mother's life or to prevent irreversible impairment of a major bodily function (Prebeck 2022). The law "specifically rules out any exception for mental health—even in instances of threatened self-harm. . . . Anyone performing the procedure—including prescribing medication—could be charged with a Class C felony, including prison time and a fine of up to $10,000" (Farmer 2022).

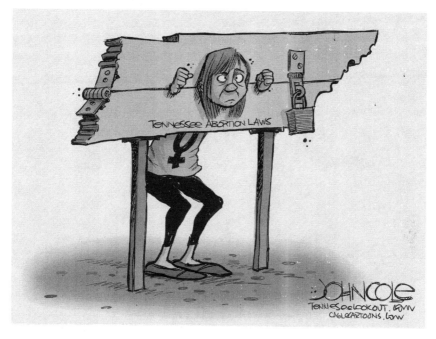

FIGURE 4.3. Tennessee Abortion Laws. © 2022 John Cole, published in the *Tennessee Lookout*. Reprinted with permission of Cagle Cartoons, Inc.

Figure 4.3 depicts Tennessee's approach to abortion regulation, and figure 4.4 shows the development of abortion restrictions and protections over time. Noteworthy is the rapid growth in abortion restrictions since 2016 and the absence of any abortion protections since 2014.

Other Differences between New Mexico and Tennessee

In addition to their diametrically opposite approaches to regulating abortion, Tennessee and New Mexico differ in other ways: partisanship, female representation, and religiosity. From 2019 to 2022, Tennessee had a Republican trifecta with a Republican governor, a Republican senate (27/6 in 2021), and a Republican house (73/26 in 2021) (Ballotpedia 2023a; Ballotpedia 2023b). During that period, New Mexico had a Democratic trifecta with a Democratic governor, Democratic senate (40/75 in 2021) and Democratic house (27/42 in 2021) (Ballotpedia 2020).

In 2020, Tennessee ranked forty-eighth in the nation in the percentage of state legislators who were female (16.7 percent). Only West Virginia

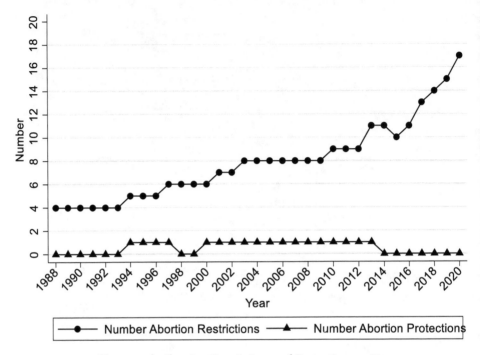

FIGURE 4.4. Tennessee's Abortion Restrictions and Protections, 1988–2020

(12.7 percent) and Mississippi (15.5 percent) had smaller proportions of women lawmakers (Center for American Women and Politics 2021). In contrast, 43.8 percent of New Mexico's 2021 state legislators were women, the seventh highest in the nation (Center for American Women and Politics 2021).

In addition to political differences, Tennesseans report being more religious than New Mexicans. In 2016, 73 percent of adults in Tennessee reported being highly religious. The corresponding percentage for New Mexico was 57 percent. One component of being highly religious is attending worship services at least weekly. Fifty-one percent of Tennessee adults report doing so, compared with 36 percent of New Mexicans (Lipka and Wormald 2016).

The combined populations of New Mexico and Tennessee make up less than 3 percent of the population of the United States. Nonetheless, these two states exemplify the wide variation in abortion regulation among the 50 states and the District of Columbia. New Mexico is representative of blue Democratic states, and Tennessee is representative of red Republican states.

Organization of Chapter

This chapter began with case studies of abortion regulation in two states, New Mexico and Tennessee. Both before and after *Dobbs*, these states chose very different paths in regulating abortion. With insights from these cases, expectations from theory, and findings from published research, the second section describes factors that may explain these state differences: politics, religion, and advocacy groups. Using an original database that spans more than three decades, the third section analyzes the determinants of state abortion regulations, both enacted and enforced. The fourth section discusses the implications of these findings for public policy and future research.

Explaining State Differences

Theoretical Expectations

Chapter 1 discussed the insights that regulatory politics, morality politics, and feminist politics offer for understanding abortion regulation. Because abortion is a highly salient issue of low technical complexity, the hearing room scenario from regulatory politics predicts that politicians and advocacy groups[7] are important participants in state abortion policy-making. Morality politics anticipates the involvement of religious groups. Feminist or gender politics suggest the importance of women's representation, as well as echoing the importance of religious groups. Both feminist and regulatory politics suggest that the determinants of specific abortion policies are likely to vary by the topic being considered. For example, the determinants of parental consent regulations may differ from regulations that apply to facilities that provide abortion services.

Findings from Previous Studies

Previous studies on state abortion policies showed that politics, interest groups, religion, and socioeconomic factors explain many of the differences in state abortion regulation (Camobreco and Barnello 2008; Patton 2007; Strickland and Whicker 1992). Most empirical studies have examined specific abortion restrictions, focusing cross-sectionally on one or two types of restrictions, such as abortion funding for low-income women or parental involvement requirements (Jones et al. 2018; Medoff and Dennis 2011; Joyce et al. 2009; Meier and McFarlane 1993). The scant literature addressing state abortion protections suggests that their political dynamics differ from those surrounding restrictions (Wilson 2020; Kreitzer 2015; Mooney and Lee 1995).

Political Forces

For political forces, previous studies demonstrated the partisan influence of elected officials, as well as the impact of female legislators. Republican legislatures are associated with more abortion restrictions (e.g., Norrander and Wilcox 2001b; Strickland and Whicker 1992). Several studies demonstrated the importance of the percentage of female legislators for state abortion policymaking (Patton 2007; Medoff 2002; Norrander and Wilcox 1999; Strickland and Whicker 1992), particularly, the percentage of Democratic women legislators (Kreitzer 2015; Medoff 2002). Past research has measured interest group activity by the size of state membership in national advocacy groups (Medoff 2002), as well as by financial contributions to those organizations (Norrander and Wilcox 1999).

Religion

The influence of religion on state abortion policies has also been examined. One study showed a positive relationship between the percentage of both Catholics and Protestant fundamentalists in the state population and the likelihood that a state would fund abortions for low-income women (Meier and McFarlane 1993). Several studies found a direct relationship between the percentage of adherents to anti-abortion denominations and the number of state abortion restrictions (Kreitzer 2015; Camobreco and Barnello 2008; Patton 2007).

Socioeconomic Conditions

Other studies have tested the influence of socioeconomic conditions on state abortion policymaking. One cross-sectional investigation found that state per capita income was negatively related to the number of abortion restrictions (Stricker and Whicker 1992), and another study found no relationship between the percentage of women in white-collar positions and the number of state abortion restrictions (Medoff 2002). Yet another study found that the percentage of women in the labor force was positively related to the likelihood of state abortion funding (Meier and McFarlane 1992). Public opinion polls over time (1995–2019) show that education is positively related to the likelihood of having a pro-choice position on abortion policy, particularly for college graduates (Pew Research Center 2022b).

Enacted versus Enforced Laws

Few studies have considered the distinction between enacted and enforced abortion laws (e.g., Meier and McFarlane 1993). For some types of abortion restrictions, this difference is not trivial. For example, courts have enjoined a fifth of the 30 enacted waiting period state laws, meaning that six states with waiting period laws cannot enforce them (Guttmacher Institute 2022c).

Explanations for State Differences in Abortion Regulation

Both the literature review and the theoretical framework suggest that politics, religion, and socioeconomic factors influence how states regulate abortion. Political factors include the abortion positions of state politicians, the partisanship of governors and both houses of state legislatures, the representation of women in the state legislatures, as well as their party makeup, and interest group spending. State religious composition may be important, especially in terms of anti-abortion religious adherents. Socioeconomic forces include educational attainment, unemployment, and income.

Political Explanations

Across the country, the structure of state governments is similar. Mimicking the federal government, each state has three branches of government: executive, legislative, and judicial. Each state has a governor who administers state government and initiates a policy agenda. Each state has a legislature, made up of two houses, except for Nebraska.[8] All states have a judiciary that includes both trial and appellate courts (Weissert and Weissert 2019).

Political Parties. Like the federal government, political parties have pivotal roles in state governments. Governors, the states' chief executives, run as partisans. In 2023, 23 governors were Democrats, and 27 were Republican (Ballotpedia 2023a). Like the US Congress, state legislatures are organized by the dominant political party in each chamber. In 2023, Democrats controlled 19 state houses, and Republicans controlled 28, with two states (Alaska and Pennsylvania) sharing powers among both partisans (Ballotpedia 2023b). In 2023, Republicans controlled 32 state senates, and Democrats controlled 18 as well the District of Columbia (Ballotpedia 2023c).

Partisanship. Political partisanship is particularly important in abortion politics. Each major political party includes abortion in its platform. The Democratic platform is pro-choice (Democratic National Committee 2020), whereas the Republican platform is anti-abortion (Republican National Committee 2016). State politicians follow suit most of the time, but not absolutely.

Abortion Positions of Elected Officials. The abortion positions of state governors and each house of the state legislature is an annual determination made by NARAL Pro-Choice America (NARAL Pro-Choice America 1989–2021)[9] From 1988 to 2021, governor's offices were held by Republicans who were anti-abortion 76 percent of the time, and by Democrats who were pro-choice 69 percent of the time. During the same period, the correlation between governors' political parties and whether they were identified as anti-abortion or pro-choice was 0.62.

Figure 4.5 shows how closely Democratic and Republican governors adhere to their respective political party positions. Although the percent fluctuates somewhat over time, there is a clear upward trend in the percentage of Democratic governors who are pro-choice and the percentage of Republican governors who are anti-abortion. For Democrats, the lowest percentage was 45 in 1994, with a high of 96 percent in 2020. For Republicans, the lowest was 53 in 1998, with a high of about 97 percent in the period from 2011 to 2014, after which there was a sharp decline before rising again to 88 percent in 2020. Overall, there is a clear upward trend in the adherence of governors to their party's stated position on abortion.

In addition to the NARAL assessments, data on party control of state governments are available for 1988–2021. These include the governor's po-

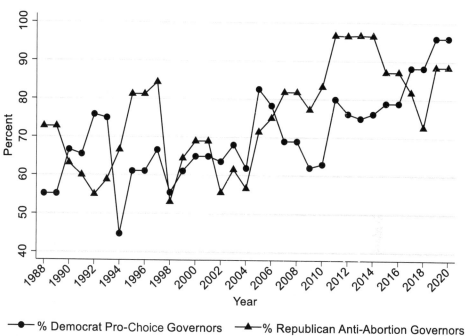

FIGURE 4.5. Party and Position of State Governors, 1988–2020

litical party and each house of the legislature (National Council of State Legislatures 2022). Both types of data were coded and included in the database constructed by the authors.

Female Lawmakers. Not only does the partisanship of state legislatures vary, but so does the gender composition of state lawmakers. In 2021, women accounted for 31.1 percent of all state legislative seats. Within state houses (lower chambers or assemblies), 32.1 percent of all representatives were women. Of those, 66.6 percent (1,158) were Democrats; 32.9 percent (572) were Republicans, 0.3 percent were Independents, and 0.1 percent were Progressives. In 2021, women state senators accounted for 28.4 percent of all state senators. Their partisan breakdown in 2021 was 64.3 percent Democratic, 33.4 percent Republican, and 2.3 percent Nonpartisan[10] (Center for American Women and Politics 2021). The representation of women has increased over the last three decades, rising sharply in recent years, as we can see in figure 4.6. In 1988, only 16 percent of state legislators were female. By 2019, that number had nearly doubled. Thirty percent of elected state legislators were women.

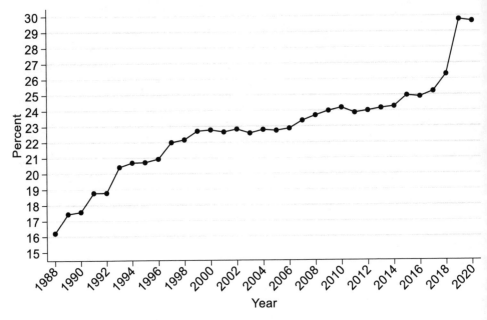

FIGURE 4.6. Average Percentage of Female Legislators per State, 1988–2020

Since 1988, the majority of women legislators have been Democrats, but that partisan proportion has fluctuated over time. As shown in figure 4.7, the proportion of Democratic female legislators rose steadily from a low of about 56 percent in 1996 to 68 percent in 2009. It dropped sharply in 2011, only to rebound in 2018.

Interest Groups and Political Action Committees. Both interest groups and political action committees (PACs) lobby the executive and legislative branches of state governments as they do the federal government (Weissert and Weissert 2019). Diverse organizations of interest groups work both to promote and to thwart state abortion legislation, including explicitly pro-choice and anti-abortion groups, representatives of religious groups, civil rights groups, women's health advocates, and more. Their activities range from working to influence legislators, making donations to political campaigns, and sometimes, drafting legislation. One anti-abortion group, Americans United for Life (AUL), describes itself as the "legal architects of the pro-life movement" (Goldman 2021, 99).[11] Each year, AUL sends a packet of model bills to state legislators (Americans

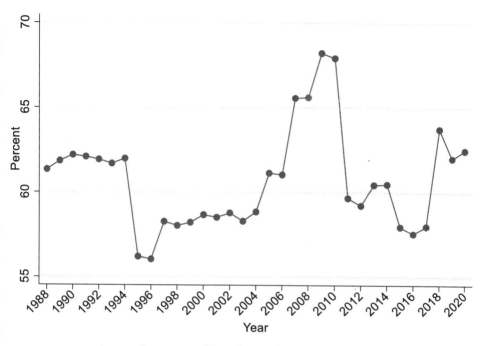

FIGURE 4.7. Average Percentage of Female Legislators Who Are Democrats per State, 1988–2020

United for Life 2010–2021), so that this prepackaged legislation can be introduced by anti-abortion state lawmakers.

Acknowledging that interest groups and PACs exercise influence in multiple ways (Baumgartner and Leech 1998),[12] we measured interest group activity by donations by pro-choice or anti-abortion groups to state political candidate campaigns (National Institute on Money in Politics 2020).[13] Groups supporting the anti-abortion position spend money to elect anti-abortion candidates and to encourage the passage of abortion restrictions. Similarly, pro-choice groups spend money to elect pro-choice candidates and counter anti-abortion strategies. For example, pro-choice groups may financially support efforts to enjoin restrictions that have been passed.

In addition to specialized pro-choice or anti-abortion groups, other groups with broader agendas than just abortion also spend money on influencing abortion regulation. However, ascertaining the identities of

Opposes abortion rights, with few or no exceptions	Supports abortion rights, with some limits	Supports abortion rights, with few or no limits	No clear position
• African Methodist Episcopal Church • Assemblies of God • Roman Catholic Church • Church of Jesus Christ of Latter-day Saints • Hinduism • Lutheran Church-Missouri Synod • Southern Baptist Convention	• Episcopal Church • Evangelical Lutheran Church in America • United Methodist Church	• Conservative Judaism • Presbyterian Church (U.S.A.) • Reform Judaism • Unitarian Universalist • United Church of Christ	• Islam • Buddhism • National Baptist Convention • Orthodox Judaism

FIGURE 4.8. Major Religious Groups' Positions on Abortion. *Source*: Pew Research Center 2016

these groups as well as the amounts of their donations is exceedingly difficult. Only political expenditure data for interest groups which are known to focus on abortion policy are included in the analysis. As a result, these fiscal data undoubtedly represent an undercount of the actual amount of money used to sway the direction of state abortion regulations (Diep 2019).

Religious Explanations

Major religious groups have different views on abortion (Masci 2016). Examples of denominations that oppose abortion rights with few exceptions (figure 4.8) include the Roman Catholic Church, the Church of Latter-Day Saints (Mormons), and Assemblies of God. The United Church of Christ, the Presbyterian Church (U.S.A.), and Reform Judaism, on the other hand, are examples of faith groups that support abortion rights, with very few exceptions (Masci 2019).

States vary greatly in their religious compositions as well as in their religiosity (Grammich et al. 2019; Lipka and Wormald 2016). Religious composition refers to the proportions of state residents identifying with various religious denominations, and hundreds of denominations exist in the United States (Grammich et al. 2012). Religiosity refers to congregants' degree of involvement in those religions: how often people attend religious services,[14] whether they are members of specific religious congregations, or if they regularly participate in the specific congregations.

Our analysis uses religious adherents, which includes both members of a denomination as well as regular participants who may not be formal members (Grammich et al. 2012).

Socioeconomic Explanations

Across the states and throughout the study period (1988–2020), socioeconomic conditions varied greatly. In our analysis of the determinants of state abortion regulations, we use three measures of socioeconomic conditions: educational attainment measured by the percent of the state population with a bachelor's degree or higher, median state income, and state unemployment rates (all socioeconomic data come from the US Bureau of the Census, various years).

Each of these varies by state and across time. The highest educational achievement in our data set is the District of Columbia in 2018, when 60.4 percent of the population had a bachelor's degree or more. West Virginia had the lowest percent at 11.1 in 1988 and 1989, followed by Alabama at 11.6 percent. West Virginia and Mississippi had the lowest median incomes in various years below $40,000 in constant 2019 dollars, with Maryland and the District of Columbia having the highest, over $90,000. The state unemployment rate (2.1 percent) was lowest in Hawaii in 2017, and highest (13.9 percent) in Michigan in 2009.

Analyzing Determinants of State Policies

Measures of state abortion regulation (protections and restrictions) were collected from multiple sources. Initial data collection began with the annual *Who Decides?* reports (NARAL 1988–2021). Since 2001, data coded from *Who Decides?* reports have been supplemented with data from the Guttmacher Institute (2001–2022) and other sources (e.g., Center for Reproductive Rights) to verify information on the adoption and enforcement of state abortion regulations.

Even when they address the same topic (e.g., parental consent), state abortion laws vary. Consequently, the way that different sources aggregate and categorize state abortion regulations may vary.

Both patients and providers encounter abortion restrictions and protections in their entirety, so first we examine aggregate restrictions and protections. Our panel consists of data for all 50 states plus the District of

Columbia over the years 1988 through 2020 ($N = 1,683$). Our multivariate analysis uses political forces, socioeconomic factors, and religious composition to predict state abortion policy adoption. Descriptive statistics for our dependent and independent variables used in the multivariate analysis (1988–2020) appear in table 4.1.

We look first at the factors that affect enacted and enforced restrictions. Because our data include all states over time with a dependent variable that is a count of the total number of restrictions, we use a cross-sectional time-series Poisson count model. We report our results in table 4.2. We use fixed effects to control for any state differences that are not accounted for by the independent variables included in our model, and we include a time trend variable to account for the steady cumulative increase in restrictions over time. We report incidence rate ratios, which indicate the percentage change in the dependent variable for a one-unit increase in each independent variable, along with standard errors and significance levels for our independent variables. Incidence rate ratios greater than one indicate a positive impact on the number of abortion regulations, whereas a ratio less than one indicates a negative impact.

Findings

Abortion Restrictions. The abortion positions of elected officials matter for the passage of restrictions, both enacted and enforced. States with pro-choice governors and legislatures enact and enforce fewer abortion restrictions than states dominated by anti-abortion officials. A pro-choice governor leads to about a 5 percent decrease in the number of restrictions, enacted and enforced, whereas a pro-choice house leads to about a 15 percent decrease. In our models, the strong correlation between the positions of the house and senate leads to the senate position being significant at only the 0.10 level, with a pro-choice senator leading to about an 8 percent decrease in the number of restrictions. When we remove the house position from the model, a pro-choice senate is significant at the 0.001 level for predicting fewer abortion restrictions at a rate of about 15 percent for both enacted and enforced restrictions.

When the abortion positions of elected officials are replaced with political party affiliation, the results are similar: Democratic control of the governor's office and either chamber of the legislature leads to fewer abor-

TABLE 4.1
Descriptive Statistics

Variable	Mean	Standard deviation	Minimum	Maximum
Abortion policies				
Number of restrictions	6.97	4.69	0	22
Number of enforced restrictions	5.06	3.97	0	19
Number of protections	1.27	1.67	0	10
Number of enforced protections	1.26	1.67	0	10
Governor's position on abortion				
Anti-abortion	0.48	0.50	0	1
Mixed	0.13	0.34	0	1
Pro-choice	0.39	0.49	0	1
House position on abortion				
Anti-abortion	0.55	0.50	0	1
Mixed	0.19	0.39	0	1
Pro-choice	0.27	0.44	0	1
Senate position on abortion				
Anti-abortion	0.51	0.50	0	1
Mixed	0.23	0.42	0	1
Pro-choice	0.26	0.44	0	1
Governor party				
Democrat	0.46	0.50	0	1
Independent	0.02	0.13	0	1
Republican	0.53	0.50	0	1
House party				
Democrat	0.52	0.50	0	1
Republican	0.46	0.50	0	1
Equally divided	0.01	0.11	0	1
Senate party				
Democrat	0.48	0.50	0	1
Independent	0.001	0.02	0	1
Republican	0.50	0.50	0	1
Equally divided	0.02	0.13	0	1
Political spending				
Anti-abortion interests ($1,000s)	4.588	50.27	0	1,635.4
Pro-choice interests ($1,000s)	15.899	86.478	0	1,435.8
Legislature				
Percent of women legislators	22.73	8.11	2.1	54.0
Percent Democrat women	60.71	18.44	0	100
State controls				
Percent with bachelor's degree	26.29	6.52	11.10	60.40
Median income ($1,000s, 2019 dollars)	59.92	9.84	36.55	95.57
State unemployment rate	5.57	1.84	2.10	13.90
State population (logged)	6.54	0.45	5.66	7.60
Religion				
Anti-abortion adherents (1,000s)	718.83	831.44	7.63	5,058.28

Note: Number of observations $N = 1,683$.

TABLE 4.2

Cross-Sectional Time-Series Poisson Count Models Predicting Number of Restrictions,
1988–2020

Independent variables	Number of abortion restrictions incidence rate ratios (robust standard errors)	Number of enforced restrictions incidence rate ratios (robust standard errors)
Political Positions		
State governor's position on abortion: base is anti-abortion		
Mixed	0.972	0.971
	(0.022)	(0.025)
Pro-choice	0.949*	0.950
	(0.026)	(0.032)
State house position on abortion: base is anti-abortion		
Mixed	0.968	0.973
	(0.025)	(0.028)
Pro-choice	0.850***	0.848***
	(0.045)	(0.052)
State senate position on abortion: base is anti-abortion		
Mixed	0.958	0.968
	(0.025)	(0.029)
Pro-choice	0.924*	0.929
	(0.043)	(0.048)
Religion		
Religious adherents (millions)	1.754**	1.908**
	(0.501)	(0.498)
State controls		
Median state household income	0.997	0.994**
($1,000s, 2019 dollars)	(0.003)	(0.003)
State unemployment rate	0.994	0.99*
	(0.004)	(0.005)
Percent of population with a bachelor's	1.003	1.004
degree	(0.011)	(0.014)
State population (logged)	0.675	3.204
	(0.595)	(3.098)
Legislature		
Percent of women legislators	1.001	1.003
	(0.004)	(0.005)
Percent of women legislators who are	0.995***	0.995***
Democrats	(0.001)	(0.001)
Political spending		
Political spending by anti-abortion	1.266***	1.134***
interests	(0.064)	(0.046)
Political spending by pro-choice	0.908*	0.893**
interests	(0.046)	(0.047)
Time control		
Time trend (1988–2020)	1.037***	1.044***
	(0.005)	(0.006)
Observations	1,683	1,650[a]
Wald chi-squared (16 degrees of freedom)	1,579.07***	3,124.46***

Note: *** $p<0.01$, ** $p<0.05$, * $p<0.1$.
[a]Vermont was dropped because it had zero enforced restriction throughout our time period.

tion restrictions than in Republican-controlled states. A Republican governor results in about 6 percent more restrictions; Republican control of the house or the senate leads to about 18 percent and 9 percent increases in the number of restrictions, respectively.

Finally, we consider the impact on restrictions under Democratic versus Republican control of all three bodies of government. Under a Republican trifecta, the number of abortion restrictions is about 12 percent higher compared with periods of divided government, whereas under a Democratic trifecta, the number of restrictions is about 10 percent lower.

The religious composition of the state also has a very large and significant effect on the number of state abortion restrictions. For each addition million adherents of religious groups that are opposed to abortion, the number increases by about 75 percent for enacted restrictions and 91 percent for enforced restrictions. Religiosity has the largest impact on state adoption of abortion restrictions.

The percentage of women legislators is not significant in predicting the number of abortion restrictions, but the percentage of women legislators identifying as Democratic has a small (0.5 percent) negative effect on the number of restrictions.

Our analysis shows that spending by both anti-abortion and pro-choice interest groups affects the number of abortion restrictions. Anti-abortion spending leads to an increase in state abortion restrictions, whereas pro-choice spending reduces the number of state abortion restrictions. An additional million dollars in anti-abortion spending leads to about a 27 percent increase in enacted restrictions and a 13 percent increase in enforced restrictions. An additional million dollars in pro-choice spending leads to about a 9 percent and 11 percent reduction in enacted and enforced restrictions, respectively.

Except for a very small effect for median state income, socioeconomic conditions have no effect on state abortion restrictions. Neither levels of education nor state unemployment rates are significant in predicting the number of restrictions. A $1,000 increase in median income causes less than 1 percent decrease in the number of enforced restrictions, significant at the 5 percent level. Our control for state population is insignificant, although the time trend variable captures the increase in restrictions over time, an increase of about 4 percent per year.

Abortion Protections. We use the same set of independent variables to predict the number of abortion protections adopted across states over time. Here, because the number of protections is much sparser, with many states over time having no enacted legislation to protect abortion rights, we use a zero-inflated Poisson count model to account for the large number of zero protections. We also report enacted and enforced protections, although the number of enjoined protections is very small. These results appear in table 4.3.

As with restrictions, the position or party of elected officials affects the passage of legislation to protect abortion rights. For example, a pro-choice governor leads to about a 32 percent increase in the number of protections, whereas a pro-choice senate leads to about an 81 percent increase, with the house position being insignificant. Again, if we replace political position with party, Republican control results in a 13 percent decrease in protections for the governor, a 19 percent decrease for the house, and a 32 percent decrease for the senate, all significant at the 0.01 level. Finally, under trifecta Democratic or Republican control, we find that Democratic control is not significant, but Republican control leads to a 54 percent reduction in the number of protections compared to periods of divided government. Politics matter significantly for the number of abortion protections.

Just as state religiosity causes more abortion restrictions in a state, it also leads to fewer protections being enacted and enforced by states. For each additional million anti-abortion religious adherents in a state, the number of protections is about 25 percent lower.

Again, except for a small effect for median income, socioeconomic factors are insignificant in predicting the number of abortion protections. A $1,000 increase in state median income leads to a less than 1 percent increase in the number of protections, significant at the 5 percent level. Education levels and the rate of unemployment are both insignificant predictors of protections.

A higher percentage of women legislators, as well as a higher percentage of Democratic women, lead to more state protections. More specifically, a 1 percent increase in the number of women legislators leads to about a 2 percent increase in the number of protections, and a 1 percent

TABLE 4.3
Cross-Sectional Time-Series Zero-Inflated Poisson Count Model Predicting Number of Protections, 1988–2020

Independent variables	Number of abortion protections incidence rate ratios (robust standard errors)	Number of enforced protections incidence rate ratios (robust standard errors)
Political Positions		
State governor's position on abortion: base is anti-abortion		
Mixed	1.027	1.043
	(0.074)	(0.076)
Pro-choice	1.325***	1.343***
	(0.080)	(0.083)
State house position on abortion: base is anti-abortion		
Mixed	1.089	1.079
	(0.114)	(0.114)
Pro-choice	1.061	1.055
	(0.119)	(0.121)
State senate position on abortion: base is anti-abortion		
Mixed	1.674***	1.660***
	(0.149)	(0.149)
Pro-choice	1.809***	1.810***
	(0.167)	(0.170)
Religion		
Religious adherents (millions)	0.752***	0.749***
	(0.039)	(0.039)
State controls		
Median state household income ($1,000s, 2019 dollars)	1.008**	1.007***
	(0.003)	(0.003)
State unemployment rate	1.008	1.007
	(0.011)	(0.011)
Percent of population with a bachelor's degree	0.995	0.996
	(0.004)	(0.004)
State population (logged)	2.147***	2.181***
	(0.126)	(0.131)
Legislature		
Percent of women legislators	1.020***	1.020***
	(0.005)	(0.005)
Percent of women legislators who are Democrats	1.008***	1.008***
	(0.003)	(0.003)
Political spending		
Political spending by anti-abortion interests	1.291	1.299
	(0.258)	(0.263)
Political spending by pro-choice interests	0.885	0.871
	(0.129)	(0.128)
Time control		
Time trend (1988–2020)	1.038***	1.038***
	(0.003)	(0.003)
Constant	0.0008***	0.0007***
	(0.0003)	(0.0003)

(*continued*)

TABLE 4.3
Continued
Inflate model (predicts probability of zero protections)

Independent variables	Number of abortion protections Coefficients (robust standard errors)	Number of enforced protections Coefficients (robust standard errors)
State governor's position on abortion: base is anti-abortion		
Mixed	0.650	0.669
	(0.486)	(0.494)
Pro-choice	−0.058	−0.023
	(0.522)	(0.525)
State house position on abortion: base is anti-abortion		
Mixed	−1.034*	−1.071*
	(0.615)	(0.626)
Pro-choice	−3.289***	−3.286***
	(1.009)	(1.026)
State senate position on abortion: base is anti-abortion		
Mixed	0.723	0.711
	(0.627)	(0.632)
Pro-choice	1.486	1.46
	(0.914)	(0.926)
Religious adherents (millions)	−0.074	−0.078
	(0.531)	(0.545)
Median state household income ($1,000s)	−0.031	−0.032
	(0.025)	(0.025)
State unemployment rate	−0.803**	−0.801**
	(0.341)	(0.362)
Percent of population with a bachelor's degree	0.056	0.056
	(0.047)	(0.048)
State population (logged)	−1.464**	−1.425**
	(0.68)	(0.689)
Percent of women legislators	−0.331***	−0.332***
	(0.057)	(0.058)
Percent of women legislators who are Democrats	0.01	0.01
	(0.022)	(0.023)
Political spending by anti-abortion interests	−18.612	−18.677
	(21.432)	(22.022)
Political spending by pro-choice interests	3.206**	3.235**
	(1.3)	(1.359)
Time trend (1988–2020)	−0.012	−0.013
	(0.031)	(0.032)
Constant	18.945***	18.758**
	(7.002)	(7.350)
Observations	1,683	1,683
Nonzero observations	908	907
Zero observations	775	776
Wald chi-squared (16 degrees of freedom)	970.38***	960.04***

Note: *** $p<0.01$, ** $p<0.05$, * $p<0.1$.

increase in Democratic women legislators leads to just under a 1 percent increase in protections.

Unlike restrictions, neither pro-choice nor anti-abortion spending by interest groups is significant in predicting the number of protections. Finally, our control for state population is significant, indicating that more populous states enact more abortion protections. Additionally, our time trend is also significant capturing the increase in the number of protections over time.

Table 4.3 includes a model for enforced protections. Fewer protections are enjoined than restrictions, so the results in these models are very similar. Finally, table 4.3 also includes the portion of the models that predicts the number of observations having zero protections. Here, we find that when the house leans pro-choice, there are less likely to be zero protections in the state. In addition, with a higher percentage of women legislators there are less likely to be zero protections. States with higher median income, higher unemployment, and larger populations are marginally less likely to have zero protections. Only pro-choice spending yields the opposite prediction—more spending predicts a greater likelihood of zero protections. Perhaps these are states where interest groups are spending to try to get protections but have not succeeded.

Overall, our results indicate that political leadership of a state, as well as state religiosity, have large and significant impacts on the passage and enforcement of abortion restrictions and protections. Pro-choice governors and legislatures adopt fewer abortion restrictions and more abortion protections than anti-abortion officials. In addition, having more women, particularly Democratic women, leads to fewer restrictions and more protections in the states. Finally, religiosity matters. More religious adherents to anti-abortion denominations in a state lead to more abortion restrictions and fewer abortion protections being adopted.

In addition to predicting the number of state abortion restrictions, in table 4.4, we model the probabilities of whether state restrictions decrease, stay the same, or increase from the previous year. We use a cross-sectional time-series ordered probit model. In column 1, we report the model coefficients, and in columns 2–4, we report the marginal effects for the three possible outcomes. The most important predictors are the governor's position on abortion, the percent of women legislators as well

TABLE 4.4
Cross-Sectional Time-Series Ordered Probit Model of Changes in Restrictions

Independent variables	(1) Coefficients	(2) Marginal effect: restrictions decrease (standard errors)	(3) Marginal effect: restrictions same (standard errors)	(4) Marginal effect: restrictions increase (standard errors)
Political Positions				
State governor's position on abortion: base is anti-abortion				
Mixed	-0.13	0.01	0.03	-0.04
	(0.08)	(0.01)	(0.02)	(0.03)
Pro-choice	-0.22***	0.02***	0.05***	-0.07***
	(0.08)	(0.01)	(0.02)	(0.02)
State house position on abortion: base is anti-abortion				
Mixed	0.06	-0.006	-0.01	0.02
	(0.10)	(0.01)	(0.02)	(0.03)
Pro-choice	-0.02	0.002	0.004	-0.01
	(0.13)	(0.01)	(0.02)	(0.04)
State senate position on abortion: base is anti-abortion				
Mixed	-0.11	0.01	0.02	-0.03
	(0.08)	(0.01)	(0.02)	(0.03)
Pro-choice	-0.17	0.018	0.03*	-0.05*
	(0.10)	(0.01)	(0.02)	(0.03)
Religion				
Religious adherents	-0.01	0.001	0.01	-0.002
	(0.03)	(0.003)	(0.01)	(0.01)
State controls				
Median household income ($1,000s)	0.006	0.0006	0.0001	-0.002
	(0.004)	(0.0004)	(0.001)	(0.001)

	(1)	(2)	(3)	(4)
State unemployment rate	0.01	−0.001	−0.002	0.003
	(0.02)	(0.002)	(0.003)	(0.005)
Percent bachelor's degree	0.004	−0.0004	−0.001	0.001
	(0.01)	(0.001)	(0.001)	(0.002)
State population (logged)	0.05*	−0.02*	−0.03*	0.05*
	(0.08)	(0.01)	(0.02)	(0.03)
Legislature				
Percent of women legislators	−0.02***	0.002***	0.004**	−0.006***
	(0.004)	(0.0004)	(0.001)	(0.001)
Percent of women legislators who are Democrats	−0.004**	0.0004**	0.001**	−0.001**
	(0.002)	(0.0002)	(0.0004)	(0.0006)
Political spending				
Anti-abortion political spending (millions)	−0.28	0.03	0.06	−0.09
	(0.36)	(0.04)	(0.07)	(0.11)
Pro-choice political spending (millions)	−0.65**	0.07**	0.13**	−0.20**
	(0.26)	(0.03)	(0.05)	(0.08)
Time control				
Time trend (1989–2020)	−0.003	0.00003	0.0001	−0.0001
	(0.004)	(0.0004)	(0.001)	(0.001)
cut1	−1.74***			
	(0.55)			
cut2	0.65			
	(0.53)			
Wald chi-squared	204.5***			
Observations	1,632	1,632	1,632	1,632

Note: *** $p<0.01$, ** $p<0.05$, * $p<0.1$.

as the percent of women who are Democrats, and the pro-choice interest group spending.

If a state has a pro-choice governor instead of anti-abortion governor, the probability that restrictions decrease goes up by 2 percent, the probability they stay the same goes up by 5 percent, and the probability that restrictions increase goes down by 7 percent, all significant at the 0.01 level. For a $1 million increase in pro-choice interest group spending, the probability that restrictions decrease goes up by 6 percent, whereas the probability that restrictions increase goes down by 19 percent. Similarly, as the percent of women legislators and percent of Democratic women legislators increase by 1 percent, restrictions are more likely to decrease or stay the same, and less likely to increase.

Figure 4.9 shows how the probability that restrictions decrease, stay the same, or increase changes as the percent of women legislators in the state rises. When the percent of women legislators increases from none to 55 percent, the probability that restrictions decrease goes from about zero to 15 percent, and the probability that restrictions increase declines from about 45 percent to 10 percent. The effect on the change in restrictions as the percent of Democratic women in the state legislature changes shows a similar pattern, although the impact is much smaller.

Postscript on State Abortion Regulations and COVID-19

Even during the COVID-19 pandemic, states continued to issue both abortion restrictions and protections. In 2020, 11 states (Alabama, Alaska, Arkansas, Iowa, Kentucky, Louisiana, Ohio, Oklahoma, Tennessee, Texas, and West Virginia) issued abortion restrictions related to COVID-19; all of these were enjoined. Twelve states (California, Hawaii, Illinois, Maryland, Massachusetts, Michigan, Minnesota, New Jersey, New Mexico, New York, Oregon, and Virginia) issued abortion protections (Jones et al. 2020).

State COVID-19 laws related to abortion appear to be a continuation of state regulatory practices. Table 4.5 shows that states that issued additional COVID-19 abortion restrictions are states that had higher numbers of restrictions over a long period (33 years) as well as in 2020. The overall average number of abortion restrictions in states that adopted new COVID-19 restrictions was 14.3 compared with 6.9 for states that did

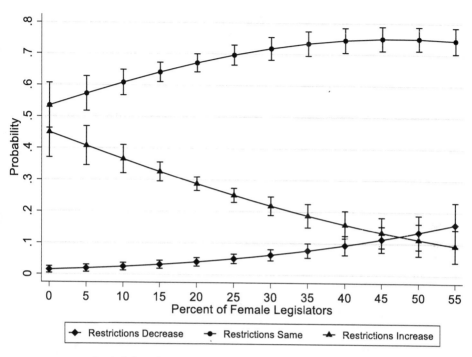

FIGURE 4.9. Probability that Abortion Restrictions Will Decrease, Increase, or Stay the Same by State Percentage of Female Legislators

not adopt COVID-19 restrictions. In 2020, the average number was 17.1 versus 9.8.

Similarly, states with higher average protections seem to have been more likely to issue COVID-19 abortion protections. The overall average number of protections for states that adopted new COVID-19 abortion protections was 7.1 compared with 1.2 for states that did not adopt COVID protections. In 2020, the average number was 6.3 compared with 1.8. For both restrictions and protections, the difference in the mean number of abortion regulations for states with and without new COVID-19 policies is statistically significant at $p < 0.001$. In short, regulating abortion remained dynamic even during the COVID-19 pandemic.

Contraceptive Access and State Abortion Regulations

Contraceptive access is an additional factor that affects state abortion rates. Some states guarantee that a woman's contraceptive prescription will be filled. Are states that have fewer restrictions and more protections

TABLE 4.5
COVID-19 Policy: Difference in Mean Number of Restrictions and Protections

Regulations	Number of states with no new abortion COVID-19 policies	Number of states with new abortion COVID-19 policies	Mean with no COVID-19 policies	Mean with COVID-19 policies	Difference in means
Abortion restrictions, 1988–2020	1,668	15	6.9	14.3	7.4*
Abortion restrictions, 2020	40	11	9.8	17.1	7.3*
Abortion protections, 1988–2020	1,667	16	1.2	7.1	5.9*
Abortion protections, 2020	39	12	1.8	6.3	4.5*

Note: *$p<0.001$.

more likely to guarantee access to contraception? In table 4.6, we show the average number of restrictions and protections for states with and without the contraception prescription guarantee policy. Since the first enactment of this type of policy in 2004, states that have required that contraceptive prescriptions be filled have had on average four fewer restrictions and 3.4 more protections compared with states with no contraceptive guarantee, both differences statistically significant at $p < 0.001$.

Conclusion

Politics, religion, and money largely explain the vast differences in state abortion regulation. Similar factors affect both the enactment and the enforcement of abortion restrictions. However, the determinants of state abortion protections differ from those for abortion restrictions.

Elected officials' abortion positions matter for the passage of both restrictions (enacted and enforced) and protections. States with pro-choice governors and legislatures enact and enforce fewer abortion restrictions (e.g., New Mexico) than states dominated by anti-abortion elected officials (e.g., Tennessee). Pro-choice politicians are also more likely to enact abortion protections. Similarly, when we consider partisanship, Democratic party control of the governor's office and either chamber of the legislature leads to fewer abortion restrictions and more protections than in states under Republican control. Over time, elected officials' stated abortion positions are somewhat better predictors of how states regulate abortion than is their respective political parties. The reason for this dis-

TABLE 4.6
*Contraceptive Prescription Policy: Difference in Mean
Number of Restrictions and Protections*

Regulations	Number of states that guarantee contraception prescriptions	Number of states that do not guarantee contraception prescriptions	Mean with guarantee	Mean with no guarantee	Difference in means
Abortion restrictions, 2005–2020	98	718	5.6	9.6	−4.0*
Abortion protections, 2005–2020	98	718	4.8	1.4	3.4*

Note: *p<0.001.

crepancy is that some politicians, namely pro-choice Republicans and anti-abortion Democrats, have crossed party lines on abortion policies. However, this crossing-over phenomenon has nearly disappeared in recent years.

Women legislators also count in state abortion policymaking. The percentage of women in state legislatures is not a significant predictor of abortion restrictions. But the proportion of female legislators who are Democratic is negatively related to the number of state abortion restrictions. More women are being elected to state legislatures, and female state women lawmakers have been increasingly Democratic (Carroll and Sanbonmatsu 2013). Over time, more Democratic female representation may thwart the growth in abortion restrictions.

Women legislators play a pivotal role in the adoption of state abortion protections. The percentage of female legislators is significantly related to the number of state protections. The percentage of women legislators who are Democratic is also an important predictor of state abortion restrictions.

A state's religious composition, namely, the number of religious adherents of denominations firmly opposed to abortion, is a powerful predictor of the number of abortion restrictions, both enacted and enforced. A larger population faithful to these precepts also suppresses the number of state abortion protections.

The impact of interest group spending differs for state abortion restrictions and protections. Our analysis shows that both anti-abortion and pro-choice interest group expenditures are associated with more state abortion restrictions, but not more protections. Whereas anti-abortion groups spend money to encourage the passage of restrictions, pro-choice groups may also spend to counter that strategy or to enjoin restrictions that have been passed. A caveat here is that our data likely represent an undercount of interest groups' spending on abortion.[15]

States tend to follow similar patterns in policy areas related to abortion. During the COVID-19 pandemic, states that restricted access to abortion were already highly restrictive (e.g., Tennessee), whereas states that protected abortion rights during the pandemic were already highly protective (e.g., New Mexico). Similarly, states that guaranteed contraceptive access tend to be states that protect abortion rights.

CHAPTER 5

After the Policymakers Go Home

Effects of State Abortion Regulations

Across the United States, women seeking abortion and providers offering those services face very different regulations. These differences have become even more pronounced since the *Dobbs* decision permitted states to ban abortion altogether. For a woman living in a state that still permits abortion, her state of residence determines whether public or private insurance will cover the procedure or medication, if she must travel to a physical clinic to obtain a medication abortion, and even what kind of patient information she will hear. If she is a minor, the state determines whether and how she must involve her parents in her abortion decision.

Not only do abortion patients encounter onerous restrictions, but abortion providers also face very different regulations depending on the state in which they are located (Cohen and Joffe 2020). For example, 17 states require that abortion clinics meet the standards of ambulatory surgical centers (ASC), even though "surgical centers tend to provide more invasive and risky procedures and use higher levels of sedation" (Guttmacher Institute 2022j). Of these states, 14 mandate this level of facility for clinics only offering medication abortion. These requirements are not just inconvenient; they are expensive, too.

In addition to regulations for abortion facilities, personnel requirements for abortion clinics differ by state. Ten states mandate that a clinician performing an abortion must have either admitting privileges at a local hospital or an alternative arrangement with another provider.[1] Before the *Dobbs* decision allowed Mississippi to ban all abortions, this state even mandated the clinician to be either a board-certified obstetrician-gynecologist or eligible for certification (Guttmacher Institute 2022j), a medically unnecessary restriction (Nippita and Paul 2018).[2]

New York and Pennsylvania

Only 81 miles separate New York City and Philadelphia, the most populous cities in New York and Pennsylvania, but vast differences separate how abortion services are delivered in these states. Women seeking abortion services in Pennsylvania must listen to a health provider deliver the state's informed consent script. After satisfying that demand, the state of Pennsylvania requires women to wait for 24 hours before they receive an abortion, including medication abortion. Minors seeking abortion services are required to get parental consent prior to either a surgical or medication abortion (Guttmacher Institute 2022c; Guttmacher Institute 2022e).

In New York State, however, there is no mandated state script for abortion counseling. The state does not impose a waiting period between the time a woman requests an abortion and when she receives that service. Minors seeking abortion are not required to involve their parents, although standard counseling protocols do encourage adolescents to discuss their abortion decisions with their families (Guttmacher Institute 2022c; Guttmacher Institute 2022e).

The Commonwealth of Pennsylvania restricts both private and public insurance for abortion.[3] But across Pennsylvania's northern border, the state of New York mandates that all private health insurance plans cover abortion services (Guttmacher Institute 2023e). Here, the state pays for abortions for Medicaid-eligible women. But neither Pennsylvania nor New York is among the 19 states requiring women to be in the physical presence of their clinicians when they take pills for medication abortion (Guttmacher Institute 2023c).

Pennsylvania imposes structural requirements comparable to those for surgical centers on all abortion providers offering surgical abortion services, even private physicians' offices. State regulations specify both the size of the room where the procedure occurs as well as the width of the corridor. Abortion providers in Pennsylvania must have a transfer agreement with a local hospital. The state of New York, on the other hand, does not impose additional requirements on abortion providers beyond standard medical and clinic licensing (Guttmacher Institute 2022j).

Arizona and California

More than 2,000 miles away, the bordering states of Arizona and California offer an even starker contrast in regulating abortion services. After the *Dobbs* decision, the Arizona legislature imposed a 15-week gestational ban on abortion (Arizona Daily Independent News Network 2022).[4] Women who obtain abortion services in the Grand Canyon State must receive medically incorrect state-mandated counseling, which includes disproven claims of fetal pain and the dubious possibility of reversing a medication abortion. After a required session, patients seeking abortion must wait 24 hours before receiving the medication or the surgical procedure. Minors requesting abortion services in Arizona must present notarized parental consent forms (Guttmacher Institute 2022e).

In contrast, the state of California does not require additional counseling on top of the standard counseling and informed consent offered by licensed abortion providers. Abortion patients are not subjected to a waiting period. The Golden State does not mandate parental involvement, but California providers routinely encourage minors to talk to their families about their abortion decisions.

Abortion providers in Arizona must comply with Targeted Regulation of Abortion Providers (TRAP) requirements, and the state prohibits the inclusion of abortion in some of the private health insurance markets. Arizona does not fund abortions for Medicaid-eligible women and forbids health insurance policies offered by the state health exchange from covering abortion. Arizona also prohibits abortion coverage in the plans it offers to state employees (Guttmacher Institute 2023e; NARAL Pro-Choice America 2021).

The state of California funds abortions through its Medicaid program, Medi-Cal. The Golden State requires that all private health insurance plans include abortion coverage. More recently, the state prohibited insurance plans from imposing copayments, deductibles, or other cost-sharing requirements for abortion and abortion-related services. In the past, these added charges significantly increased the price of abortion (Guttmacher Institute 2023e; Beam 2022a; Beam 2022b; Kyrylenko 2022).

Abortion providers in California are not subjected to TRAP laws and special inspections. The state of California does not have medically unnecessary TRAP laws that impose stringent regulations only on abortion providers. Medical providers who offer abortion services in California do not receive additional state inspections simply because they offer pregnancy terminations (Guttmacher Institute 2022j). The state of California even has a website to facilitate access to abortion (State of California 2023).

Organization of Chapter

To illustrate the very different regulatory environments faced by both women seeking abortion and providers offering these services across different states, this chapter first presented brief case studies of two pairs of bordering states. The second section discusses some of the research findings from published studies about the impact of abortion regulation in the US states. Using an original database compiled by the authors, the third section analyzes the multifarious effects of state abortion regulation. The fourth section discusses caveats in interpreting the outcomes of state abortion regulation: the variation in the same categories of state restrictions and differences in enforcement and compliance. The final section summarizes what we know about the impact of state abortion regulation.

Previous Work Analyzing the Impact of State Abortion Regulation

Effect on State Abortion Rates. Much of the work addressing the impact of state abortion regulations analyzes the effect of the enactment of these laws on state abortion rates. For example, Meier et al. (1996) found that despite the myriad state abortion regulations, only one type of abortion regulation affected abortion rates: whether the state funded abortions for low-income women. A more recent study (Gius 2019) showed that mandatory state ultrasound laws had no effect on state abortion rates.

Other Impact Measures. In addition to the impact on state abortion rates, abortion restrictions have shown other effects. Haas-Wilson (1993) found that both the presence of parental involvement laws and the lack of state funding for abortion services decreased the number of providers in a state. Llamas et al. (2018) published a thorough review of the public health impacts of state abortion restrictions. More recently, McKetta and Keyes (2019) demonstrated that abortion restrictions increased state infant mortality rates, finding that restrictive abortion laws contributed to the differential mortality between Black and white women and children. Vilda et al. (2021) reported that states with higher abortion restrictiveness scores had a 7 percent increase in maternal mortality rates.

Individual State Restrictions. Colman and Joyce (2011) examined the effect of the 2004 Texas TRAP laws on both abortion rates and out-of-state travel. Two years following the implementation of the TRAP laws, second-trimester abortions in Texas had declined by over 50 percent. During "the same period, abortions to residents of Texas obtained out of state almost quadrupled," but the rise in late abortions obtained out-of-state "did not offset the decline in abortions obtained in Texas" (Coleman and Joyce 2011, 795). Moreover, the average price of a second-trimester abortion "increased by more than $400 (39 percent) between 2001 and 2006" (Coleman and Joyce 2011, 795).

In terms of its impact on the abortion rate, the 2004 Texas TRAP laws greatly exceeded the effects of a parental consent requirement in Texas (Joyce et al. 2006). This result and other state-level findings (e.g., Jacobsen and Royer 2011) led researchers to speculate that supply-side abortion restrictions are more potent than demand-side restrictions (Joyce 2011). More recently, a study on the impact of TRAP laws suggested that future work should prioritize "the specific TRAP laws that may have a uniquely strong effect on state-level abortion rates and other outcomes" (Austin and Harper 2017, 128).

Impacts from Demand- and Supply-Side Restrictions. In a 23-state study of hospital discharges following abortion, Rolnick and Vohries (2012) found that complications were lower in states with at least one demand-side abortion restriction, specifically lack of funding or mandatory waiting period, than in states without these restrictions. This seemingly incongruous result can be explained by women traveling across state lines for abortion.

Both making plans for an out-of-state abortion and accruing funds for travel take time, which can easily extend the gestational age of the pregnancy. As a result, women traveling to other states for abortion are more likely to have second-trimester procedures. These later abortions have higher rates of complications than early abortions, which are counted in the abortion occurrence statistics of states where the procedures were performed.

In a more recent study, Gonzalez et al. (2020) examined the effects of two demand-side abortion restrictions on the timing of abortions. The lack of abortion funding for Medicaid-eligible women was associated with a 13 percent increase in the abortion rate after the first trimester. Parental involvement laws showed no effect on gestational age at abortion.

Impacts for Individual Women. The prospective Turnaway Study collected data on nearly 1,000 women who visited 30 abortion facilities across the United States from 2008 to 2010. For five years, researchers followed both women who had been able to secure abortions and those who had been turned away because they had missed the gestational limit for pregnancy termination in the state in which they had sought services. Given the large size of this natural experiment, researchers were able to compare physical health, mental health, and socioeconomic outcomes for women who received a wanted abortion and those who were denied a pregnancy termination. In every category, women who requested but were denied an abortion fared worse than women who were able to access abortion services (Slusky 2022; Foster 2020; Biggs et al. 2017; Dobkin et al. 2014).

Racial and Ethnic Differences. The racial and ethnic differences in abortion rates and abortion gestational age are well-documented (Jones and Jerman 2017b; Jones and Jerman 2017c; Dehlendorf et al. 2013). Both African American and Hispanic women have higher abortion rates than do non-Hispanic white women. Several studies have shown that these differences are exacerbated by state regulations. In a study on the demand for abortion in Texas, Brown et al. (2001) showed that travel distances to abortion clinics were more of a deterrent for Hispanic women than for Black and white women. More state abortion restrictions are likely to exacerbate racial disparities in gestational age at abortion as well as other adverse outcomes (Hing et al. 2022; Dehlendorf and Weitz 2011). A recent longitudinal study of state TRAP laws demonstrated a differential effect on African American teens: "Black women first exposed to TRAP laws before age 18 are 1 to 3 percentage points less likely to initiate and complete college" (Jones and Pineda-Torres 2021, 1).

Impact on Life Cycle and Welfare. Recent work by economists has also examined the broader effects of liberalized access to abortion since *Roe v. Wade*. Myers (2017) found that abortion access, not contraception, has allowed large numbers of women to delay marriage and motherhood. In "states where abortion was legalized and young women could obtain an abortion without involving a parent, the likelihood of becoming a mother before age 19 declined by a third and the likelihood of a shotgun marriage declined by more than one-half" (Myers 2017, 2222). The findings of Jones and Pineda-Torres (2021, 1) also suggest that "modern abortion restrictions are harming women's efforts at economic advancement and are perpetuating racial inequality."

Analyzing the Effects of State Abortion Regulation (1988–2020)

To answer some of the questions raised by the literature and in public policy debates, we conducted our own analyses. Specifically, we wanted to know the effect of the decline in the number of abortion providers on state abortion rates, the effect of increased availability of contraception on state abortion rates, the effect of TRAP laws on state abortion rates, and whether state abortion restrictions disproportionately affect women of color.

The way that abortion data are collected in the United States makes answering these questions less than straightforward (NAS 2018, 23, 26). The Centers for Disease Control and the Guttmacher Institute both collect state-level abortion data. Both of these sources "provide estimates of the number and rate of abortions, the use of different abortion methods, the characteristics of women who have abortions, and other related statistics. However, both sources have limitations" (NAS 2018, 26).

The CDC abortion surveillance system is a voluntary system to which the states report annually (NAS 2018, 26; Saul 1998). National abortion surveillance reports generally follow within two to three years. Three states (California, Maryland, and New Hampshire) do not contribute data to this system (Centers for Disease Control and Prevention 2021).

The Guttmacher Institute's abortion census is also voluntary. Unlike the CDC, the Guttmacher Abortion Provider Census (APC) "solicits information from all known abortion providers throughout the United States, including in the states that do not submit information to the CDC surveillance system" (NAS 2018, 26). For 2020, the latest year reported by Guttmacher, information was obtained directly from 52 percent of abortion providers. Data for non-respondents were imputed or gathered from alternative sources such as state health department reports (Jones et al. 2022a).

Given the differences in data collection, it is not surprising that the CDC's reported abortion data provide lower counts than those from Guttmacher. In 2020, the most recent year reported by Guttmacher, the CDC reported approximately 67 percent of the number of abortions reported by the Guttmacher Institute for that year[5] (Jones et al. 2022a; Jones et al. 2019). That percentage was similar for 2017:

> Both data collection systems report descriptive statistics on women who have abortions and the types of abortion provided, although they define demographic variables and procedure types differently. Nevertheless, in the aggregate, the trends in abortion utilization reported by the CDC and Guttmacher closely mirror each other—indicating decreasing rates of abortion, an increasing proportion of medication abortions, and the vast majority of abortions (90 percent) occurring by 13 weeks' gestation. (NAS 2018, 26)

Estimating Annual State Abortion Rates

Both the Guttmacher Institute's and CDC's abortion data were used to develop the annual state-level estimates of the abortion rate used in our analysis. For years when the Guttmacher Institute reported those rates, those figures were used directly. For years when Guttmacher did not report those rates, we calculated the annual rate of growth (or decline) in each state's abortion rate reported by the CDC. We then applied this rate

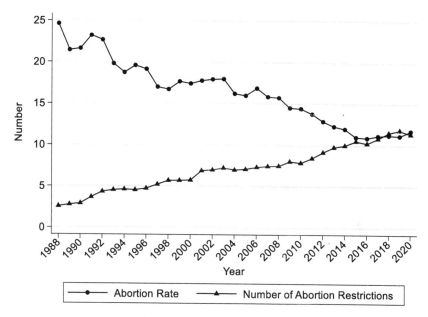

FIGURE 5.1. Average Abortion Rate and Number of Abortion Restrictions per State, 1988–2020

of change to the Guttmacher data to estimate the state abortion rate missing in the Guttmacher time trend. This procedure assumes that the bias in CDC abortion rate data is consistent from year to year. Other researchers have used a similar process (Meier et al. 1996; Meier and McFarlane 1994).

Figure 5.1 shows the relationships between state abortion restrictions and state abortion rates over time. The average number of state abortions per 1,000 women aged 15–44 steadily declined from 24.6 in 1988 to 11.2 by 2017, a more than 50 percent decline. During the same period, the average number of state restrictions increased from about 2.5 to 11, a 340 percent increase! Abortion rates and restrictions have remained relatively steady since 2017, with a slight increase (0.60) in the average abortion rates from 2019 to 2020 and slight decrease (0.46) in the average number of abortion restrictions in the same period.

The reasons for the decrease in state abortions until 2017, as well as the very modest recent increase, are not fully understood. This steep decrease "has been attributed to several factors, including the increasing use of contraceptives, especially long-acting methods (e.g., intrauterine devices and implants); historic declines in the rate of unintended pregnancy; and increasing numbers of state regulations resulting in limited access to abortion services" (NAS 2018, 28) The abortion rate was decreasing long before the current level of abortion restrictions, and has recently increased in the face of a slight decrease in those restrictions.

Availability of Abortion Providers over Time

In addition to new and more effective contraceptive methods, greater contraceptive use, and state abortion restrictions, another factor that affects the rate of abortions is the availability of abortion providers. The number of providers varies dramatically across states and over time. The lowest number of abortion providers per state is one provider each in North and South Dakota throughout most of the study period (1988–2020). The highest number of abortion providers is in California: 608 abortion clinics at its peak in the end of the 1980s.

Overall, the state average number of abortion providers has declined over time, as shown in figure 5.2, from a high of 51 to a low of 31. New York and California stand out as the states with the largest number of providers across our study period. California dropped from its peak of 608 providers in 1988 to 419 in 2017, the year with the most recent consistent data. During the same time, New York fell from its peak of 305 in 1988 to 218 in the mid-2010s, before rising again to 252 in the later 2010s. The state with the next largest number of providers is Florida, which had its largest number (143) of providers in the late 1980s, falling to 85 by the late 2010s. These states also have among the largest state populations, so the larger number of providers is not surprising. The number of providers may increase or decrease with changes in state populations.

Controlling for population, there has been a steady decline over time in the state average number of providers, as shown in figure 5.2, from about 11 providers per million people to just under five by 2017.[6] Per population size, the states with the largest average number of providers per year in descending order are Hawaii, District of Columbia, Vermont, California, Connecticut, and Alaska. The states at the bottom, with the lowest average number of providers per million people per year in ascending order are Kentucky, Mississippi, Missouri, Wisconsin, North Dakota,

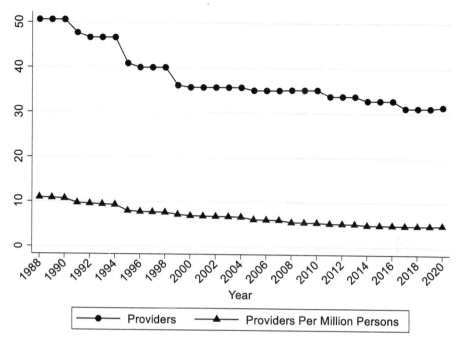

FIGURE 5.2. Average Number of Abortion Providers per State

South Dakota, Oklahoma, West Virginia, Arkansas, Louisiana, Indiana, and Minnesota, followed closely by South Carolina, Ohio, Alabama, Utah, and Texas. Each of these states had on average fewer than three providers per million people per year across our time period, 1988–2020. By 2020, 24 states had fewer than three providers per million people, with an additional 10 under four providers per million people.

The number of providers in a state is sensitive to public policy. For example, in the 16 states that funded abortion beyond the limits of the Hyde Amendment, in 2020. the average number of abortion providers was 75. In contrast, the average number of abortion providers in states that restricted funding was 20. For states that forbid abortion from being covered in their health insurance marketplaces,[7] the average number of abortion providers was 16. States without this restriction had an average of 41 abortion providers. Similarly, states with the median number (six) or more of abortion restrictions in 2020 had an average of 20 providers, whereas those states with fewer than six restrictions had a mean of 53 providers.

When there is a need for abortion but few or no nearby providers, individuals will cross state lines to seek abortion services. This cross-state activity may also increase where there is a discrepancy in number and degree of regulations between one state and neighboring states. States with fewer restrictions and more protections, along with states with more providers, may attract people seeking abortion services. Abortion rates are reported by the CDC and Guttmacher in two forms: occurrence and residence. We provide an analysis of both. Because data on occurrence are more complete, we start with an analysis of abortion rate occurrence.

We model the state rate of abortion occurrence using cross-sectional time-series regression analysis. Our main independent variables are the providers per population, along with a number of measures of restrictions and protections. Because the number of providers is potentially endogenous, meaning that causality could go in both directions with the abortion rate also predicting the number of providers, we use a two-stage model, which takes potential endogeneity into account and adjusts for it in the results. This method entails the use of instrumental variables (in addition to all the independent variables in the model that predict abortion rates, we use the position of the state governing bodies along with state dummy variables as instruments) to first predict the number of providers, and then use the predicted number of providers in the model to predict rate of abortion occurrence. The use of this method adjusts for the potential endogeneity problem and provides a more accurate and robust prediction of the rate of abortion occurrence, which is the dependent variable of interest.

For our measures of regulations, first we subdivide the number of abortion restrictions by regulations that affect women's demand for abortion[8] and regulations that affect the ability of the state or providers to provide abortion services.[9] We expect both types of restrictions to lead to a lower rate of occurrence. We also include our measure of the number of state abortion protections,[10] along with a dummy variable that controls for whether or not the state guarantees that a woman's birth control prescription will be filled. Because availability of contraception may reduce the need for abortion, we expect a negative relationship between this measure and the rate of abortion in the state, and a positive relationship between protections and the rate of occurrence.

In addition, we include our previous controls for state median income, unemployment, and level of education, along with the state reproductive-aged population (15–44 years old). Because most abortion clinics are in metropolitan areas, we expect a higher population to lead to a higher rate of occurrence. We include the number of religious adherents opposed to abortion because this may dampen the rate of occurrence. Finally, we control for the racial makeup of the state with the percent of the population that is African American, Hispanic, or Other, using the percent white as the base of comparison.

The results in Model 1 of table 5.1 show that the number of providers is important to the provision of abortions. Each additional provider per 1 million people increases the abortion rate (number of abortions per 1,000 women aged 15–44) of occurrence by almost two. Restrictions, particularly restrictions that impact a woman's demand for abortion, lead to lower rates of occurrence. Each additional demand-side restriction reduces the rate of occurrence by about 0.27. Guaranteed access to birth control prescriptions also reduces abortion rates by over three abortions per 1,000 reproductive age women. This finding suggests that the availability of contraception reduces the demand for abortion services.

A higher percent of the population with bachelor's degrees reduces abortion rates in a state, as does a higher number of religious adherents in the state. States with larger populations have higher rates of abortion; a $\log_{10}$ unit increase in population aged 15 to 44 results in an 11-point increase in the rate of abortion. For example, an increase in the reproductive-age population from the mean of about 1.47 million to about 14.7 million reproductive-age people results in an increase of 11 abortions per 1,000 reproductive age women. Finally, a 1 percent increase in the population of African Americans of a state leads to about a 0.8 increase in the abortion rate compared with the white population. The Hispanic population in our model is not statistically significantly different from whites, whereas all other racial categories as a group show a rate about 0.3 lower than whites.

We explore the relationship between supply restrictions and abortion rates further by looking specifically at the impact of TRAP laws on abortion rates, rather than all supply restrictions. TRAP laws impose requirements on facilities and equipment of providers, beyond what is necessary to ensure patient safety. Although supply restrictions overall do not have

TABLE 5.1

Two-Stage Least-Squares Cross-Sectional Time-Series Regression Models of the Rate of Abortion Occurrence and Residence

Independent variables	(1) Occurrence Coefficients (standard errors)	(2) Occurrence Coefficients (standard errors)	(3) Residence Coefficients (standard errors)
Providers per millions of population	1.765*** (0.115)	1.781*** (0.114)	1.029*** (0.104)
Number of restrictions on the demand for abortion	−0.274** (0.127)	−0.266** (0.118)	−0.092 (0.163)
Number of restrictions on the supply of abortion	−0.162 (0.195)		
TRAP laws		−0.648** (0.257)	−0.158 (0.352)
State guarantees filling of birth control prescriptions	−3.036*** (0.822)	−3.053*** (0.823)	−2.792*** (1.07)
Number of abortion protections	−0.199 (0.211)	−0.263 (0.211)	−0.343 (0.336)
Median state income ($1,000s), 2019 dollars	0.047 (0.037)	0.041 (0.038)	0.223*** (0.049)
State unemployment rate (%)	−0.032 (0.092)	−0.008 (0.093)	0.033 (0.123)
Population with a bachelor's degree (%)	−0.586*** (0.086)	−0.587*** (0.086)	−0.283*** (0.097)
Population aged 15–44, $\log_{10}$	11.302*** (2.348)	11.265*** (2.307)	6.385*** (1.435)
Religious adherents (millions)	−4.298*** (1.105)	−4.192*** (1.096)	−2.634*** (0.777)
State African American population (%)	0.771*** (0.073)	0.758*** (0.072)	0.32*** (0.046)
State Hispanic population (%)	0.051 (0.08)	0.069 (0.079)	0.247*** (0.057)
State population of all others (%)	−0.321*** (0.085)	−0.317*** (0.084)	−0.294*** (0.066)
Time trend (1988–2020)	0.275*** (0.065)	0.301*** (0.063)	−0.011 (0.069)
Constant	−58.516*** (14.033)	−58.484*** (13.785)	−35.997*** (8.43)
Observations	1,635[a]	1,635	983

Note: *** $p<0.01$, ** $p<0.05$, * $p<0.1$. Because we are primarily interested in the second stage predicting abortion rates above, the first stage estimates for the instrumented model are not reported here.

[a] Observations are less than 1,683 because of random missing values on the dependent and some independent variables. Model 3 is further impacted by missing data on the dependent variable, abortion rate by residence.

a statistically significant impact on abortions rates, TRAP laws do. In Model 2, we replace our overall measure of supply restrictions with just TRAP laws, which ranges from zero to three.[11] The models are very similar, with the important difference in the impact of TRAP laws. More specifically, on average an additional TRAP law causes about a 0.6 decrease in the rate of abortion. If we look more specifically at the number of TRAP laws (zero to three) that states enact, the impact on abortion rates for states with three TRAP laws (Alabama, Arizona, Arkansas, Florida, Illinois, Indiana, Kansas, Kentucky, Louisiana, Mississippi, Missouri, Oklahoma, South Carolina, Tennessee, Texas, and Utah) is particularly strong, decreasing the abortion rate by about 3.4 abortions per 1,000 women ages 15 to 44.

In Model 3 of table 5.1 we look at the impact of the same independent variables on the abortion rate by state of residence instead of occurrence. Here, the number of observations is much smaller because of missing data on this measure. We only have data from 1988 through 2014, with some states missing in this period due to a lack of reporting. Here, there are some interesting differences between abortion rates by residence versus occurrence. Although state restrictions do not have a significant impact on rates by state of residence, median state income and the percent of the population that is Hispanic are both statistically significant.

This difference in the prediction of the rate of occurrence versus residence could be capturing the crossing of state lines by women in highly restrictive states seeking abortions in states with fewer restrictions. For example, women in Texas, with a median state income of about $67,000 in 2019 and who faced 18 state abortion restrictions, may choose to travel to New Mexico, which has seven restrictions and a median state income of about $53,000. These women receiving abortion services in New Mexico would be counted in the abortion rates by residence in a state with a higher median income. Similarly, Texans may choose to travel to another state that has a lower Hispanic population, like Colorado, which is about 22% Hispanic compared with 40% in Texas.

Race and ethnicity are likely to influence the impacts of abortion regulation. In order to test the differential impact of abortion regulations on minority populations, we analyzed how the interaction between minority populations and abortion restrictions affects abortion rates. We find that restrictions on the demand for abortion affect both African American and Hispanic women similarly, relative to whites. For states in the middle population range, an additional restriction on the demand side causes a significant reduction in the abortion rate. More specifically, for each additional demand restriction, abortion rates decrease as the population

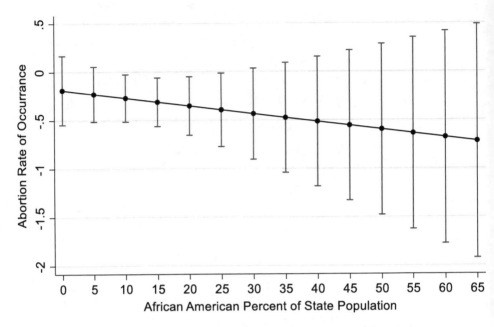

FIGURE 5.3. Average Marginal Effects of an Increase in Demand Restrictions on State Abortion Rates by State Percentage of African Americans

of African Americans increases, and the impact is significant for the population between about 10 and 25 percent. This includes states across the south, as well as Midwest and Northeastern states. We see the same effect for the Hispanic population, significant in the range from about 10 percent to 30 percent, which includes states such as Arizona, California, Colorado, Florida, Nevada, New Jersey, New York, and Texas, among others. This is depicted graphically in figures 5.3 and 5.4.

Although we find no significant difference over the range of state Hispanic populations for supply-side restrictions, in figure 5.5 we find a relatively large significant effect for African Americans, particularly for states with African American populations greater than about 20 percent. These states include Alabama, Delaware, Georgia, Louisiana, Maryland, Mississippi, North and South Carolina, and the District of Columbia. As the percentage of African Americans in a state increases, abortion rates decrease from about a half to over two abortions per 1,000 women aged 15–44. These results illustrate the potential differential effects that supply and demand restrictions on abortion may have on states with larger minority populations.

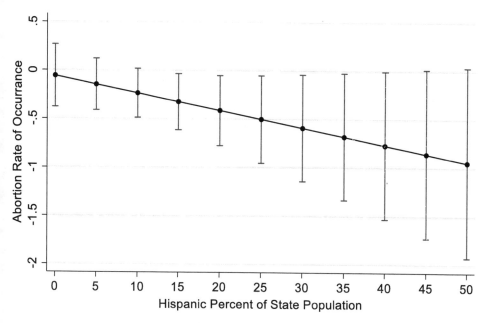

FIGURE 5.4. Average Marginal Effects of an Increase in Demand Restrictions on State Abortion Rates by State Percentage of Hispanics

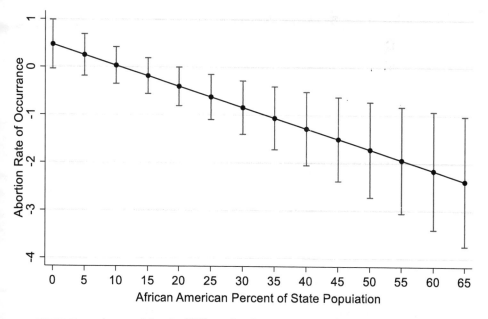

FIGURE 5.5. Average Marginal Effect of an Increase in Supply Restrictions on State Abortion Rates by State Percentage of African Americans

Caveats for Interpreting Impacts

Previously reported studies as well as our own analyses provide substantial evidence of the impacts of state abortion regulations. Nonetheless, it is important to mention some caveats. First, not all state laws are identical, even when they are placed in the same category (Gius 2019). For example, TRAP laws can include many different regulations, ranging from specifying the width of clinic hallways to requiring a specific certification for clinicians (Guttmacher Institute 2022j). Our quantitative analysis does show the importance of TRAP provisions because it is measured from one to three. Nonetheless, a three-point measure does not reflect all of the differences in state TRAP laws.

Similarly, not all state sonogram requirements or informed consent regulations are the same. Some state sonogram laws require the pregnant woman to look at the sonogram; others just provide the option. Some state informed consent laws mandate that women be given incorrect information, for example, that medication abortion can be reversed or that abortion increases the risk of cancer, whereas others follow standard medical counseling protocols. If laws in the same category are considerably different, they are likely to have different effects. However, most quantitative studies, including ours, can only measure the presence of a mandatory sonogram law.

The second caveat is the variation in how states enforce abortion regulations. For example, some states may inspect abortion clinics frequently to enforce TRAP laws or other state licensure requirements. In other states with TRAP laws, enforcement may be more lenient and specific requirements for abortion clinics may even be ignored or overlooked by those charged with enforcement. In other states, however, enforcement can be quite strident depending on who is in the governor's office or who is running the state health department (Joffe 2018).

Despite the importance of this topic, published research thus far has paid scant attention to the enforcement of state abortion regulations. Some work has focused on judicial bypass, a compliance alternative for state parental involvement laws. However, we found only one scholarly article addressing differences in how states perform clinic inspections to monitor compliance with TRAP laws (Joffe 2018). Following its lead, we rely on journalistic accounts from two states, Ohio and Arizona, to show differences between states and across time in enforcement practices.[12]

State Practices in the Judicial Bypass Alternative

Judicial bypass is an enforcement alternative to state parental involvement laws. Chapter 2 explained that in multiple cases, the US Supreme Court has ruled that states with parental involvement laws must provide a confidential judicial bypass option for minors seeking abortion, but not wanting to involve their parents. However, systematic information about the use of this alternative is sparse.

One well-designed study that used Arkansas data found that about 10 percent of adolescents obtaining abortions used the judicial bypass to get permission for this procedure (Joyce 2010). This proportion cannot be meaningfully extrapolated to national data because Arkansas is less populous and less urbanized than many other states. Moreover, more recent work has shown wide variation in the granting of judicial bypasses for minors in other states, even in states with demographic profiles similar to Arkansas (Altindag and Joyce 2017).

For many adolescents, the prospect of going before a judge to discuss an unintended pregnancy is "overwhelming" as well as "logistically complicated" (Kavanaugh et al. 2012, 163). Some states require that a minor seeking abortion without parental involvement must have her judicial bypass hearing in her home county, "not the county where the clinic is located" (Cohen and Joffe 2020, 49). By design, this local requirement is likely to compromise confidentiality, especially in small towns and rural counties. The aim, of course, is to discourage young women from pursuing these alternatives; anecdotal information suggests that this tactic is successful (Cohen and Joffe 2020).

In sum, how states comply with the judicial bypass requirement for parental involvement laws (parental consent or parental notification) certainly affects the impact of this type of abortion restriction. However, quantitative studies of the impact of these regulations only include the presence of these laws, not how states implement the judicial bypass option. Parsing out the effects of different judicial bypass practices would be useful future research that could inform state policymakers.

State Practices in Enforcing TRAP Laws

TRAP laws became a mainstay of restrictive state abortion regulation in the decade following the 2010 election, "which brought a significant increase in Republican governorships and control of state legislatures—and strong pressure for favorable legislation from anti-abortion groups which had worked assiduously for Republicans' elections" (Joffe 2018, 3). In addition to enacted TRAP laws, anti-abortion politicians in various states have "brought pressure on state bureaucracies to more frequently inspect abortion clinics to ascertain that these facilities were complying with both existing and new laws" (Joffe 2018, 4–5).

At least one qualitative study has documented the burden of complying with the enforcement of state TRAP laws. Here 50 individuals from nine states, primarily from the Midwest and the South, were interviewed. Respondents noted the financial costs and time burdens of converting abortion clinics into ambulatory surgery facilities, a practice that is not required for much riskier procedures.[13] They also reported that compliance involves more interaction with state bureaucracies, which takes more staff time. Clinic workers discussed the disruption caused by repeated inspections as well as the dilemmas of inspectors from state health departments who were trying to be professional but were answering to political appointees with anti-abortion agendas (Joffe 2018).

Because of security issues associated with abortion provision, this research did not identify specific states or clinics (Joffe 2018). However, journalistic accounts of state practices provide useful detail. The cases below discuss TRAP enforcement practices in Arizona and Ohio.

Abortion Clinic Inspections in Arizona and Ohio

The TRAP laws in Arizona include private physicians' offices that provide abortion services, so these private practices are subject to state inspection. Anecdotal information from one Arizona doctor's experience indicates that the inspections have been getting more rigorous. In 2012, the state inspection took five hours. Two years later, the same type of inspection lasted for 16 hours (Sieg 2014).

These types of inspections are state-specific. If the same doctor had a private practice in California, for example, her office would not be inspected as an outpatient clinic facility just because abortions were part of her practice. By offering even medication abortions in Arizona, however, this doctor's private practice office must comply with structural standards comparable to those for surgical centers (Guttmacher Institute 2022j). Since 2015, Arizona doctors offering abortion services as part of their practices have also been subject to surprise state inspections, which disrupt patient services and staffing (Joffe 2018; Bennett 2014).

In Ohio, considerable evidence suggests that the state treats abortion clinics differently from other types of health facilities and that the number of citations can increase for abortion facilities when a governor is anti-abortion. Ohio health department officials "are supposed to issue a license and inspect every outpatient surgery facility in the state annually. Outpatient facilities offer plastic, eye or endoscopy surgeries as well as abortions, among other types of medical care" (Seitz 2014). However, nearly all of the abortion clinics in Ohio at the time of this reporting had expired licenses because the state health department had neither approved nor denied their annual applications.

In all but one of these cases, the Ohio Department of Health had inspected the surgical abortion facility, but the health department had never issued a report to notify the clinic if the annual licenses were valid. Abortion providers paid a $1,750 inspection and license renewal fee but never heard back from the state about the clinic's renewal. Some clinics waited months or even years to learn if the state had renewed or denied their licenses (Seitz 2014).

This differential enforcement has been aimed at abortion clinics. In 2014, a journalistic investigation reviewed records of the 135 outpatient surgery clinics in six of Ohio's largest counties, each of which had at least one abortion clinic. The health department issued license renewals for all but eight of these clinics, all of them abortion clinics. That year, only one abortion clinic in Ohio was issued a timely license. Not surprisingly, there has been a large drop in abortion providers in Ohio, dropping from 53 in 1988 to 14 in 2020.

The variation in administrative practices and enforcement mechanisms in both TRAP laws and parental involvement laws has been ignored in most studies that analyze the effects of abortion regulation. At this point, the lack of data about these compliance issues is a good reason for doing so. However, compliance with and enforcement of abortion regulations is an area that merits more data collection and analysis.

Conclusion

State abortion regulations are consequential. These laws can fund, delay, or prevent women from accessing abortion services. Our analysis shows that states with more restrictions have lower abortion rates. However, women from restrictive states also travel in great numbers to less restrictive states to procure abortion services. For example, in 2020, out-of-state women accounted for 50.8 percent of abortions occurring in Kansas and 30.3 percent of those occurring in New Mexico (Centers for Disease Control and Prevention 2021, Table 2). Our analysis suggests that women travel to states with fewer abortion restrictions; the presence of abortion protections does not appear to be an important draw.

Certain types of restrictions have more impact on state abortion rates than others. Demand-side laws attempt to influence patients seeking abortion services and supply-side laws apply to facilities and health personnel who provide these services. In contrast to previous findings, our analysis shows that demand-side restrictions have more impact on the abortion rates of occurrence than do supply-side restrictions. However, if we focus only on TRAP laws—aimed directly at abortion providers—there is a strong and significant negative effect on state abortion rates.

State abortion restrictions affect some groups of women more than others. Because abortion rates are higher among African American and Hispanic women, women in these groups are already more susceptible to state abortion restrictions. However, an additional interaction seems to be occurring. Our analysis shows that additional demand restrictions in states with high percentages of African American or Hispanic women have a disproportionate effect on the state's overall abortion rate. This also holds for the impact of supply restrictions in states where there is a large percentage of African American women, but not Hispanic women. Without state-level abortion rates by race and ethnicity, we do not know the cause of this enhanced impact of additional demand and supply restrictions. This pattern suggests that restrictions may have a disproportionate effect on women of color. These findings merit further investigation and data collection.

The availability of reproductive health services also affects state abortion rates. States that mandate access to birth control prescriptions reduce their abortion rates significantly. States with a higher density of abortion providers have higher abortion rates, especially for occurrence, showing that they are drawing women from other states. The number of abortion providers in a state is also sensitive to state abortion regulations. Since 2010, state anti-abortion regulations have increasingly targeted providers.

Our analysis rests on enacted and enforced state abortion regulations. Although we have discussed the importance and impact of compliance and enforcement on state abortion rates and numbers of providers, we do not have systematic data for those caveats.

CHAPTER 6

How Abortion Is Regulated in Western Europe

A Comparison with the United States

Given the rapidly changing abortion landscape in the United States, it is instructive to look at another region to see alternative models of abortion regulation. This chapter focuses on abortion regulation in the 18 countries of Western Europe. All Western European countries regulate the practice of abortion to some degree. Collectively, these countries have the world's lowest regional abortion rate, but they vary widely in their use of regulations.

The first section addresses Irish abortion law, discussing how it has evolved over the last four decades and highlighting the 2018 referendum that legalized early abortion in the Emerald Isle. Ireland is featured here because it was one of the last holdouts in Western Europe without a liberalized abortion law. This case shows how the rise of secularization in an economically prosperous country can affect abortion regulation. The second section discusses why Western Europe serves as a good comparator for the United States. The third section describes the types of abortion restrictions found in the 18 Western European countries and analyzes their relationship to national abortion rates. The chapter concludes by comparing abortion regulation in Western Europe with abortion restrictions and protections in US states, including COVID-19 provisions.

The Evolution of Irish Abortion Policy, 1983–2018

On May 25, 2018, voters went to the polls to decide if abortion would be legalized in the Republic of Ireland. Along with Malta (Coi 2022; Benavides 2019), Andorra (Bernhard 2022), and Northern Ireland[1] (Carroll 2022; Glennie et al. 2021), the Republic of Ireland was one of the last criminal abortion holdouts in Western Europe (Levels et al. 2014). The issue at hand was whether to repeal the Eighth Amendment to the Irish Constitution. Passed by referendum in 1983, this amendment established the "right to life of the unborn" (Government of Ireland 2022).

Before the inception of the Eighth Amendment, the 1861 Offenses Against the Person Act already prohibited the practice of abortion in Ireland (Carnegie and Roth 2019, 110). The Eighth Amendment went further by precluding travel for abortion and ensuring that any change in abortion policy had to occur through another Constitutional referendum (Glennie et al. 2021, 8). By 1986, the Eighth Amendment proscribed even the transmission of abortion information because the Irish High Court ruled that it was illegal to provide information that would help women to access abortions in Britain (Gilmartin and Kennedy 2019, 129).[2]

1992 Referendum

The right to travel abroad for abortion was challenged in 1992. That year, the Irish High Court, prevented a pregnant 14-year-old girl who had been raped from leaving the country for an abortion (Gilmartin and Kennedy 2019). Deeming the girl's life to be in danger through risk of suicide, the Irish Supreme Court overturned the decision and allowed the pregnant teenager's parents to take their daughter abroad for a pregnancy termination. Figure 6.1 shows the famous Martyn Turner cartoon from the *Irish Times* depicting the incident.

Because of the Eighth Amendment, the Irish Supreme Court's 1992 decision precipitated a referendum on the right to travel for an abortion. In November 1992, the Irish electorate voted to guarantee a woman's right to travel, resulting in the adoption of the Thirteenth Amendment to the Irish Constitution (Glennie et al. 2021, 8). Beginning in 1993, Irish women could legally travel abroad for abortions. During the years that followed, at least 150,000 Irish women left the country for pregnancy

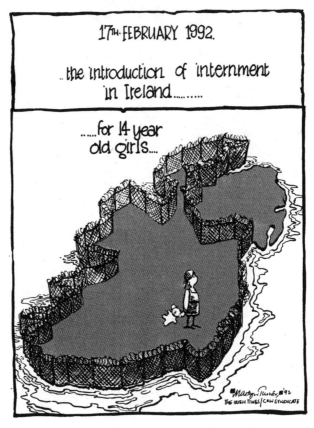

FIGURE 6.1. The Introduction of Internment in Ireland. © 1992 Martyn Turner, published in the *Irish Times*. Reprinted with permission of the artist.

terminations.[3] Traveling, however, required time and money. These resources, of course, were scarcer for low-income women and for migrant women, who also faced issues with their visa status (Gilmartin and Kennedy 2019, 128)

In 1995, the Regulation of Information Act allowed doctors, advisory agencies, and individual counselors to give information about abortion services available abroad to women requesting these facts. This policy change allowed abortion activists to focus on access—how to travel to and access abortion services in the United Kingdom and elsewhere (Gilmartin and Kennedy 2019, 135). But more than two decades would pass before another abortion referendum occurred.

2018 Referendum

The wording of the 2018 referendum ballot was simple: "Do you approve of the proposal to amend the Constitution contained in the undermentioned Bill?"[4] (RTE 2018). The ballot did not reference the Eighth Amendment, nor did it mention abortion. Nonetheless, nearly everyone in the country knew what was at stake: continuing a near total ban on abortion or permitting abortion up to 12 weeks.

In the months and weeks leading up to the referendum, both sides campaigned vigorously. Dozens of pro-choice groups formed. One of the most effective was Anna Cosgrave's Repeal Campaign that kept selling out of Repeal sweaters. Anti-abortion groups, including the Pro-Life Campaign, Youth Defence, and the Iona Institute, also clamored with demonstrations and marches (AlmostAttorneyatLaw 2017). On May 25, 64.1 percent of Irish voters cast ballots, the third highest turnout for a referendum since the adoption of the Irish constitution in 1937 (McDonald et al. 2018).[5]

When the results were tallied, nearly two-thirds of those voting opted for changing the law. This victory was definitive across most segments of society. Both men and women voted for repeal, as did both urban and rural voters. Majorities in every age group, except those 65 and over, voted to legalize abortion, and all but one of Ireland's 43 parliamentary constituencies[6] voted to repeal the Eighth Amendment (McDonald et al. 2018). The long-time campaign and careful community organizing of abortion rights activists had paid off (Gilmartin and Kennedy 2019).

Increasing Secularization

Although the winning margin was higher than expected, this policy change had been anticipated. Both the increasing secularization of the Irish population[7] and the declining reputation of the Catholic Church were important factors in this shift. For years, the predominant Irish Catholic Church held firm in its resolve not to change the law, even though more than 6,000 Irish women left the country each year to obtain abortion services. By 2018, however, the Church was increasingly in disrepute, especially regarding gender issues. Both the Magdalene laundry scandal revelations and the 2012 death of Dr. Savita Halappanavar damaged public regard for the Church as an institution (Harrison 2013).

The laundry scandal showed the Catholic Church's callous disregard for the plight of thousands of women confined to servitude for over a half century. In "Irish lore, the laundries were synonymous with so-called 'fallen women'—unmarried mothers" (Dalby 2013a), a designation that stigmatized anyone who entered these facilities. During the period 1922–1996, more than 14,000 women were held, often against their will, by four orders of Catholic nuns in at least 10 facilities. These women and young girls were forced to work long hours for no pay, a situation abetted by the Irish government (Government of Ireland 2013).

After decades of trying, advocates for these enslaved women, known as "Maggies," convinced the United Nations Committee Against Torture to request the Irish government to investigate what had transpired in these laundries and what the state's role had been. That report, released in February 2013, showed that young girls and women were sent to these facilities for many reasons, including poverty, mental illness, and petty crime, not just unwed pregnancy. The average age was 23, but the youngest girl to enter was nine years old. The median stay was seven months, but some women were kept in servitude for decades (Government of Ireland 2013). The Irish prime minister issued an official apology for the state's collusion with the Catholic laundries a few weeks after the report was issued (Dalby 2013a, 2013b).

The other focusing event in the most recent Irish abortion struggle was the preventable death of Dr. Savita Halappanavar, a 31-year-old Indian immigrant dentist, living in Galway, Ireland. In October 2012, Dr. Halappanavar was pregnant with her first child. When she began to experience severe back pain, she and her husband reported to the Galway Hospital. After admitting Dr. Halappanavar to the hospital, "doctors refused to intervene after she was diagnosed with an incomplete miscarriage at approximately 16 weeks of pregnancy" (Carnegie and Roth 2019, 111) because that would have been considered an abortion (McFarlane 2015). Hospital staff "told her and her husband that they could not do anything to expedite her miscarriage because a fetal heartbeat was still present and this was a 'Catholic country.'" Dr. Halappanavar died of sepsis from "medical mismanagement of her condition" seven days after being hospitalized (Carnegie and Roth 2019, 111).[8]

Both the Halappanavar tragedy and the laundry scandal revelations damaged the reputation of the Catholic Church. Another indicator of the Church's waning influence was the 2015 Irish referendum on gay marriage (McFarlane 2015). Sweeping "aside the opposition of the Roman Catholic Church" (Hakim and Dalby 2015), Ireland became the first country in the world to approve gay marriage by referendum. The measure had passed comfortably: 62 percent of those who voted supported legalizing gay marriage (Hakim and Dalby 2015). Three years later, the vote for legalizing abortion was even higher with 66.4 percent voting to repeal the Eighth Amendment.

This referendum was about very circumscribed conditions for legal abortion. Pregnancy terminations would be legal only up until 12 weeks since a woman's last menstrual period, really 10 weeks of gestation. Nonetheless, this referendum meant that the Republic of Ireland had joined nearly all Western European countries, most of which liberalized their abortion laws between 1960 and 1990 (Levels et al. 2014).

Abortion Regulation in Western Europe

Western Europe was selected a comparator for US abortion regulation for several reasons. First, Western European countries collectively have the lowest regional abortion rate in the world, a fact which offers the potential for policy learning in the US states. Socioeconomic and political similarities are the second reason. Most Western European countries are wealthy democracies, and their populations have fertility aspirations similar to those in the United States.

Comparing policy sectors between North American and Western European countries is a common practice in comparative health policy analysis (Wong 2014; Marmor et al. 2005; Parsons 1995); abortion policy is no exception. A series of case studies covering changes in abortion regulation from policy formulation to policy implementation in the United States, Western Europe, Eastern Europe, and Japan was published in the mid-1990s (Githens and McBride 1996). Another compilation of country studies from roughly the same period of time described the relationship between the women's movement and abortion policy (McBride 2001). A 2014 study reviewed Western European legal developments in abortion policy from 1960 to 2010. This study, however, did not quantify the total bundle or intensity of abortion restrictions, making cross-national comparisons difficult (Levels et al. 2014).

Global Abortion Regulations

To put US and Western European abortion regulations in context, this section reviews the status of global abortion policies. Across the world, national abortion policies vary greatly. These laws are consequential; they affect both the safety and availability of abortion services (Kulczycki 2015). For patient safety, the most important attribute of a national abortion policy is legality, that is, whether most pregnancy terminations in a country take place legally. Over a quarter of the world's women live in countries where highly restrictive laws make most induced abortions illegal. On the other hand, global data collected before the *Dobbs* decision indicated that more than 60 percent of the world's population lives in countries with liberalized abortion laws, where at least early abortion is legally available on broad grounds (Kulczycki 2015, 188).

One of the many controversies surrounding the regulation of abortion is whether highly restrictive abortion laws, making most abortions illegal, thwart the incidence of abortion. Recent global evidence shows that highly restrictive abortion laws are related positively to abortion rates. In other words, countries with the most restrictive abortion laws also tend to have the highest abortion rates (Sedgh et al. 2012, 625).

Restrictive abortion laws, however, do not cause high abortion rates. This positive relationship is due to changing fertility preferences in developing countries, which tend to have restrictive abortion laws. As women or couples increasingly prefer to have smaller families, the incidence of induced abortion increases. Higher abortion rates are only temporary. As modern contraception becomes more available in that country or region, birth control replaces induced abortion as the dominant method of fertility control (Denton 2015, 207).

Eastern Europe, with a relatively high abortion rate, provides a stark contrast to this generalization. Most countries in this region do have liberalized abortion laws, but abortion rates are relatively high in this region.

The reason for this anomaly is historical. For years, modern contraception was severely lacking in these post-Soviet societies, but abortion services were readily available (Kulczycki 2015, 176).[9]

The practice of abortion and the use of contraception in Western Europe stand in sharp contrast to Eastern Europe. Here too, abortion services are largely accessible and fertility preferences low. Unlike Eastern Europe, Western European countries have one of the lowest regional abortion rates in the world (Guttmacher Institute 2022d) because modern contraceptive prevalence is relatively high. Nevertheless, contraceptive prevalence among Western European countries varies greatly. In 2020, the percentage of women ages 15–49 using modern contraceptive methods ranged from 45.9 in Greece to 82.2 in Norway. Despite the region's relatively high contraceptive prevalence, abortion is practiced throughout Western Europe (United Nations Population Division 2021).

Abortion Policy in Western Europe

Brief History

After a wave of abortion liberalization or reform from 1960 to 1980, Western European laws have been mostly stable. Politically, abortion cuts across the dominant cleavage of Western European party systems, usually based on the socioeconomic divides in each country. To maintain their coalitions, political parties in Western Europe are reluctant to take a stand on abortion, an issue that touches on secular and religious divides (Outshoorn 1996). Unlike "American politicians, Western European party elites try to prevent the issue from gaining agenda status because they know that abortion has the potential to divide electoral party politics" (McFarlane 2015, 59).

As a result, stable abortion compromises have existed in most Western European countries for decades (Outshoorn 1996). Three exceptions are Germany, Spain, and Ireland. In the first case, the reunification of Germany required the conciliation of West and East German abortion laws (Kamenitsa 2001). In the second case, Spain's abortion law was liberalized in 2010 by the socialist government then in power, allowing abortion without restriction up to the fourteenth week of pregnancy.[10] The subsequent conservative government tried to tighten Spain's liberal abortion law, but eventually backed down in the face of significant domestic and international opposition (Bhatia and Naili 2015; Kassam 2014). As explained earlier in this chapter, Ireland legalized early abortion through a 2018 national referendum.

Currently, abortion is legal in every Western European country except for Andorra and Malta. However, legality and accessibility can be very different. Pregnancy termination is legal in most Western European nations, but access to abortion, abortion regulations, and abortion rates vary widely in the region.

Abortion Rates by Country

In 2020,[11] the mean abortion rate among Western European countries was 10.4 abortions per 1,000 women aged 15–49, the lowest regional abortion rate in the world. Nonetheless, considerable variation in the incidence of induced abortion exists in this region. Overall, the lowest abortion rate (by definition, the abortion rate is the number of abortions per 1,000 reproductive age women; reproductive age is 15–44 in the United States and 15–49 in Europe[12]) was 3.1 for Luxembourg, and the highest was 19 for Sweden (Abort Report EU 2022).

Within different regions of Western Europe, abortion rates also fluctuate. In Southern Europe, Italy's 2020 abortion rate was 5.5 per 1,000 women aged 15–49; Spain's was 10.3, and Greece's was 15. In central Western Europe, the 2020 French abortion rate was 15.4, but adjacent countries had much lower rates: 8.4 in Belgium, 6.8 in Switzerland, and 5.9 in Germany. Abortion rates in the Scandinavian countries also exhibited wide variation, with a low of 7.7 in Finland to the Swedish rate of 19 (Abort Report EU 2022).

Abortion Restrictions in Western European Countries

All Western European countries regulate the practice of abortion. Like US states, Western European countries have both abortion restrictions and abortion protections. Also, like US states, Western European nations have both demand-side and supply-side abortion regulations.

WAITING PERIODS

Eight of the 18 Western European countries require a waiting period between the time a woman requests an abortion and the procedure itself. The length of these waiting periods varies considerably from a low of 72 hours (three days) in Germany, Ireland, Luxembourg, Portugal, and Spain, to a high of 168 hours (seven days) in Italy. The Netherlands has a waiting time of five days and Belgium's waiting period is six days.

MANDATORY COUNSELING

Eight Western European countries (Austria, Belgium, Finland, Germany, Greece, Italy, the Netherlands, and Spain) require specific abortion counseling before women can receive abortion services. Three countries (Luxembourg, France, and Switzerland) require abortion counseling for minors, but not for older women. Among the countries that mandate abortion counseling, there is no uniform protocol for what it entails.

Specific abortion counseling may be more extensive than informed consent, which means that women seeking abortion—like any other health service—are fully informed of their treatment options.[13] Compelling women to undergo counseling, whether they want it or not, risks manipulation and may undermine personal freedom (International Planned Parenthood Federation 2019, 12).

Although five Eastern European countries report that their abortion counseling is designed to manipulate a woman or girl into continuing through a pregnancy, this type of systematic persuasion at the national level is not reported among Western European countries. More common are inconsistencies in the requirements for and capacity to provide abortion counseling, especially in Italy and Greece. Noteworthy is the German requirement for abortion counseling, which is more women-centered than what is required for abortion counseling in many other countries (International Planned Parenthood Federation 2019).[14]

PARENTAL INVOLVEMENT

Eleven of the 18 Western European countries require parental involvement in a minor's decision to have an abortion. The age of consent varies from 14 years of age in Austria to 16 years in five countries (Germany,

Iceland, the Netherlands, Norway, and Portugal) and 18 years of age in five countries (Denmark, Greece, Italy, Luxembourg, and Spain). Countries that do not require parental consent or notification for minors are Belgium, Ireland, Finland, France, Sweden, Switzerland, and the United Kingdom (International Planned Parenthood Federation 2019).

MEDICAL REFUSAL OR CONSCIENTIOUS OBJECTION BY HEALTH CARE WORKERS

In 14 Western European countries, health care workers have the right to conscientiously object to rendering or participating in abortion services. Conscientious objection restrictions can have serious implications for access to abortion services (Abort Report EU 2022) because there may not be enough physicians and other health care workers to provide the services. The negative impact of medical refusal for the delivery of abortion services is substantiated in reports from six of the countries with this provision: Austria, France, Germany, Italy, Portugal, and Spain (International Planned Parenthood Federation 2019).

LACK OF PROVIDERS

In the most recent country survey conducted in 2018 by International Planned Parenthood's European Network, respondents from eight Western European nations (Austria, France, Germany, Ireland, Italy, Luxembourg, Portugal, and Spain) reported that they did not have "sufficient trained and willing service providers" for abortion services (International Planned Parenthood Federation 2019). Italy, Luxembourg, and Portugal reported that many physicians refuse to provide abortion care.

Total Restrictions

Three (Germany, Italy, and Spain) of the 18 countries have all five of these restrictions. However, there is no straightforward relationship between national abortion rates and the number of restrictions. The abortion rate in these countries varies from 5.5 per 1,000 women aged 15–49 in Italy to 10.3 in Spain. Four countries (Austria, Luxembourg, Netherlands, and Portugal) have four of these restrictions. Again, no direct relationship exists between national abortion rates and the number of restrictions; the highest rate is 15 in Austria and the lowest is 3.1 in Luxembourg.

Within the three Western European countries (Belgium, Greece, and Ireland) with three abortion restrictions, a wide range of abortion rates exists. The highest rate is 15 in Greece; the lowest is 5.3 in Ireland. The three countries with only two restrictions each (Denmark, France, and Norway) also show wide variance. Their abortion rates vary from 15.4 in France to 9.7 in Norway. Similarly, abortion rates of the three countries (Finland, Iceland, and the United Kingdom) with one abortion restriction each range from 7.7 in Finland to 18.2 in the United Kingdom. The two countries (Sweden and Switzerland) with no abortion restrictions have very different rates: 6.8 in Switzerland and 19 in Sweden.

Abortion Protections in Western European Countries

In addition to restrictions, Western European countries have also enacted measures to assist or facilitate abortion. Table 6.2 shows two abortion protections that were in place before COVID-19 and four measures adopted by some European countries to facilitate access to abortion during the COVID-19 pandemic.

FUNDING

Nearly all Western European countries fund abortion, at least in part, for their residents through the first three months or 13 weeks of pregnancy. The German health system is the least generous in this respect, usually covering only the initial visit but not the procedure itself. However, the state does cover the cost of the procedure for low-income women (Abort Report EU 2022; International Planned Parenthood Federation 2019).

According to the International Planned Parenthood Federation (2019), Finland, France, Norway, and the United Kingdom each fund both medication and surgical abortions for everyone. However, women seeking abortion services often face extra costs even if they are eligible for free services under the country's law. In Finland, for example, women seeking abortion services must pay a 35 € hospital fee in a public hospital and a 94 € fee in a private hospital. In France, women pay for abortion services up front, and then they are fully reimbursed by the national health insurance system for the cost of the procedure or medication. Both low-income women and minors without parental consent are exempted from having to advance funds for abortion. Norwegian national

TABLE 6.1

Abortion Rates and Abortion Restrictions in Western European Countries, 2020

Country	Abortion rate (number of abortions per 1,000 women age 15–49)	Waiting period (yes=1, no=0)	Waiting time (hours)	Mandatory counseling (yes=1, no=0)	Medical refusal (yes=1, no=0)	Parental involvement (yes=1, no=0)	Lack of providers (yes=1, no=0)
Austria	15	0	0	1	1	0	1
Belgium	8.4	1	144	1	1	1	0
Denmark	11.4	0	0	0	1	0	0
Finland	7.7	0	0	1	0	0	0
France	15.4	0	0	0	1	0	1
Germany	5.9	1	72	1	1	1	1
Greece	15	0	0	1	1	1	0
Iceland	12.8	0	0	0	0	0	0
Ireland	5.3	1	72	1	1	0	1
Italy	5.5	1	168	1	1	1	1
Luxembourg	3.1	1	72	0	1	1	1
Netherlands	8.9	1	120	1	1	1	0
Norway	9.7	0	0	0	1	1	0
Portugal	6.5	1	72	0	1	1	1
Spain	10.3	1	72	1	1	1	1
Sweden	19	0	0	0	0	0	0
Switzerland	6.8	0	0	0	0	0	0
United Kingdom	18.2	0	0	0	1	0	0

Sources: Abortion rates are from Abort Report EU (2022) and US Census (2021b); restrictions data are from International Planned Parenthood Federation (2019, 2012).

TABLE 6.2

Abortion Rates and Abortion Protections in Western European Countries, 2020

Country	Abortion rate (number of abortions per 1,000 women age, 15–49)	Funding (partial=0, full=1)	Gestational limit (weeks)	Extended gestation limits during COVID-19 (yes=1, no=0)	Telemedicine for abortion available during COVID-19 (yes=2, partial=1, no=0)	Facilitated access during COVID-19 (yes=1, no=0)	Early medical abortion available during COVID-19 (yes=1, no=0)
Austria	15	0	16	1	0	1	1
Belgium	8.4	0	15	0	1	1	1
Denmark	11.4	0	12	0	2	0	1
Finland	7.7	1	12	0	0	1	1
France	15.4	1	14	0	2	1	1
Germany	5.9	0	14	0	1	1	1
Greece	15	0	12	0	0	0	1
Iceland	12.8	0	23	0	0	0	0
Ireland	5.3	0	12	0	2	1	1
Italy	5.5	0	12	1	0	1	1
Luxembourg	3.1	0	14	0	0	0	1
Netherlands	8.9	0	24	0	0	0	1
Norway	9.7	1	12	0	0	0	0
Portugal	6.5	0	10	0	1	0	1
Spain	10.3	0	14	0	0	1	1
Sweden	19	0	18	0	2	0	1
Switzerland	6.8	0	12	0	0	0	0
United Kingdom	18.2	1	24	0	2	1	1

Sources: Abortion rates are from Abort Report EU (2022) and US Census (2021b); restrictions data are from International Planned Parenthood Federation (2019, 2012).

health insurance covers the entire cost of abortion services for all women living in Norway.[15]

GESTATIONAL LIMITS

Depending on their length, gestational limits can be considered restrictions (short intervals) or protections (long intervals). Because women may not be aware that they are pregnant for several weeks, lower gestational limits can curtail their opportunities to seek abortion. Conversely, higher gestational limits provide more time to make decisions and obtain services. Table 6.2 shows that gestational limits in Western European countries vary from a low of 10 weeks since last menstrual period (LMP)[16] in Portugal to a high of 24 weeks LMP in the Netherlands and the United Kingdom (Fontaine 2019; International Planned Parenthood Federation 2019). It should be noted that in cases of fetal malformation, most Western European countries either waive the gestational limit or extend it to at least 24 weeks.[17]

The relationship between gestational limits and abortion rates, however, is not straightforward.[18] For example, the two countries with the highest gestational limits, the Netherlands and the United Kingdom, have very different abortion rates. For 2020, the abortion rate for the Netherlands was 8.9, below average for Western European countries. At 18.2, the United Kingdom's abortion rate was more than twice as high.

COVID-19 Protections

COVID-19 brought new challenges for abortion services around the world. In the United States, states enacted both restrictions (11 states) and protections (12 states) (Liptak 2021b; Capello 2020; Jones et al. 2020). In Western Europe, many countries put protections in place to facilitate access to abortion during the COVID-19 pandemic. These measures included making early medical abortion available (15 countries), facilitating access through policy changes (10 countries) and enhancing telemedicine (eight countries). In addition, both Austria and Italy extended their gestational limits. Among the protections, the length of gestational limits and the availability of telemedicine have the highest correlations with abortion rates, 0.48 and 0.36, respectively (Abort Report EU 2022; Bojovic et al. 2021).

Impact of Abortion Restrictions and Protections

Difference of Means

Among the restrictions and protections, only waiting periods show a statistically significant effect on the mean abortion rate of countries. Table 6.3 shows the mean abortion rate for countries with and without the various restriction and protections, the difference in the means and the significance levels. With a mean difference of 6.4, significant at the 0.01 level, only waiting periods are related to lower abortion rates.

Table 6.4 shows the correlations between the abortion rate and each of the restrictions and protections listed in tables 6.1 and 6.2. All the restrictions have a negative relationship with abortion rates, with waiting period (0.69) and waiting time (0.60) being the strongest. No other relationship exceeds a correlation of 0.5; indeed, most correlations are quite low.

Regression Analysis

To further explore the effects of restrictions and protections, we use ordinary least-squares regression models for Western Europe (table 6.5) and US states (table 6.6) for the latest year of available data to predict abortion rates. Taken together in total, neither restrictions nor protections are significant in predicting abortion rates in Europe. To further explore the potential impact of these regulations, we looked at them individually. Among all the restrictions and protections explored alone and in combination, waiting time and gestational limits were the only restrictions that were statistically significant in affecting abortion rates. On the protection side, neither telemedicine nor funding were significant. In Model 1 of table 6.5, we include restrictive policies, along with several other variables that have been used to predict abortion rates. We use a measure of abortion providers (lack of providers), the percent of the population that is religious (Catholic and Orthodox), income (per capita), education (percentage of females with the equivalent of a bachelor's degree), and the percentage of contraceptive coverage (modern contraceptive prevalence). We also included a control for the reproductive aged (15–44) population, the same range used in the United States.

The results show that waiting periods, gestational limits, and contraceptive prevalence are all statistically significant in explaining abortion

TABLE 6.3

Comparison of Mean Abortion Rates for Western European Countries with and without Various Restrictions and Protections, 2020

Regulation	Number of countries without regulation	Number of countries with regulation	Mean without regulation	Mean with regulation	Difference	Standard error	t-value	p-value
Restrictions								
Waiting period	10	8	13.1	6.74	6.36	1.65	3.85*	0.00
Counseling	10	8	10.82	9.59	1.23	2.27	0.54	0.60
Medical refusal	4	14	11.58	9.90	1.68	2.71	0.62	0.55
Parental involvement	7	11	11.54	9.46	2.08	2.28	0.91	0.38
Lack of providers	10	8	11.79	8.38	3.42	2.13	1.60	0.13
Protections								
Funding (partial or full)	14	4	9.57	12.75	-3.19	2.62	-1.2	0.24
Facilitated abortion during COVID-19	8	10	10.84	9.82	1.02	2.28	0.45	0.66
Early medical abortion during COVID-19	3	15	9.77	10.37	-0.61	3.06	-0.20	0.85
Telemedicine during COVID-19	10	8	9.48	11.26	-1.78	2.25	-0.79	0.44
Extended gestational limits during COVID-19	16	2	10.27	10.25	0.03	3.63	0.01	0.99

Note: * significance $p<$o.o1.

TABLE 6.4
Correlations

Variables	(1)	(2)	(3)	(4)	(5)	(6)	(7)	(8)	(9)	(10)	(11)	(12)	(13)	(14)	(15)	(16)	(17)
(1) Abortion rate	1.00																
(2) Waiting period	-0.69	1.00															
(3) Waiting time (hours)	-0.60	0.89	1.00														
(4) Counseling	-0.13	0.33	0.46	1.00													
(5) Medical refusal	-0.15	0.48	0.43	0.21	1.00												
(6) Parental involvement	-0.22	0.25	0.19	0.25	0.40	1.00											
(7) Gestational limits	0.48	-0.13	-0.05	-0.03	-0.16	-0.05	1.00										
(8) Extended gestation-COVID-19	-0.00	0.04	0.26	0.40	0.19	0.28	-0.08	1.00									
(9) Lack of providers	-0.37	0.55	0.36	0.10	0.48	0.25	-0.30	0.40	1.00								
(10) Funding	0.29	-0.48	-0.43	-0.21	-0.04	-0.40	0.06	-0.19	0.06	1.00							
(11) Telemedicine during COVID-19	0.36	-0.10	-0.16	-0.49	0.14	-0.52	0.06	-0.29	0.29	0.17	1.00						
(12) Early medication abortion during COVID-19	0.05	0.40	0.36	0.40	0.48	-0.05	-0.07	0.16	0.40	-0.12	0.37	1.00					
(13) Facilitated abortion during COVID-19	-0.11	0.35	0.33	0.35	0.33	-0.25	-0.18	0.32	0.58	0.21	0.23	0.50	1.00				
(14) Modern contraceptive prevalence	-0.20	-0.11	-0.27	-0.43	-0.26	-0.12	0.18	-0.43	0.02	0.41	0.12	-0.32	-0.13	1.00			
(15) Religion (%)	-0.36	0.55	0.48	0.31	0.50	0.24	-0.43	0.39	0.45	-0.47	-0.23	0.38	0.35	-0.65	1.00		
(16) Per capita income	-0.38	0.04	-0.04	-0.40	-0.14	-0.15	0.02	-0.13	0.04	-0.05	0.05	-0.28	-0.36	0.61	-0.25	1.00	
(17) Female education (% with a bachelors)	-0.24	-0.08	-0.14	-0.53	-0.33	-0.20	0.18	-0.51	-0.32	-0.07	-0.06	-0.50	-0.58	0.39	-0.29	0.61	1.00

TABLE 6.5
Regression Models of Abortion Rates in Western European Countries, 2020

Independent Variable	(1) Coefficients (robust standard errors)	(2) Coefficients (robust standard errors)
Waiting time (hours)	−0.052***	−0.043***
	(0.015)	(0.013)
Gestational limit (weeks)	0.500***	0.511***
	(0.125)	(0.098)
Lack of providers (yes=1, no=0)	0.886	−0.743
	(2.772)	(2.761)
Telemedicine during COVID-19 (yes=2, partial=1, no=0)		2.706
		(1.540)
Funding (all=1, some=0)		1.734
		(1.265)
Percent religious	−0.050	−0.043
	(0.044)	(0.049)
Per capita income ($1,000s)	0.007	0.006
	(0.041)	(0.044)
Modern contraceptive prevalence (% coverage)	−0.277*	−0.323**
	(0.143)	(0.127)
Female education (% with a bachelors)	−0.098	−0.108
	(0.082)	(0.066)
Reproductive age (15–44) population ($\log_{10}$)	0.304	−1.147
	(1.130)	(0.910)
Constant	26.865***	37.398**
	(14.735)	(13.092)
Observations	18	18
R-squared	0.87	0.93
F-statistic	15.09***	43.78***

Note: *** $p<0.01$, ** $p<0.05$, * $p<0.1$.

rates in Western Europe. For a country with a waiting period of 100 hours (the mean), abortion rates go down by five abortions per 1,000 women aged 15–49 compared with a country without a waiting period. Each additional week added to the gestational limit results in a 0.5 increase in the abortion rate. Therefore, a country that has a 20-week limit compared with a country with a 10-week limit would increase its abortion rate by about five abortions per 1,000 women of reproductive age.

In our analysis, a lack of providers does not affect national abortion rates, but this finding may be related to this being a weak measure.[19] It was found that income, education, and religion do not impact abortion rates. However, modern contraceptive prevalence, ranging from about 46 percent to 82 percent, does reduce the abortion rate. Specifically, an additional 10 percent coverage reduces the abortion rate by about three abortions per 1,000 women aged 15–49. In Model 2 of table 6.5, we include the two protection policies, funding and telemedicine access during COVID-19. Although full funding does not impact the rate, telemedicine has a positive effect just below the 0.10 level of significance. A country that offered abortion services during COVID-19 had abortion rates about 2.7 times higher than countries that did not offer these services. If we exclude lack of providers from Model 2, telemedicine becomes significant at the 0.08 level and education becomes significant at the 0.03 level.

Finally, in table 6.6, we offer a comparison, analyzing factors that affected 2020 abortion rates in the 50 US states and the District of Columbia. Model 1 includes our previous measures of both number of restrictions and number of protections, along with a similar set of controls used in table 6.5 including income, education, reproductive age population, and religious adherence, along with racial composition—known to be a factor in US rates. The number and variety of US state restrictions and protections prevents us from including them individually in such a small sample ($N=51$).

When included together, neither restrictions nor protections were significant in predicting rates because they have a particularly high correlation by 2020, at 0.73 (unlike Europe, where the correlation between aggregate restrictions and protections is only 0.03). Due to this multicollinearity, they are insignificant. Among the controls, education, religious adherents, and racial composition of the states are all statistically significant in predicting abortion rates. States with a higher number of religious adherents have lower rates, whereas states with higher percentages of African American and Hispanic populations have higher rates. Oddly, higher education has a positive effect on rates. Because these are rates of occurrence (rather than residence) it includes women who cross state lines to receive services in less restrictive states. But in addition, education is highly correlated with median income (0.84) as well as abortion protections (0.54) and restrictions (−0.55). These strong correlations inflate the standard errors of the coefficients, making them insignificant.

In Models 2 and 3, we separate restrictions and protections so we can see their individual effects. We drop education from the model because of its high correlations with multiple variables. Here, median income is now significant at the 0.05 level (Models 2 and 3), as well as protections—

TABLE 6.6
Regression Models of Abortion Rates in US States, 2020

Independent Variable	(1) Coefficients (robust standard errors)	(2) Coefficients (robust standard errors)	(3) Coefficients (robust standard errors)	(4) Coefficients (robust standard errors)	(5) Coefficients (robust standard errors)
Number of abortion restrictions	-0.139 (0.224)	-0.291* (0.174)		-0.525*** (0.182)	
Number of abortion protections	0.146 (0.45)		0.691** (0.271)		1.123*** (0.316)
Median household income ($1,000s) (2019 dollars)	-0.195 (0.119)	0.239** (0.108)	0.238** (0.1)		
Population with a bachelor's degree (%)	0.829*** (0.258)				
Reproductive age (15–44) population ($\log_{10}$)	3.529 (2.463)	3.426 (2.962)	1.192 (3.095)	4.516 (3.007)	0.894 (3.567)
Religious adherents (millions)	-2.344*** (0.751)	-2.627*** (0.802)	-2.301*** (0.811)	-3.042*** (0.947)	-2.682*** (0.889)
Black population (%)	0.393*** (0.085)	0.48*** (0.141)	0.497*** (0.143)	0.515*** (0.185)	0.542*** (0.188)
Hispanic population (%)	0.291*** (0.068)	0.262*** (0.06)	0.269*** (0.056)	0.284*** (0.088)	0.308*** (0.086)
Other non-white population (%)	0.152** (0.068)	-0.002 (0.056)	-0.012 (0.05)	0.073 (0.045)	0.062** (0.029)
Constant	-30.834** (13.604)	-28.348* (14.638)	-19.6 (15.849)	-18.471 (17.298)	-4.958 (19.496)
Observations	51	51	51	51	51
R-squared	0.775	0.689	0.697	0.638	0.642
F-statistic	12.24***	11.80***	12.40***	11.49***	13.71***

Note: *** $p<0.01$, ** $p<0.05$, * $p<0.101$.

each additional protection increases the rate by 0.69, significant at the 0.05 level (Model 3). Number of restrictions just misses significance ($p = 0.101$), with each additional restriction resulting in a reduction of 0.29 in the abortion rate. In both models, the impact of the other independent variables is similar to Model 1.

Finally, Models 4 and 5 drop both median income and education because median income is also correlated with restrictions (-0.61) and protections (0.57). Here, both restrictions and protections are highly significant, both at the 0.001 level. Unfortunately, the strong correlations among restrictions, protections, income, and education prevent an independent assessment of their impacts, but clearly these factors, along with religious adherence and racial makeup, are important in predicting abortion rates in US states.

Conclusion

The 18 nations[20] of Western Europe have the lowest regional abortion rate in the world. Within these countries, however, national abortion rates vary widely. Western European countries also differ greatly in religiosity, contraceptive prevalence, and income levels. Our analysis shows that contraceptive prevalence reduces abortion rates.

As in US states, all Western European nations regulate the practice of abortion. Many of these restrictions are similar: waiting periods, mandatory counseling, conscientious objection by health workers, parental involvement, and gestational limits. One important difference between gestational limits in US states and Western Europe is that most Western European countries waive gestational limits in cases of fetal malformations. Often these unfortunate situations are not discovered until late in pregnancy (Hern 2021). How these circumstances are handled is regarded as a medical matter outside the scope of abortion regulation.

Both US states and some Western European countries have institutional requirements, but these regulations differ greatly. Most institutional requirements in Western Europe require women to obtain abortion services at a higher-level facility than is necessary for good care, so these requirements can cause bottlenecks and extended waiting times. US TRAP laws, on the other hand, try to put private abortion providers out of business by mandating unnecessary and costly requirements for clinics.

Many US states and eight Western European countries require a waiting period between the time that a woman requests abortion services and when she receives them. In our analysis, waiting periods were the only Western European restriction that had a statistically significant impact on national abortion rates. In the United States, nearly 97 percent of states with mandatory waiting periods also require specific abortion counseling, often with medically inaccurate information (Daniels et al. 2016). No country in Western Europe requires health care providers to transmit incorrect facts to abortion patients.

Western European countries also have abortion protections, but there are marked differences from those in US states. All Western European countries provide partial or full funding for abortion. In contrast, only 17 American states fund abortion for low-income women. Research has shown that the lack of funding for abortion services can deter access to abortion (Meier et al. 1996) or at least increase waiting periods.

During the COVID-19 pandemic, two Western European nations extended gestational limits for pregnancy terminations—an abortion protection not found in any US state during that period. Eight countries in this region also extended telemedicine services. As explained in this book's introduction, using telemedicine to proscribe medication abortion would have defied US FDA regulations at the time.

What are the impacts of these different policies? In terms of abortion rates, the 2020 US abortion rate of 14.4 (Guttmacher Institute 2022d) is higher than that in all but five Western European countries (Austria, France, Greece, Sweden, and the United Kingdom), none of which have waiting period restrictions. Overall, Sweden and the United Kingdom are among the least restrictive Western European countries. A comparison of US and British data suggests that abortions take place earlier in the United Kingdom than in the United States. In 2020, 88 percent of all abortions in the United Kingdom occurred at under 10 weeks gestation. For 2020, the corresponding US percentage was 80.0. The increased use of medical abortion is a major reason for this difference (Kortsmit et al. 2022).

Table 6.7 shows that the majority of abortions in most Western European countries are medication abortions. In 2020, the two countries with the highest abortion rates in Western Europe also had among the highest rates of medication abortions: 85 percent of abortions in the United King-

TABLE 6.7
Medical Abortions in Western Europe and the United States, 2020

Country	Number of abortions	Number of medical abortions	Percentage of abortions that are medical abortions	Notes
Austria	30,000	N/A	N/A	Most physicians would like to order but cannot. Only available in hospitals and Ob/Gyn clinics
Denmark	14,188	11,209	79	
Finland	8,707	8,533	98	
France	221,000	159,120	72	
Germany	99,948	28,943	29	
Greece	N/A	N/A	N/A	
Iceland	1,049	829	79	
Ireland	N/A	N/A	N/A	
Italy	66,413	23,005	35	
Luxembourg	500	500	100	
Netherlands	32,233	9,992	31	
Norway	11,726	10,905	93	
Portugal	14,928	10,094	68	
Spain	93,131	33,886	36	
Sweden	36,151	33,982	94	
Switzerland	11,143	8,803	79	
United Kingdom	210,860	179,231	85	73% in 2019
United States	930,160	474,382–492,985	51–53	

Sources: Abort Report EU (2022) for the number of abortions, Abort Report EU (2022) and Department of Health and Care (2020) for number of medical abortions, and CDC (Kortsmit et al. 2022) and Guttmacher (Jones et al. 2022a) for US data.

dom and 94 percent of abortions in Sweden were medication abortions (only Finland (98 percent) and Luxemburg (100 percent) had medication abortion rates higher than Sweden's). In the United States, the corresponding figure was 51 to 53 percent. Because medication abortion is used for early abortions, these numbers suggest that in many Western European countries, pregnancy terminations take place at earlier gestational ages than in the United States.

CHAPTER 7

The *Dobbs* Decision and Beyond

On June 29, 2022, the US Supreme Court ruled on *Dobbs v. Mississippi Women's Health Organization*. Tossing aside the principle of *stare decisis*, the Court overturned almost a half century of settled law established by *Roe v. Wade* in 1973 and reaffirmed by *Planned Parenthood of Southeastern Pennsylvania v. Casey* in 1992. Writing for the majority, Justice Alito stated that "the right to abortion was not deeply rooted in the country's history and traditions" (Gerstein and Ward 2022). In addition to the Court's skewed historical interpretation, the ruling was scathing in its interpretation of past legal reasoning:

> *Roe* was egregiously wrong from the start. Its reasoning was exceptionally weak, and the decision has had damaging consequences. And far from bringing a national settlement of the abortion issue, *Roe* and *Casey* have inflamed debate and deepened division. The majority concluded that both decisions must be overruled.[1]

Legal scholar Mary Ziegler noted that it is "close to unprecedented or unprecedented" for the Supreme Court of the United States to "undo [...] rights that were viewed as constitutionally central for half a century" (Reed 2022). She observed the unrelenting tone of the draft that showed little respect for opposing viewpoints (Reed 2022). This stance may not be characteristic of legal stewardship or even legal scholarship, but it is consistent with morality politics.[2] In this arena, there are absolute wrongs and absolute rights, a posture not subject to compromises or negotiation (Haider-Markel 2020; Mooney 2001).

Even before the May 2 *Politico* leak (Gerstein and Ward 2022; Shear and Liptak 2022), the composition of the Supreme Court made the final *Dobbs* vote count predictable. After all, three of the justices were nominated by President Trump in his single term so they could overrule *Roe* (Ziegler 2020; Mangan 2016; Vaida 2016). Justice Alito had been nominated by President George W. Bush in 2006 in part because of his anti-abortion views.[3] Chief Justice Roberts, appointed by Bush in 2005, also came to the high court with an anti-abortion record (*On the Issues* 2022; McFarlane 2006).

Six justices (Alito, Barrett, Gorsuch, Kavanaugh, Roberts, and Thomas) signed on to the majority opinion. Three justices vigorously dissented (Breyer, Kagan, and Sotomayor). Because she was replacing Justice Breyer, retiring at the end of the Court's summer term, newly confirmed Justice Brown Jackson was not involved in these deliberations.

The *Dobbs* ruling showed that the long-term judicial strategy of the anti-abortion forces had paid off (NARAL Pro-Choice America 2022; Ziegler 2020). By the end of 2020, a solid majority of US Supreme Court justices were firmly in the anti-abortion camp. In May 2021, the Court announced that it would hear Mississippi's petition, which had already been ruled unconstitutional by two lower federal courts.

Thirteen months later, the highest court in the land had vacated both *Roe* and *Casey.* States now had more latitude to tighten controls on women living within their borders. After *Dobbs,* states had an even freer rein to regulate and even prohibit abortion within their borders. They were also freer to regulate abortion providers or prohibit abortion altogether (NARAL Pro-Choice America 2022).

The short-term policy impacts are clear. Not only are pre-viability bans constitutional, but abortion is now illegal or nearly illegal in about half of the American states (Kitchener et al. 2023). Just three months after the *Dobbs* ruling, at least 66 clinics in 15 states had stopped offering abortion services (Kirstein et al. 2022). The number of legal abortions dropped by 6 percent in the first two months following the Dobbs decision (Sanger-Katz and Miller 2022).

For much of the country, the policy change was immediate, or close to immediate.[4] By June 2022, 12 states had already enacted trigger ban laws (Idaho, Kentucky Louisiana, Mississippi, Missouri, North Dakota, Oklahoma, South Dakota, Tennessee, Texas, Utah, and Wyoming) automatically imposing total criminal bans on abortion that would go into effect were *Roe* to be overturned (NARAL Pro-Choice America 2022; Nash and Cross 2022). Nine states already had criminal bans on the books, unchanged from pre-*Roe* days, which again became enforceable (Alabama, Arizona, Arkansas, Michigan, Mississippi, Oklahoma, Texas, West Virginia, and Wisconsin) (Nash and Cross 2022). Four more states had passed similar criminal abortion bans: Alabama (2019), Arkansas (2021), Louisiana (2019), and Oklahoma (2021). Four states (Alabama, Louisiana, Tennessee, and West Virginia) had amended their state constitutions to clarify that they did not include the right to abortion (NARAL Pro-Choice America 2022), and three more states (Iowa, Kansas, and Kentucky) were in the process of amending their constitutions to reflect their anti-abortion stance (NARAL Pro-Choice America 2022). As depicted in figure 7.1, these anti-abortion actions largely reflected the preferences of Republican elected officials in the states.

Pending the *Dobbs* Decision

Anticipating the *Dobbs* decision, some states were already pushing the limits of abortion restrictions. As discussed in Chapters 1 and 3, this pattern of adopting more abortion restrictions before consequential Supreme Court decisions is not new (Patton 2007). This time, however, the types of restrictions being implemented were unprecedented.

On September 1, 2021, Texas passed SB 8, effectively banning most abortions. The gestational limit was only six weeks—a time when many women do not even realize they are pregnant. The means of enforcement for SB 8 were radical: deputizing ordinary citizens to sue abortion providers and others, and even offering a financial bounty to citizens who sue those providers. Abortion providers sued, but the US Supreme Court declined to intervene, so this law went into effect (Feuer 2021).

While the *Dobbs* decision was pending, other states followed Texas's

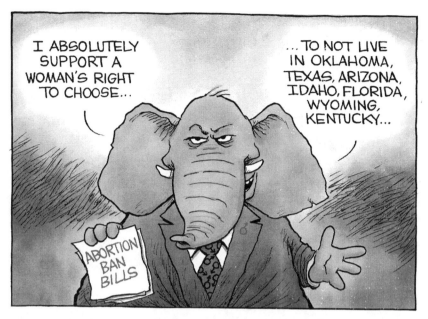

FIGURE 7.1. GOP's Right to Choose. © 2022 Christopher Weyant, published in the *Boston Globe*. Reprinted with permission of Cagle Cartoons, Inc.

lead and enacted more stringent abortion restrictions. Despite acknowledging that the law passed by the Idaho legislature was probably unconstitutional, Governor Brad Little signed a bill in March 2022 making abortion illegal after six weeks gestation (Levin 2022). Idaho put its own spin on enforcement. Rather than empowering any private citizen to sue to enforce the law as Texas did, the Idaho law specified that family members of the fetus, including family members of a rapist—but not a rapist himself—could sue abortion providers. Relatives could exercise this privilege for up to four years after the procedure, for a minimum of $20,000 in damages (Levin 2022).

Other states introduced, and sometimes passed, new types of restrictions. In March 2022, South Dakota enacted new abortion regulations. One new provision, immediately enjoined, required three trips for a medication abortion: "one trip for receiving the first dose of the medication, a second trip 24 to 72 hours after the first trip for the second dose, and a third trip two weeks later to confirm the abortion was successful" (Slavin 2022; Todd 2022).

In April 2022, the Wyoming legislature passed a law that would ban abortion altogether if *Roe v. Wade* were vacated (Better Wyoming 2022). A Missouri lawmaker introduced a bill to ban pregnant women from leaving the state to obtain abortion services (Ollstein and Messerly 2022). Another Missouri legislator submitted a bill to make it a crime to terminate ectopic pregnancies, which are never viable and can be fatal for women without medical intervention (de Graf et al. 2022; Kaufman 2022).[5]

Not to be outdone, the Oklahoma legislature passed, and the governor signed, the strictest ban in the country following the May 2 *Politico* leak. This law allowed citizens to sue "anyone, anywhere who 'aids or abets' a patient in terminating a pregnancy." In addition, the bill banned "abortion from conception, even before an egg implants in the uterus," apparently taking aim at some forms of contraception. This law went into effect as soon as Oklahoma's governor signed it, ending the practice of legal abortion in the Sooner State even before the *Dobbs* ruling (Glenza 2022; Murphy 2022).

Three months before the *Dobbs* decision, the split partisanship of Kentucky's state government was on full display. On March 30, 2022, the Republican-led Kentucky legislature passed a bill not only emulating Mississippi's 15-week ban, but also restricting access to medication abortion and making it more difficult for minors to obtain abortion services (Stracqualursi 2022b). Democratic governor Andy Beshear vetoed the bill, saying it was unconstitutional, but two weeks later, the Kentucky legislature overrode his veto (Stracqualursi and Musa 2022). Within a week, a federal judge temporarily blocked enforcement of the law, and the two remaining abortion clinics in the state resumed services (McCammon 2023a; Stracqualursi 2022a). Due to the *Dobbs* decision and Kentucky's trigger ban, these clinics were forced to stop providing services by early August (ACLU Kentucky 2023).

Even before the *Dobbs* decision, the situation on the ground had rapidly deteriorated for women who lived in restrictive states to seek abortion services. Following SB 8's passage in Texas, abortion clinics in surrounding states reported huge influxes of patients from the Lone Star State (Associated Press 2022b; White et al. 2022). For months, Oklahoma had been a haven for Texas women seeking abortion—that is, until the Oklahoma legislature passed a similar ban. Thereafter, women from both states scrambled to get appointments in Arkansas, New Mexico, Colorado, Kansas, and elsewhere (Luthra 2022a; Miller 2022). By the late summer of 2022, 75 percent of abortion patients at the University of New Mexico Center for Reproductive Health were from Texas, but women were also traveling from Oklahoma and elsewhere. The greatly increased demand had pushed scheduled appointments out by weeks; this wait meant that some women would become ineligible for medication abortion (McCullough 2022).

Following the *Dobbs* Decision

Throughout the United States, the *Dobbs* ruling means that more women than ever are traveling across state lines to access abortion services. Situated near many states with abortion bans and restrictions, North Carolina had the largest increase (37 percent)[6] in abortions following *Dobbs* (Kelly 2023; Society of Family Planning 2023) and before the state legislature overrode the governor's veto of the 12 week ban in 2023 (Kitchener et al. 2023). According to economist Caitlin Myers, there have been dramatic changes in the availability of services, especially in Texas, Louisiana, Mississippi, Arkansas, Oklahoma, and Idaho (Simmons-Duffin 2023; Myers et al. 2019).

Women seeking these health services are not just going to other states. Clinics in both Canada and Mexico are also providing procedural and medication abortion services for US women. But these services are not free. US women accessing abortion services in Canada must pay $400 or more for a surgical procedure, and they may have to wait a week or considerably longer to secure an appointment. Indeed, the abrupt change in US abortion policy has focused attention on uneven access and waiting times in Canada (Beaumont 2022; Sahagian 2019).

Planning for an influx of US patients, "both private and public clinics in Mexican border cities have been expanding services" (Beaumont 2022). The Mexican Supreme Court ruled in 2021 that it was unconstitutional for states to criminalize abortion. But access to surgical abortion in Mexico varies by state. These procedures are available in Sinaloa, Coahuila, and Baja California, but only up to 12 weeks of pregnancy. US women are also traveling to Mexico to obtain medication abortion (Beaumont 2022).

Travel, however, takes money—in short supply for many women who experience unintended pregnancy. Medication abortion does not necessarily require travel, and throughout the United States, women are ordering abortion pills online. For example, a recent study shows the demand for online abortifacients increased dramatically following the passage of Texas SB 8 (Aiken et al. 2022b).

Not surprisingly, this demand has expanded since both the *Dobbs* leak and the *Dobbs* ruling. It is considerably cheaper for women to pay $105–$150 to Aid Access, the only telemedicine service that openly provides pills in states with abortion bans, than to travel. Indeed, the largest increases in requests for telemedicine medication abortion have come from women living in states with total abortion bans (Aiken et al. 2022c; Bazelon 2022a; Bazelon 2022b; Bhatia et al. 2022).

In January 2023, the FDA finalized regulations to allow pharmacies to dispense abortion pills if they have been prescribed by a medical provider. Those regulations have been challenged by a lawsuit brought by anti-abortion activists (Durkee 2023). Not only is the distribution of abortion pills being litigated, but in Texas and other states, some legislators are trying to figure out how to stop women from accessing medication abortion (Schreiber 2022). Chasing abortion pills across state lines is reminiscent of late nineteenth and early twentieth century enforcement of the Comstock law, forbidding the transport of all objects of fertility control across state lines (Mohr 1978, 196–199). For now, most of the punitive legislation is focused on abortion providers, but that singular focus is likely to widen (Cohen et al. 2022).

Exacerbating Racial and Class Divides

In the United States, the incidence of abortion is concentrated among low-income women. And, as explained in Chapter 1, women who experience unintended pregnancy are disproportionately women of color. It is likely that both the selective enforcement and vigorous prosecution of current and future punitive state laws will exacerbate racial and class divides (Hing et al. 2022; Williamson 2022; Solazzo 2018).

The case of Lizelle Herrera is just the start (Martinez 2022). In April 2022, this 26-year-old mother was arrested and held with $500,000 bail in Starr County, Texas. Her crime? Telling a staff member in a south Texas hospital that she had self-managed an abortion. In doing so, Ms. Herrera had not broken any Texas law (Goldberg 2022). However, the county sheriff referred this case to the District Attorney after a health care worker apparently violated the code of patient confidentiality to report her (Kitchener, 2022).

After protests and publicity generated by local reproductive justice advocates, namely, the Frontera Fund (2022), the charges against Lizelle Herrera were dropped (Klibanoff 2022). Her case, however, serves as a warning, reminding other young women that they may not be able to trust the health care system to protect them from the political fallout of abortion politics, including criminal charges (Baker 2022). "Even mistakes quickly resolved or retracted can have a chilling effect," noted legal scholar Mary Ziegler (2022).

For those who have watched state abortion policy unfold since *Roe,* Lizelle Herrera's arrest had an eerie similarity to the Rosie Jimenez tragedy (Martinez 2022; Cohen and Joffe 2020, 84–85). Ms. Jimenez was also a young, single Latina mother in Texas's Rio Grande Valley. She had dreams for herself and her daughter; she was working and going to college. But Rosie Jimenez died in 1977 of a botched abortion performed in McAllen, Texas, shortly after the Hyde Amendment went into effect (Chavez 2021; Garcia-Ditta 2015).

At the time of her death, Ms. Jimenez had an up-to-date Medicaid card in her wallet. The Texas Medicaid program would have paid for her abortion only a month earlier, but a doctor told her that she would have to pay in full for the procedure because Medicaid no longer covered abortions. Lacking resources, trying to go to school, and caring for her four-year-old daughter, Rosie opted for a cheaper alternative offered by an unlicensed midwife. Within a week, she was dead from an infection caused by an abortion performed in unsanitary conditions. Rosie Jimenez was the first CDC documented case of a death caused by the Hyde Amendment (Garcia-Ditta 2022; National Network of Abortion Funds 2011).

A half-century later, the demographics are similar. Low-income women bear and will continue to endure the brunt of the *Dobbs* decision. Fully half of abortion patients in the United States live below the federal poverty level,[7] and "another quarter live between 100 percent and 199 percent of the poverty level" (Cohen and Joffe 2020, 86).[8] They are disproportionately women of color, and many are struggling just to get by. Most often, they do not have $500 in savings even for an early medication abortion (Cohen and Joffe 2020). This fact alone pushes them into later-gestation procedures as resource-strapped women with unintended pregnancies try to amass the necessary funds. Tragically, as suggested by the analysis in Chapter 4, the need for many abortions could be averted with better access to contraception. But as Chapter 4 also indicates, the same political and religious forces that restrict abortion services also work to limit access to birth control.

Protecting Reproductive Rights

In some states, recent developments in abortion regulation and reproductive rights have been starkly different from those in Texas, Oklahoma, and Idaho. Even before the *Dobbs* ruling, many states had protected the right to choose. Fifteen states (California, Connecticut, Delaware, Hawaii, Illinois, Maine, Maryland, Massachusetts, Nevada, New Jersey, New York, Oregon, Rhode Island, Vermont, and Washington), as well as the District of Columbia, had codified the right to abortion in state law before June 2022. Twelve states (California, Connecticut, Delaware, Hawaii, Illinois, Maine, Maryland, Massachusetts, Nevada, New York, Rhode Island, and Washington) had passed laws explicitly permitting abortion prior to viability or when necessary to protect the life or health of the pregnant person. Nine states (Alaska, California, Florida, Iowa, Kansas, Massachusetts, Minnesota, Montana, and New Jersey) had established that their constitutions protected the right to abortion. But even in those states, anti-abortion politicians have been determined to roll back access to abortion (NARAL Pro-Choice America 2022).

Further regulations to protect state abortion rights also include a handful of states aiming to address the high cost of abortion. In recent years, California, Illinois, New York, and Oregon enacted laws banning private insurance fees for abortion.[9] Each of these states already required private health insurance plans to cover abortion services. Even so, these plans were charging co-pays and deductibles to women seeking abortion services. In California, for example, this practice added an average of $553 to the patient's cost of a medication abortion and an $887 charge for a procedural abortion (Beam 2022b; Kyrylenko 2022). Other states are likely to eliminate or at least reduce of out-of-pocket costs for women with private insurance coverage.

In April 2022, Connecticut passed what lawmakers said could be a model for other states seeking to safeguard abortion rights. Anticipating that women seeking abortion might travel there from more restrictive states, this law shields abortion providers and patients from lawsuits initiated by states that have banned or plan to ban abortion, even outside their own borders (CBS New York Team 2022; Keating 2022; Nir and Zernike 2022).

In April 2022, Michigan governor Gretchen Whitmer filed a lawsuit requesting that the state supreme court overturn the state's 1931 abortion law, which would automatically go into effect if *Roe v. Wade* were vacated. Michigan's pre-*Roe* abortion ban was among the country's harshest. Under that statute, abortion was felony manslaughter, and there were no exceptions for rape or incest (El Sayd 2022).

Governor Whitmer's lawsuit also asked the court to recognize a constitutional right to an abortion under the Due Process clause of the Michigan Constitution, "which provides a right to privacy and bodily autonomy" (Executive Office of the Governor, Communications Division 2022). Her lawsuit pointed out that Michigan's 1931 abortion law "violates Michigan's Equal Protection Clause due to the way the ban denies women equal rights because the law was adopted to reinforce antiquated notions of the proper role for women in society" (Executive Office of the Governor, Communications Division 2022). It is noteworthy that a January 2022 poll found that nearly 80 percent of Michiganders supported a woman's right to choose (Eggert 2022; El Sayd 2022).

Initially, the Michigan Supreme Court agreed to take up procedural questions in this case against Michigan's dormant abortion law (Boucher 2022), but ultimately, the court allowed a ballot initiative to go forward. In November 2022, nearly 57 percent of those voting in the Michigan election supported the creation of a state constitutional right to reproductive freedom, including decisions "about all matters relating to pregnancy," such as abortion and contraception.

In January 2023, the court dismissed the governor's lawsuit because voters had already decided the question (Pluta 2023).

Four other states had abortion on the November 2022 ballot. More than 52 percent of Kentucky voters rejected an amendment that would have stated there was no right to abortion, or any requirement to fund abortion, in the state constitution. Nearly 77 percent of those voting in Vermont supported "a constitutional right to personal reproductive autonomy." Almost 67 percent of California voters supported amending the state constitution to protect a person's reproductive freedom "in their most intimate decisions," including the right to abortion and contraceptives. Nearly 53 percent of Montana voters rejected enacting a law "making any infant 'born alive' at any gestational age a legal person, a protection that already exists under a federal law passed 20 years ago" (*New York Times* 2022a).[10] In August 2022, Kansas voters rejected (59 to 41 percent) an anti-abortion amendment designed to eliminate the state's constitutional protections for abortion rights (Doan 2022; Sanchez and Boston 2022).

It is too early to know many of the consequences of the *Dobbs* decision. We do know that some states and their politicians will go as far with abortion regulation as the Supreme Court will let them. The *Dobbs* decision showed that the Court itself is not immune from an absolute win, characteristic of morality politics. This stance is not the stable political compromise on abortion that many Western European countries have struck (Outshoorn 1996). Instead of recognizing that abortion is an issue that could threaten the political order, US politicians—especially in the GOP (Emba 2022)—have exploited the issue to garner votes.

Conclusion

The *Dobbs* decision upended abortion regulations in the United States. Going beyond the question posed by Mississippi's 15-week abortion ban, the majority of the Court, three of them appointed by President Trump, signed on to vacate both *Roe* and *Casey*. Given the composition of the Court, the outcome was not unexpected.

Anticipating a change, both red and blue states prepared for this outcome. Many Republican states passed trigger bans that would end legal abortion services in their states if *Roe* were overturned. Many blue states, on the other hand, passed legislation protecting abortion rights for both patients and providers. After the leak and actual *Dobbs* ruling, states have scrambled to pass new pro-choice and anti-abortion legislation, a phenomenon that is likely to continue for some time.

This book has examined how abortion is regulated in America, as well as the forces that have led to state abortion restrictions and protections. Within the constraints of available data, we have analyzed the consequences of those policies. Among common medical services, abortion is one of the most regulated health services in the United States and undoubtedly, the most politicized.

Chapter 1 began with a description of the landscape of abortion services in the United States including patient characteristics, types of providers, and techniques of abortion. The number of providers is declining in the United States, but there are great regional differences. The mix of abortion providers has also changed, mainly due to new technology. More than half of abortions in the country are now medication abortions (Jones et al. 2022b), a technology that lends itself to being woman-controlled.

Chapter 1 also discussed the theoretical constructs we used to guide our analysis of abortion regulation. Most regulatory decisions about abortion, especially at the state level, emanate from hearing room politics where politicians and citizens' groups vie for media spotlight. Messages are simple and succinct, seldom reflecting the complexity of the issue at hand. Given the abortion issue and morality politics, religious fervor adds to the intensity and absoluteness of hearing room debates. Opposing groups, particularly religious ones, frame the issue in stark, uncompromising terms. In this setting, politicians often confuse these public pronouncements with private behavior, so they end up promoting public policies that are more extreme than the actual preferences of their constituents (McFarlane and Meier 2001).

Because only women experience pregnancy, many consider abortion a women's issue (Sommer and Forman-Rabinovici 2021; Htun and Weldon 2018). Consequently, advocates for women's issues as well as female legislative representatives are important influences on abortion policy. Neither women's advocates nor women legislators are necessarily like-minded, but our analysis in Chapter 4 showed that the presence of women in state legislative chambers increases the odds of passing abortion protections. Examples from the Republic of Ireland and Texas's Rio Grande Valley attest to the potency of women's groups in shaping abortion policy.

Contrary to Justice Alito's assertion in the *Dobbs* decision, the practice of abortion has a long history in the United States. Because "past patterns illuminate present policies" (Morone 1998, xii), Chapter 2 began with a brief history of US abortion policy. Chapter 2 also covered more than 40 US Supreme Court cases related to abortion that have been decided since *Roe v. Wade*, showing the sensitivity of those decisions to the composition of the Court.

Even with these judicial bounds, states maintain considerable discretion in regulating abortion, demonstrated by the variation in state restrictions and protections. State policies affect both the supply of and the demand for abortion services: they can discourage health care providers from offering abortion services and they can support, delay, or prevent women from terminating unwanted pregnancies. The weightiness of these policy impacts underscores the need to understand the dynamics of state abortion policymaking.

Chapter 3 described the many forms of abortion regulation, including denying funding, requiring in-person visits for dispensing pills, specifying the physical layout and staffing of abortion clinics, and even subsidizing services trying to dissuade women from pregnancy termination. In many states, abortion providers face double regulatory burdens as providers of medical care and as providers of abortion services. Some states, however, have laws that protect women who seek abortion services and safeguard those who provide them.

The breadth and scale of abortion regulation is staggering. Government controls on abortion continue to expand because states keep coming up with new ideas. Fueling this regulatory frenzy, national organizations such as Americans United for Life distribute model bills to the states each year. Our analysis of state abortion policymaking in Chapter 4 showed the importance of partisanship, religion, and money. Abortion politics marry the unstable, combative, and divisive politics of regulation (Smith and Larimer 2017) with the conflictual and uncompromising politics of morality issues (Haider-Market 2020).

Chapter 5 showed the consequences of this regulation. This is a cultural war where young women and low-income women—and their children—are collateral damage (Cohen and Joffe 2020; Foster 2020). The irony is that most abortions could be prevented if contraception were more accessible. Yet, as Chapter 4 showed, the same political forces that fight to curtail the practice of abortion tend to be against easing access to contraception. Many women with private health insurance do not face that battle, but women at the bottom of the economic ladder do. Birth control pills can cost $50 a month or more, putting them out of reach for women struggling to get by (National Women's Health Network 2017). Many low-income women are unable to access subsidized birth control services. In Texas, for example, the most uninsured state in the country (Kaiser Family Foundation 2023), less than half of the population living below the federal poverty level is covered by Medicaid.

In Chapter 6, we looked outside the US borders for insight and policy alternatives. With the world's lowest regional abortion rate and similar socioeconomic conditions as the United States, the 18 countries of Western Europe offer comparators to the US states. Nearly all Western European countries have liberalized abortion laws, but each of them regulates the practice of abortion. For example, some countries mandate parental involvement for minors seeking abortion; others require a waiting period between the initial request and the procedure, or before dispensing medication. These requirements, of course, have counterparts in individual US states.

But stark differences exist. For the most part, abortion funding is not a policy lever in Western European countries. Except for Germany,[1] each country's national health system covers abortion like any other health service. This is true even in the Republic of Ireland, where abortion was only legalized in 2018. Despite the historical contentiousness of the issue, denying funding for abortion was never on the table in the Irish referendum. There are also other policy divergences. Nowhere in Western Europe are abortion patients required to listen to medically inaccurate state-mandated scripts. Moreover, medically unnecessary regulations do not target clinics that offer abortion services in Western European countries.

Chapter 7 covered the *Dobbs* decision and its aftermath. The ruling overturning *Roe* and *Casey* opened the door for states to adopt new legislation and enforce existing legislation that had previously been blocked by the Court. Many states, anticipating the overturn of *Roe*, passed trigger bans that went into effect once the ruling was announced. And in the aftermath, states continue to push forward with anti-abortion and pro-choice legislation.

Revisiting Myths about Abortion Regulation

We close with the three myths that obfuscate policymaking in abortion regulation. As explained in Chapter 1, these myths are inaccurate or partially accurate at best. These fictions are powerful because lawmakers, advocates, the media, and the public often deliberate as if they were true. As a result, the realities of real people's lives, especially concerning unintended pregnancy, are neglected or ignored.

The first myth is that **abortion policy mirrors public opinion**. The US Supreme Court vacated both *Roe* and *Casey* in 2022, yet most Americans—then and now—favor legal abortion. According to the American National Election Studies (ANES) survey conducted in November 2022 following the election, as shown in table C.1, 47 percent of respondents opposed the Supreme Court's decision to overturn *Roe v. Wade*, whereas only 34 percent favored that decision. Nearly a fifth (19 percent) of the 1,500 respondents neither favored nor opposed overturning *Roe*. Because public opinion varies by state, table C.1 also shows the percentages in favor and opposed in the 10 most populous states. Although the sample sizes in each state are relatively small, with the exception of Florida, the most

TABLE C.1

Public Opinion on the Overturning of Roe v. Wade, *2022*

State	N	Favor overturning *Roe* (%)	Oppose overturning *Roe* (%)	Neither favor nor oppose (%)
Total US	1,500	34	47	19
California	153	24	50	25
Florida	109	37	37	26
Georgia	63	32	48	20
Illinois	47	34	58	8
Michigan	47	30	56	13
New York	100	28	55	17
North Carolina	39	23	61	16
Ohio	56	33	49	17
Pennsylvania	67	32	51	16
Texas	145	32	51	16

Source: American National Election Studies (2022) Pilot Study, https://electionstudies.org/data-center/2022-pilot-study/.

Note: Weighted percentages.

frequent response across these states is opposition to the decision to overturn *Roe*.

Within very broad contours, some of these state public opinion responses reflect general policy positions. For example, California, a state with few restrictions and with new policies protecting the right to choose (*New York Times* 2023), has the second-to-lowest approval for the *Dobbs* decision among these states. However, the percentage of California respondents opposing overturning *Roe* is similar to the percentage of respondents in Pennsylvania and Texas, two states with among the highest number of abortion restrictions in the country. Respondents in North Carolina reported the highest disapproval of the *Dobbs* decision, even though the number of abortion restrictions in North Carolina was above the median in 2020. Polls frequently show a divergence of public opinion from national and state policies on abortion.

Not only does public opinion vary by state (Diamont and Sandstrom 2020), but it also varies by how questions are framed. Most Americans support the right to choose abortion, yet public opinion is more mixed when survey questions are nuanced in terms of the conditions under which abortion should be permitted. For example, the 2016 Cooperative Congressional Election Study (CCES) data revealed that nationally, 58 percent of respondents supported always allowing a woman to obtain an abortion as a matter of choice. Additionally, 84 percent opposed making abortions illegal in all circumstances, but a majority (63 percent) also supported prohibiting all abortions after 20 weeks of pregnancy (Cooperative Congressional Election Study 2016). Overall, the reasons for seeking abortion as well as gestational age are important factors that influence public opinion on abortion.

Religion also plays a role in public opinion on abortion. In the 2016 American National Election Studies survey, respondents were asked where they stood on the abortion issue on a scale from one to four, where one on the scale is that by law, abortion should never be permitted, two on the scale is that it should be permitted only in the case of rape, incest, or the life of the woman is in danger, a score of three refers to allowing other reasons if need is established, and four on the scale is that by law, abortion should be a matter of personal choice. A majority of respondents (59 percent) supported abortion as a matter of personal choice or if need is established (American National Election Studies 2016).

But responses varied by religious beliefs. Among respondents who said that religion is an important part of their lives, over half would severely limit or prohibit abortion: 19 percent said abortion should never be allowed and 33 percent said it should only be allowed in the case of rape, incest, or when a woman's life is in danger. In contrast, among those who said religion is not important, 80 percent supported abortion as a matter of personal choice or if need is established. But even among those who said religion is an important part of their lives, one-third (33 percent) chose category four, that by law abortion should be a matter of personal choice.

Public opinion surveys also show that abortion can be a more salient issue for some groups than others. When asked about abortion in the CCES 2016 survey, Republicans and Democrats responded nearly identically, with 60 percent of Democrats and 58 percent of Republicans saying that abortion was "very high" or "somewhat high" in importance (Cooperative Congressional Election Study 2016). Other surveys have shown that until very recently, abortion was a more potent issue for Republicans than for Democrats. With *Roe v. Wade* vacated, polls showed abortion had become more of a priority for Democratic and Independent voters for autumn 2022 and beyond. Nevertheless, the polls show that most Americans are not well-informed about the abortion regulations in their own states (Lauter 2023; Skelley et al. 2022; Tesler 2022; Yi and Thomson-DeVeaux 2022).

Public opinion and public preferences, of course, do not automatically turn into public policy. At most, public opinion about abortion reflects the broad contours of polling at a particular point in time. Issues are aired in public forums and deliberative bodies. For a highly salient issue, such as abortion, that is framed as being of low technical complexity, those deliberations take place in hearing room politics. Chapter 1 explained that among the pathologies of the hearing room is the fact that "responsiveness to less privileged citizens is quite rare," and that "politicians are responsive to citizens in direct proportion to their socioeconomic status" (Gormley 1986, 617).

Even before *Dobbs*, US abortion policy, indeed reproductive health policy more broadly, had been in this space for many years. Both birth control and abortion services were far more accessible to women of means than low-income women. The 1978 Hyde Amendment targeted poor women without affecting the access of women who had health insurance coverage (Morone 2003, 490). Our results show that states with more abortion restrictions have lower abortion rates. Given that low-income women and women of color are more likely to obtain abortions (Jones and Jerman 2017c), we can surmise that restrictions are likely to have a disproportional impact on low-income women and women of color.

Finally, there is a normative concern: is it appropriate for public opinion to decide how abortion is regulated? Certainly, this is not the case for other health services. However, morality politics[2] are likely to weigh into any discussion of abortion. In morality politics, small but very organized and vocal interest groups dominate debate and policymaking, rather than public opinion more broadly. As a result, those most impacted by the policies are unlikely to have much say.

The second myth is that **abortion regulation is only symbolic**. The essence of this myth is that abortion restrictions really do not matter. They may be on the books, but they can be overcome. Despite the obstacles, women seeking abortion services can obtain them. Even with the *Dobbs* decision, enough states allow abortion so that it is available. Believing this myth may make it easier for lawmakers to vote in favor of new abortion restrictions, even when they believe that abortion is appropriate under certain conditions.

Some conservative commentators have trivialized the impact of the *Dobbs* decision. Following the *Politico* leak, during the May 4, 2022, edition of Fox News' *Outnumbered*, co-host Kayleigh McEnany said that it is fine to allow states to regulate abortion if that is what the majority want: "Give the decision to the people." Jackie DeAngelis, a financial correspondent for Fox Business Network, added that the Supreme Court decision to overturn *Roe* will "not undo abortion in this country. States may put some more restrictions on it, but people have the right to leave. They can go live somewhere else where it's more of a free-for-all, and they can do whatever they want" (Baragona 2022). This sentiment assumes, of course, an ability to "vote with your feet," which is out of reach for most people (Hargis and Taaffe 2022; Smith and Larimer 2017; Tiebout 1956).

Other conservatives do understand abortion regulation is more than symbolic. For example, following the *Dobbs* decision, former governor of Arkansas Asa Hutchinson seemed to backtrack from his absolute support of Arkansas's trigger law, which includes no exceptions for rape or incest. He realized that the law was no longer just a symbol but would go into effect and become a tool of governance. The outgoing governor and presidential aspirant said that "the absence of a rape and incest exception would cause a lot of heartbreak if applied to the post-*Roe v. Wade* world" (Brummett 2022).

Regardless of the rhetoric, abortion restrictions do have effects. They can decrease the number of abortion providers, and they can lower state abortion rates. They force mostly low-income women to travel for abortion, and they extend gestational times. They also limit the options for pregnant women with fetal abnormalities (Megas 2017).

Abortion regulations have disparate effects on different groups of women. Our analysis shows that these restrictions may impact African American and Hispanic women disproportionately. Data limitations precluded a quantitative analysis of their effect on Native American women, but reports from the field document increased obstacles following the *Dobbs* decision (Associated Press 2023). Recognizing these barriers, the Department of Defense has changed its policies to assist military women to travel to obtain abortion services and other sensitive services, regardless of where they are stationed (Myers 2023).

The third myth is that **abortion regulation protects women**. This myth is the most long-lived. Over time, the canard has morphed a bit, but its essence is the same: women need protection from their own decisions. They need to see sonograms, hear biased counseling, and take time to rethink their decisions to seek abortion services.

As a result of the myth, the vast evidence showing that women know how to make complex decisions is disregarded. States have tried to mandate spousal consent, require parental involvement, and even fund crisis pregnancy centers—each to assist women with their allegedly poor decision-making skills. This myth was also invoked in the majority opinion in *Gonzales v. Carhart*. Writing for the majority, Justice Kennedy relied on the notion that women require protection from the harms of abortion, including the regret that some women face because of that choice. Acknowledging the lack of "reliable data" to measure the phenomenon, the majority decision, nonetheless, pivoted on abortion regret.[3]

Adhering to the myth that abortion protects women is detrimental to those it purports to safeguard. Ample evidence exists showing that abortion regulation harms women by pushing them into later-gestation abortions, increasing maternal mortality (Vilda et al. 2021) and infant mortality (McKetta and Keyes 2019), and changing their life chances (Myers 2017).

For the most part, abortion regulation in the United States is not related to medical necessity or to professional standards of care. Instead, it is a political exercise related to the preferences of those who wield power. It also reflects the vagaries of political institutions and political parties. Many Americans, especially citizens marginalized by poverty and race, do not vote regularly and cannot afford to contribute to political candidates or causes. Consequently, their voices are muted on abortion, as well as on many other issues.

Epilogue

So, what is the endgame? Unintended pregnancy has been declining, but it will not disappear, especially when many women lack access to effective contraception. For women in their reproductive years, the odds of becoming pregnant are high. Without contraception, fully 85 percent of sexually active women (or couples) can expect to get pregnant in a year (Trussell 2011).

Other aspects of human biology may make some conservatives uncomfortable. Many fetal genetic abnormalities are not discovered until later in pregnancy (Hern 2021), a time when most states no longer permit pregnancy terminations. In Western Europe, these complex and tragic situations are managed by medical specialists, not politicians. What about state abortion restrictions and IVF treatment for couples trying to conceive? US legal scholars are now debating whether these fertilized embryos are subject to state laws declaring that life begins at fertilization (Cohen et al. 2022).

Myths should not guide abortion policymaking. Instead, abortion regulation should rely on scientific evidence, medical knowledge, and compassion for pregnant women who face difficult choices. Policies that improve access to contraception and those that support women's reproductive health decisions meet these criteria.

Modern contraception, when used consistently, is highly effective in preventing pregnancy. Most abortions result from unintended pregnancies. Policies that increase access to modern birth control methods decrease abortion rates (Meier and McFarlane 1994). Even after controlling for many other factors, our analysis of state abortion regulations shows that one type of state law, mandating that contraceptive prescriptions be filled in a timely manner, lowers abortion rates. Similarly, our analysis of Western Europe shows that countries with higher contraceptive prevalence have lower abortion rates.

Women are quite capable of making complex decisions, including whether to carry a pregnancy to term or to have an abortion. Women who elect to terminate their pregnancies do not make these decisions lightly, and they understand the realities of their own lives. Most of them are already mothers (Cohen and Joffe 2020; Foster 2020; Torres and Forrest 1988). Research shows that few women who choose abortion experience abortion regret (Foster 2020; Ehrlich and Doan 2018). In fact, women who choose abortion fare better than women who are denied this choice (Foster 2020).

Regardless of their choices, women's reproductive decisions should be backed in material ways: affordable health care and, if needed, income maintenance. Most Western European countries have much more robust health and social supports than the United States and lower abortion rates. Additionally, most Western European countries treat abortion as a matter of women's health. In this context, women, in consultation with their health providers, can decide what is in their best interests.

The *Dobbs* decision greatly increased the power of states to regulate abortion. After all, the primary aim of the majority opinion written by Justice Alito was to return the authority to regulate abortion to the "people and their elected representatives" and to allow the states to "evaluate those interests differently" (US Supreme Court 2022, 1, 4). Already, the abortion regulation cleavage between the states has widened (Nash and Ephross 2022). In February 2023, 20 Democratic governors formed a network to strengthen abortion access in the wake of *Dobbs* (Barrow and Mulvihill 2023).

Nevertheless, the short-term impacts of the *Dobbs* ruling are clear: more out-of-state travel for abortions, more abortions later in pregnancy because of delays in obtaining those services, more demand for online medication abortion services, more unwanted births, higher maternal mortality (Vilda et al. 2021), and more domestic violence (Tobin-Tyler 2022). At the same time, state policies making contraception and health care services more accessible have not improved (Society of Family Planning 2023). Expanding the availability of health care, including birth control, would likely reduce the demand for abortion, yet some conservative politicians are even trying to block access to certain types of contraception (Luthra 2022b).[4]

Medication abortion, accounting for a majority of US pregnancy terminations, is now a pivotal issue in abortion politics. Nearly two-thirds of Americans oppose laws banning medication abortion, including 55 percent of Republicans (Montanaro 2023). However, in April 2023, two federal district courts issued contradictory decisions regarding the availability of mifepristone. Matthew Kacsmaryk, a conservative federal district judge from Texas, ordered the FDA "to stay its approval of mifepristone, which has been deemed safe and legal for 23 years" (Iones 2023). Thomas Rice, a federal court judge in Washington state, issued a directly contradictory decision the same day (Iones 2023). For now, mifepristone is legally available in states without abortion bans, and several Democratic governors (California, Washington State, and Massachusetts) have purchased large quantities of the drug in case it becomes unavailable (McCammon 2023b). Other pro-choice advocates continue to argue for federal preemption (Zettler and Sarpatwari 2021). Another US Supreme Court case seems likely. Meanwhile, many US women, especially those in states with abortion bans, continue to order medication abortion online (Aiken et al. 2022b).

Post-*Dobbs* abortion politics have even spilled over to Congressional appropriations for the Department of Defense (DOD) as well as military promotions. In February 2023, the DOD issued new policies "aimed at closing some of the gaps that the overturn of *Roe v. Wade* opened up in service members' ability to access reproductive health" (Myers 2023). These new policies include fully paid travel expenses for troops who have to go out of state to obtain an abortion, up to three weeks of leave to accompany a dependent or spouse for an abortion or a fertility treatment, and up to 20 weeks "to notify commanders of a pregnancy" (Myers 2023). In July 2023, in a narrow and partisan vote, the US House of Representatives voted to end these policies as they marked up the DOD appropriations bill (Demirjian 2023). Meanwhile, in the Senate, Alabama senator Tommy Tuberville was holding up hundreds of high-level military promotions because he disagreed with the DOD's abortion policy (Watson 2023).

In the wake of *Dobbs*, how do we change course? Perhaps we should take a cue from Justice Alito and take the abortion issue back to the people. The pro-choice sentiment is there. Our analysis plainly shows that states that elect pro-choice governors and legislatures have fewer abortion restrictions and more abortion protections. Additionally, states that elect substantial numbers of women legislators, especially Democratic women, have fewer restrictions and more abortion protections than states that do not.

Just how party affiliation and abortion will play out among women legislators in the post-*Dobbs* era is unknown. In Spring 2023, a bipartisan group of female state senators filibustered and stalled a near-total abortion ban in South Carolina (Zernike 2023). While filibustering, Republican senator Sandy Senn said the issue was about male control:

> Abortion laws, each and every one of them, have been about control. It's always about control, plain and simple. And in the senate, the males all have control. We, the women, have not asked for . . . nor do we want your protection. We don't need it. There is not a single thing I can do when women such as me are insulted except make sure that you get an earful. And on these divisive issues, it just needs to be on a ballot. And the men in our legislature, they're just not going to let that happen. And our legislature is overwhelmingly male. (NPR 2023)

In 2016, only 14 percent of Americans said that abortion should never be permitted. In South Carolina, this percentage was only 16 (American National Election Studies 2016). If put to a referendum, most states are unlikely to ban abortion at conception and unlikely to ban abortion without exceptions. However, it is difficult to get a referendum on abortion because many states do not allow citizens to put constitutional amendments on the ballot. That "includes most of the states with the strictest abortion bans" (Rakich and Thomson-Deveaux 2022).

Recent public opinion polls suggest that a majority of Americans consider themselves as pro-choice (55 percent). Only 35 percent say that abortion should not be allowed if the pregnancy is unwanted for any reason (American National Election Studies 2022). If there are birth defects, this drops to 20 percent. Where a woman's life is at risk, only 10 percent of respondents said that abortion should not be permitted. If we take the abortion issue back to the people, public opinion has ample room for policy prescriptions based on medical realities and the health and welfare of women. In comparison with Western Europe, on a scale from one (abortion is never justified) to 10 (abortion is always justified), one public opinion poll showed that only Portugal (4.29), Ireland (4.87), and Greece (4.58) have a lower mean than the United States (5.07) (European Values Study 2017–2022; year of survey varies by country). Similar to the United States, the majority public opinion in most Western European countries leans toward some provision for abortion.

Other US polls taken since the *Dobbs* decision also show a recent shift in public opinion toward abortion rights. In June 2023, Gallup reported that "the share of Americans who are dissatisfied with policies on abortion had hit the highest point in the 23 years the firm has asked about it—almost 7 in 10 adults" (Lauter 2023). Among Republicans, support for making abortion illegal in all cases dropped from 21 percent in September 2021 to 14 percent by December 2022, according to the Public Religion Research Institute survey. Just since 2021, this survey showed that the percentage of Americans "who say they would only vote for a candidate who agrees with them that abortion should be legal in all or most cases has risen from 15 percent in 2020 to 26 percent" (Lauter 2023). A year after the *Dobbs* ruling, the majority of US adults, including those living in states with total abortion bans, think that abortion should be legal at least through the initial stages of pregnancy (Mulvihill and Sanders 2023).

Public opinion polls do not always drive public policy. Our research has shown the importance of partisanship as well as the power of both religious forces and political donations. We have documented the potency of organizing women, for example, the Frontera Fund in south Texas and the scores of women's organizations that worked on the Irish repeal campaign.

Pro-choice advocates will have to keep in mind that all elections matter. For example, states and counties can elect prosecutors that will not vigorously enforce trigger bans (Descano 2022). Advocates will also need to work on reframing abortion as an important component of regular health care (Cohen and Joffe 2020), taking the lead from organizations such as the ACOG, AMA, and the SisterSong Women of Color Reproductive Justice Collective (Espey 2023). Only 67 percent of those who cite health care as an extremely or very important issue facing the country today also cite abortion as such (American National Election Studies 2022). If women's health is a priority, the availability of needed health services should not depend on the state where a woman lives. Eventually, fairness may demand action at the federal level rather than leaving policy to state legislatures.

APPENDIX

Sources that Cite US Supreme Court Cases as Important to Abortion Policy, along with Decision and Impact

(cites=1, does not cite=0)

Garrow	Zeigler	ACLU	Westlaw	NARAL	Oyez	Total	Year	Ruling	Case	Major points for state laws
0	0	0	1	1	0	2	1927	8–1	*Buck v. Bell*	Upheld Virginia law allowing sterilization of inmates at certain state mental institutions
1	0	0	0	1	0	2	1942	9–0	*Skinner v. State of Oklahoma*	Struck down Oklahoma law mandating sterilization as punishment for certain crimes
1	1	1	1	1	0	5	1965	7–2	*Griswold v. Connecticut*	Struck down Connecticut law banning use of contraception by married couples
1	1	1	1	0	1	5	1971	8–1	*U.S. v. Vuitch*	Rejected challenge to Washington DC law permitting abortion only for life or health
1	1	1	1	1	1	6	1972	6–1	*Eisenstadt v. Baird*	Invalidated Massachusetts law prohibiting distribution of contraceptives to unmarried people
1	1	1	1	1	1	6	1973	7–2	*Roe v. Wade*	Legalized abortion. Articulated trimester framework
1	1	1	1	0	1	5	1973	7–2	*Doe v. Bolton*	Struck Georgia laws requiring state residence and specifically accredited hospitals for abortion
0	0	1	1	1	0	3	1975	7–2	*Bigelow v. Virginia*	Upheld advertisements for legal abortion
0	0	0	1	0	1	2	1975	9–0	*Connecticut v. Menillo*	Upheld requiring physicians to perform abortions
1	1	0	1	0	1	4	1976	6–3	*Planned Parenthood v. Danforth*	Struck down partner veto, saline abortion ban (>12 weeks), and absolute parental veto. Upheld written informed consent and Missouri reporting requirements

(continued)

TABLE A.1.
Continued

Garrow	Zeigler	ACLU	Westlaw	NARAL	Oyez	Total	Year	Ruling	Case	Major points for state laws
0	0	0	0	0	1	1	1977	N/A	Guste v. Jackson	Vacated injunction against Louisiana informed consent and remanded
1	0	0	1	1	1	4	1977	7–2	Carey v. Population Services	Invalidated New York law prohibiting sale of contraception to minors
1	1	0	1	0	1	4	1977	6–3	Beal v. Doe	Upheld Pennsylvania's refusal to use Medicaid funds for non-therapeutic abortions
1	1	0	1	0	1	4	1977	6–3	Maher v. Roe	Upheld Connecticut's refusal to use Medicaid funds for non-therapeutic abortions
1	1	0	1	0	1	4	1977	6–3	Poelker v. Doe	Upheld St. Louis public hospital funding child-birth services, but not non-therapeutic abortions
0	0	0	0	0	1	1	1979	8–1	Anders v. Floyd	Remanded South Carolina case regarding viability of 25 week fetus
1	1	1	1	1	1	6	1979	8–1	Bellotti v. Baird	Struck down Massachusetts law requiring consent of both parents. Insists on judicial bypass
1	1	0	1	1	1	5	1979	6–3	Colautti v. Franklin	Struck down Pennsylvania law requiring doctor save the life of a fetus that may be viable
1	1	1	1	1	1	6	1980	5–4	Harris v. McRae	Upheld Hyde Amendment prohibiting use of federal funds for abortion (Medicaid) unless the pregnant woman's life is endangered

Description	Case	Vote	Year						
Upheld Illinois in not paying for medically necessary abortions through Medicaid program	*Williams v. Zbaraz*	5–4	1981	5	1	1	1	1	1
Upheld Utah law requiring physician to notify a minor's parent before providing an abortion	*H.L. v. Matheson*	6–3	1981	3	1	0	0	0	0
Struck down Ohio law requiring a 24-hour waiting period and elaborate reporting requirements	*City of Akron v. Akron Center for Reproductive Health*	6–3	1983	6	1	1	1	1	1
Struck down hospital requirement after 12 weeks, but upheld other restrictions	*Planned Parenthood of Kansas City v. Ashcroft*	6–3	1983	4	1	0	0	1	0
Upheld Virginia hospitalization requirement because outpatient clinics included	*Simopoulos v. Virginia*	8–1	1983	5	1	0	1	1	1
Struck down law banning unsolicited contraceptive advertising in the mail	*Bolger v. Youngs Drug Products Corporation*	8–0	1983	2	0	1	1	0	0
Supreme Court let stand a lower court ruling denying appellate standing to sue regarding Illinois abortion law	*Diamonds v. Charles*	N/A	1983	1	0	1	0	1	0
Struck down Pennsylvania restrictions, including informed consent and post-viability requirements	*Thornburgh v. ACOG*	5–4	1986	6	1	1	1	1	1
Struck down Illinois 24-hour waiting period	*Hartigan v. Zbaraz*	4–4	1987	1	0	0	0	0	0
Supreme Court let stand lower court's refusal to allow biological father to stop partner's abortion	*Doe v. Smith*	N/A	1988	1	0	1	0	0	0

(*continued*)

TABLE A.1.
Continued

Garrow	Zeigler	ACLU	Westlaw	NARAL	Oyez	Total	Year	Ruling	Case	Major points for state laws
0	0	1	1	0	0	2	1988	5–4	*Bowen v. Kendrick*	Challenged Adolescent Family Life Act (AFLA) and teaching of religion. Remanded to lower court
1	1	1	1	1	1	6	1989	5–4	*Webster v. Reproductive Health Services*	Upheld Missouri prohibition on state-employed physicians, state facilities ban, and requirement for fetal viability determination >20 weeks gestation
1	1	1	1	1	1	6	1990	5–4	*Hodgson v. Minnesota*	Upheld notification of two biological parents if judicial bypass is provided and 48-hour waiting period between notification and abortion procedure
1	0	1	1	1	1	5	1990	6–3	*Ohio v. Akron Center for Reproductive Health*	Upheld one-parent notification with judicial bypass without requiring anonymity for minor, a more stringent standard for minor bypass
1	0	1	1	1	1	5	1991	5–4	*Rust v. Sullivan*	Upheld federal regulations prohibiting health care professionals at federally funded family planning clinics from counselling or referring patients to abortion services
1	1	1	1	1	1	6	1992	5–4	*Planned Parenthood of Southeastern Pennsylvania v. Casey*	Upheld *Roe v. Wade* in principle, but replaced trimester framework with undue burden standard. Upheld 24-hour waiting period, informed consent, reporting, and parental or judicial consent. Struck down spousal consent

							Year	Vote	Case	Description
1	1	0	1	1	0	4	1993	6–3	*Bray v. Alexandria Womens Health Clinic*	Struck down the use of a federal civil rights law to protect abortion patients from protestors
1	1	0	0	1	0	4	1994	9–0	*National Organization of Women v. Scheidler*	Upheld use of federal anti-racketeering law in lawsuits against violent anti-abortion protestors
0	1	1	1	1	0	4	1994	6–3	*Madsen v. Womens Health Center*	Upheld some court-ordered restrictions on abortion clinic protests
0	0	0	0	0	0	0	1995	N/A	*Cheffer v. Reno*	Supreme Court let stand lower court ruling upholding constitutionality of Freedom of Access to Clinic Entrances Act (FACE)
0	0	1	0	1	0	1	1996	*per curiam*	*Dalton v. Little Rock Family Planning Services*	Regulation of abortion clinic protests
0	0	0	0	0	0	1	1996	5–4	*Leavitt v. Jane L.*	Upheld Utah governor's request to sever the regulations for early and late abortion
0	1	1	1	1	1	5	1997	8–1	*Schenck v. Pro-Choice Network, W. New York*	Struck down floating bubble zone for protection of abortion clinic and patients
0	1	0	1	0	1	3	1997	*per curiam*	*Lambert v. Wickland*	*per curiam.* Upheld Montana law for minor's judicial bypass
0	1	0	0	0	1	3	1997	6–3	*Mazurek v. Armstrong*	Reversed lower court ruling that might have allowed licensed physicians' assistants to provide abortion
0	1	1	1	1	1	4	2000	5–4	*Stenberg v. Carhart*	Struck down Nebraska law banning partial birth abortion, with no health of mother exception
0	0	1	0	0	1	3	2000	6–3	*Hill v. Colorado*	Upheld Colorado law

(continued)

TABLE A.1.
Continued

Garrow	Zeigler	ACLU	Westlaw	NARAL	Oyez	Total	Year	Ruling	Case	Major points for state laws
0	0	0	0	1	0	2	2001	6–3	*Ferguson v. City of Charleston*	Ruled that the Medical College of South Carolina's policy of testing women for cocaine was unconstitutional
0	0	0	1	0	0	1	2003	6–3	*Lawrence v. Texas*	Struck down Texas law criminalizing homosexual sodomy (on due process grounds)
0	0	0	0	1	1	2	2003	8–1	*Scheidler v. National Organization for Women*	Voided use of RICO Act against clinic protestors, remanded case to lower court
0	0	1	1	1	1	4	2006	9–0	*Ayotte v. Planned Parenthood of Northern New England*	Remanded to lower court New Hampshire's 48-hour notification with no health exception
0	0	1	0	0	1	2	2006	8–0	*Scheidler v. National Organization for Women*	RICO laws could not be invoked to challenge abortion clinic protests.
0	1	1	1	0	1	4	2007	5–4	*Gonzales v. Carhart*	Upheld partial birth abortion with life endangerment clause, but no health exception
0	0	0	0	0	1	1	2008	5–4	*Gonzales v. Planned Parenthood of America*	Upheld partial birth abortion with life endangerment clause, but no health exception

							Year		Case	
0	0	0	1	1	1	3	2014	9–0	*McCullen v. Coakley*	Struck down Massachusetts law to protect abortion providers from protests
0	1	0	1	1	1	4	2016	5–3	*Whole Women's Health v. Hellerstedt*	Struck down two Texas abortion restrictions
0	1	0	1	1	1	4	2018	8–0	*National Institute of Family & Life Advocates v. Becerra, 138 S. Ct. 2361*	Struck down 2 sections of California's Reproductive Freedom Act: requiring facilities to inform patients about the full range of reproductive health options as well as when they are not medically supervised
0	0	0	1	0	1	2	2019	7–2	*Box v. Planned Parenthood of Indiana and Kentucky*	Indiana law regulating providers' disposal of fetal remains was supported by rational basis, not undue burden
0	0	0	1	0	1	2	2020	5–4	*June Medical Services v. Russo*	Struck down Louisiana TRAP law
0	0	0	0	0	0	0	2021	6–3	*FDA, et al. v. ACOG, et al.*	Allows in-person requirement for medication abortion during COVID-19 pandemic
0	0	0	0	0	0	1	2021	Dismissed	*American Medical Association v. Cochran*	Challenged Trump administration restrictions on referrals made by Title X grantees
0	0	0	0	0	1	1	2021	6–3	*Dobbs v. Jackson Women's Health Organization*	Vacated *Roe v. Wade* and *Planned Parenthood of Southeastern Pennsylvania v. Casey*
Total = 26	28	23	44	36	46					

TABLE A.2
Number of Years of Existence from 1988 through 2020 for Each Abortion Restriction, by State

State	Bans specific abortion procedures	Bans abortion at viability	Requires viability testing	Bans abortion by gestation week	Bans all abortions	Requires parental consent for minor's abortion
Alabama	24	28	29	10	33	33
Alaska	24	0	0	0	0	22
Arizona	24	33	0	9	33	33
Arkansas	24	33	0	8	33	16
California	0	33	0	0	14	33
Colorado	0	0	0	0	25	20
Connecticut	0	30	0	0	0	0
Delaware	0	30	0	0	30	7
DC	0	25	0	0	16	0
Florida	23	33	0	0	0	6
Georgia	22	33	0	9	0	0
Hawaii	0	0	0	0	0	0
Idaho	23	33	0	10	1	21
Illinois	22	33	0	0	0	5
Indiana	24	33	0	10	0	33
Iowa	23	33	0	4	0	0
Kansas	23	29	23	10	7	10
Kentucky	23	33	0	4	3	33
Louisiana	24	33	31	23	30	33
Maine	0	33	0	6	0	0
Maryland	0	28	0	0	4	0
Massachusetts	0	33	0	0	31	33
Michigan	25	30	0	0	33	33
Minnesota	0	33	0	0	0	0
Mississippi	24	0	0	7	33	33
Missouri	22	33	31	1	2	33
Montana	17	33	0	1	0	8
Nebraska	24	33	0	11	0	15
Nevada	0	33	0	0	0	0
New Hampshire	9	6	0	0	9	0
New Jersey	24	0	0	0	0	0
New Mexico	17	17	0	0	33	33
New York	0	30	0	0	0	0
North Carolina	0	30	0	3	0	28
North Dakota	22	33	0	8	7	33
Ohio	26	28	26	4	2	25
Oklahoma	23	33	0	10	33	15
Oregon	0	0	0	0	0	0
Pennsylvania	0	33	22	0	0	33
Rhode Island	21	33	0	0	0	33
South Carolina	24	30	0	5	0	27
South Dakota	24	33	0	5	7	5
Tennessee	24	30	0	3	2	29
Texas	5	30	0	8	15	16
Utah	24	32	0	29	22	16
Vermont	0	0	0	0	26	0
Virginia	22	33	0	0	0	18
Washington	0	29	0	0	0	3
West Virginia	23	0	0	6	33	10
Wisconsin	23	33	0	6	29	30
Wyoming	0	33	0	0	0	23

Requires parental notification for minor's abortion	Permits official choose life license plates	Allows providers to refuse information/services/referrals for reproductive health	Mandates biased counseling before abortion	Prohibits abortion coverage in private insurance market	Requires notification/consent of husband for abortion	TRAP laws
0	8	4	31	0	0	20
12	9	30	29	0	0	20
0	12	33	8	0	0	20
17	18	30	20	0	0	20
0	0	29	11	0	0	13
23	0	33	0	0	30	7
0	18	30	11	0	0	20
26	11	33	29	0	0	14
0	8	16	0	0	0	13
22	22	29	33	0	7	20
33	14	29	16	0	0	20
0	8	29	0	0	0	20
12	0	33	33	30	0	20
33	0	29	1	0	30	18
0	15	29	30	7	0	20
25	9	32	5	0	0	14
23	2	29	29	10	0	7
0	15	28	31	33	30	20
0	20	29	33	0	28	20
2	0	29	17	0	0	12
32	18	29	1	0	0	16
0	11	31	32	0	0	18
0	0	33	28	7	0	20
33	0	33	29	0	0	20
0	19	17	30	0	0	20
1	13	33	33	29	0	20
32	17	30	26	0	4	0
18	5	33	32	10	0	17
33	0	30	12	0	0	18
17	0	0	0	0	0	0
22	9	33	0	0	0	20
0	0	29	0	0	0	14
0	0	33	0	0	0	18
0	10	29	9	0	0	20
0	8	30	30	30	30	19
17	16	30	30	0	0	20
23	19	29	16	17	0	20
0	0	29	0	0	0	0
0	14	29	33	0	30	20
0	0	32	32	32	30	20
0	20	33	28	0	30	20
28	14	33	33	0	0	20
7	18	30	30	0	0	20
23	10	29	21	4	0	20
32	12	31	31	10	30	20
0	0	0	0	0	0	0
16	12	33	29	0	0	19
0	0	29	0	0	0	14
33	0	16	18	0	0	0
0	0	33	33	12	0	20
13	0	33	0	0	0	14

(continued)

State	TRAP law requiring hospital or specialized facility	TRAP law requiring MD hospital privileges	Prohibits abortion coverage for state employees	Bans state-supported agencies from abortion counseling/ referrals	Prohibits abortion coverage in state ACA insurance market-places	Mandates waiting period before abortion procedures
Alabama	8	8	0	19	9	19
Alaska	0	0	0	0	0	0
Arizona	8	8	11	22	11	12
Arkansas	8	6	23	11	8	20
California	0	0	0	0	0	0
Colorado	0	0	33	0	0	0
Connecticut	3	0	0	0	0	0
Delaware	0	0	0	0	0	26
DC	0	0	0	0	0	0
Florida	3	8	0	0	10	5
Georgia	0	0	8	0	7	16
Hawaii	0	0	0	0	0	0
Idaho	0	0	6	0	10	29
Illinois	3	2	25	22	0	0
Indiana	6	8	0	22	10	29
Iowa	0	0	0	0	0	5
Kansas	8	8	11	20	10	29
Kentucky	8	4	23	22	0	29
Louisiana	8	8	0	30	11	26
Maine	0	0	0	0	0	0
Maryland	3	0	0	0	0	0
Massachusetts	0	0	32	0	0	28
Michigan	8	1	14	25	7	29
Minnesota	0	0	1	22	0	18
Mississippi	8	8	20	22	11	29
Missouri	8	8	7	30	11	18
Montana	0	0	0	0	0	26
Nebraska	3	0	33	23	10	28
Nevada	0	0	0	0	0	0
New Hampshire	0	0	0	0	0	0
New Jersey	0	3	0	0	0	0
New Mexico	0	0	0	0	0	0
New York	0	2	0	0	0	0
North Carolina	8	0	10	0	8	9
North Dakota	0	8	13	30	0	28
Ohio	8	0	23	24	9	28
Oklahoma	8	8	0	14	10	16
Oregon	0	0	0	0	0	0
Pennsylvania	8	0	33	26	8	28
Rhode Island	8	0	31	0	0	0
South Carolina	8	8	20	17	9	27
South Dakota	8	0	0	0	9	27
Tennessee	7	8	0	0	11	27
Texas	8	8	0	12	4	18
Utah	8	5	0	0	10	28
Vermont	0	0	0	0	0	0
Virginia	3	0	25	22	10	18
Washington	0	0	0	0	0	0
West Virginia	0	0	0	0	0	18
Wisconsin	0	3	9	24	9	25
Wyoming	0	1	0	0	0	0

Funds crisis pregnancy centers	Holds MDs liable for certain reasons for women seeking abortion	Limits abortion access during COVID-19	Requires MDs to tell patients about reversing medication abortion	Forbids abortion in state facilities	Requires sonogram before abortion	Prohibits tele-medicine abortion
0	0	1	0	0	15	4
0	0	1	0	0	0	0
0	5	0	0	33	14	4
0	4	1	2	0	2	4
0	2	4	4	0	0	0
0	0	0	0	0	0	0
0	0	0	0	0	0	0
12	0	0	0	0	0	0
0	0	0	0	0	0	0
4	0	0	0	0	10	0
5	0	0	0	0	14	0
0	0	0	0	0	0	0
0	0	0	2	0	5	0
4	3	0	0	0	0	0
1	5	0	0	0	5	4
0	0	1	0	23	4	3
11	5	0	0	23	10	3
0	3	0	2	32	4	2
7	5	1	0	30	11	4
0	0	0	0	0	0	0
0	0	0	0	0	0	0
0	0	0	0	0	0	0
11	0	0	0	0	13	7
10	0	0	0	0	0	0
0	1	1	0	20	1	4
25	2	0	0	33	11	4
0	0	0	0	0	0	0
0	0	0	2	0	12	4
0	0	0	0	0	0	0
0	0	0	0	0	0	0
0	0	0	0	0	0	0
6	0	0	0	0	0	0
0	0	0	0	0	0	0
10	5	0	0	0	10	4
11	5	0	2	32	12	4
8	3	1	0	0	7	2
4	5	1	2	0	4	4
0	0	0	0	0	0	0
25	5	0	0	32	0	0
0	0	0	0	0	0	0
0	0	0	0	0	5	4
0	4	0	2	0	3	4
0	1	1	1	0	3	4
17	0	1	0	0	11	4
0	2	0	2	0	24	0
0	0	0	0	0	0	0
0	0	0	0	0	8	0
0	0	0	0	0	0	0
0	0	1	0	0	11	4
12	0	0	0	0	8	4
0	0	0	0	0	4	0

TABLE A.3
Number of Years of Existence from 1988 through 2020 for Each Abortion Protection, by State

State	Codifies women's right to choose abortion	Improves access to emergency contraception	Funds abortions for low income women	Requires insurance coverage for abortion	Permits advance practice clinicians to provide medical or surgical abortion
Alabama	0	0	0	0	0
Alaska	0	0	31	0	0
Arizona	0	0	17	0	0
Arkansas	0	14	0	0	0
California	19	19	33	7	9
Colorado	0	14	0	0	1
Connecticut	31	14	33	0	9
Delaware	3	0	0	0	0
DC	1	12	3	0	5
Florida	0	0	0	0	0
Georgia	0	0	0	0	0
Hawaii	15	8	33	0	0
Idaho	0	0	4	0	1
Illinois	2	17	21	2	9
Indiana	0	0	3	0	0
Iowa	0	0	0	0	0
Kansas	0	0	0	0	0
Kentucky	0	0	0	0	0
Louisiana	0	0	0	0	0
Maine	20	0	3	2	0
Maryland	29	0	26	0	1
Massachusetts	2	16	33	0	1
Michigan	0	0	0	0	1
Minnesota	0	14	27	0	0
Mississippi	0	0	0	0	0
Missouri	0	0	0	0	0
Montana	0	0	26	0	5
Nebraska	0	0	0	0	0
Nevada	16	0	0	0	0
New Hampshire	0	0	0	0	6
New Jersey	0	16	33	0	1
New Mexico	0	18	27	0	0
New York	2	18	33	4	9
North Carolina	0	0	7	0	0
North Dakota	0	0	0	0	0
Ohio	0	0	0	0	0
Oklahoma	0	0	0	0	0
Oregon	3	14	33	4	6
Pennsylvania	0	1	0	0	0
Rhode Island	2	0	0	0	9
South Carolina	0	17	0	0	0
South Dakota	0	0	0	0	0
Tennessee	0	0	0	0	0
Texas	0	7	1	0	0
Utah	0	12	0	0	0
Vermont	2	0	33	0	6
Virginia	0	0	0	0	1
Washington	29	19	33	3	9
West Virginia	1	0	30	0	1
Wisconsin	0	13	0	0	0
Wyoming	0	0	0	0	0

Permits advanced practice clinicians to provide surgical abortion	Protects abortion providers, facilities, or patients	State constitution provides more protection for right to choose than US Constitution	State Supreme Court has ruled that state constitution protects right to choose separate from US Constitution	Protected abortion access during COVID-19	Guarantees women's contraceptive prescription will be filled
0	0	0	0	0	0
0	0	25	3	0	0
0	0	20	0	0	0
0	0	0	0	0	0
6	30	27	3	4	16
0	28	0	0	0	0
0	20	27	0	0	0
0	0	0	0	1	0
0	26	0	0	0	0
0	0	27	3	0	0
0	0	0	0	0	0
0	0	0	0	1	0
0	0	8	0	0	0
1	0	27	0	1	16
0	0	21	0	0	0
0	0	0	3	0	0
0	29	0	2	0	0
0	0	0	0	0	0
0	0	0	0	0	0
2	26	0	0	0	14
0	30	0	0	0	0
1	27	27	3	1	0
0	22	3	0	0	0
0	27	27	3	1	0
0	0	0	0	0	0
0	0	0	0	0	0
6	16	26	3	1	0
0	0	0	0	0	0
0	30	0	0	0	14
6	7	0	0	0	0
0	2	27	3	1	14
0	0	26	2	1	0
6	22	0	0	1	0
0	28	0	0	0	0
0	0	0	0	0	0
0	0	0	0	0	0
0	4	0	0	0	0
5	26	22	0	1	0
0	0	4	0	0	0
0	0	0	0	0	0
0	0	0	0	0	0
0	0	0	0	0	0
0	0	18	0	0	0
0	0	3	0	0	0
0	0	0	0	0	0
5	0	27	0	0	0
1	0	0	0	1	0
1	27	0	0	1	13
0	0	27	0	0	0
0	30	0	0	0	11
0	0	0	0	0	0

Introduction

1. *Dobbs, State Health Officer of the Mississippi Department of Health, et al. v. Jackson Women's Health Organization, et al.*, is the full name of this case. https://www.supreme court.gov/opinions/21pdf/19-1392_6j37.pdf.

2. As an example of its selective use of history, the majority *Dobbs* opinion makes no reference to James Mohr's acclaimed 1978 book, *Abortion in America: The Origins and Evolution of National Policy.*

3. This amicus brief from the American Historical Association discussed the reasons for nineteenth-century state anti-abortion laws (Center for Reproductive Rights 2022b).

4. *Food and Drug Administration, et al. v. American College of Obstetricians and Gynecologists, et al.* On Application for Stay. 592 U. S. ____ (2021). https://www.supreme court.gov/opinions/20pdf/20a34_3f14.pdf.

5. This requirement was part of the mifepristone REMS imposed by the FDA at the time mifepristone was approved in 2000. (See Chapter 1 for more discussion on REMS.)

6. A federal court in Hawaii was slated to hear *Chelius v. Becerra*, a case challenging the FDA's in-person pickup requirement for medication abortion because it lacks medical justification, "pandemic aside" (Fox and Cole 2021, e94(2)). The FDA announced on May 7, 2021, however, that it intended to review its restrictions on mifepristone. The plaintiffs asked the court to stay (i.e., pause) the litigation until December 1, 2021, in light of the FDA's review (ACLU 2021).

7. Scholars differ on which US Supreme Court decisions are classified as abortion cases. Appendix table A.1 shows how various authors have categorized abortion decisions.

Chapter 1 · Abortion Services in the United States and Theoretical Approaches to Their Regulation

1. Medication abortion is also called medical abortion (Mayo Clinic 2021).

2. The Centers for Disease Control and Prevention began its abortion surveillance program in 1969 (Smith and Bourne 1973; Smith 1970).

3. The abortion rate is the annual number of abortions per 1,000 women of reproductive age (15–44 years) (Centers for Disease Control and Prevention 2021; Population Reference Bureau 2011).

4. These estimates are from the Guttmacher Institute, which collects abortion data from providers, rather than from the Centers for Disease Control and Prevention (CDC), which collects data from the health departments of most states.

5. The US population was 244,498,982 in 1988 and is projected to be 339,665,118 in 2024 (US Census Bureau 2023b).

6. Unintended pregnancies are more likely than intended pregnancies to end in

abortion. Research showed that women's reasons for seeking abortion are complex and interrelated (Foster 2020; Biggs et al. 2017, 2013). Table 1.2 shows that since 2001, most unintended pregnancies have been carried to term.

7. Birth control pills, the most widely used reversible contraceptive in the United States (Guttmacher Institute 2021), are expensive. For patients without health insurance, birth control pills typically cost $20 to $50 a month. Out-of-pocket costs for women with health insurance range from $5 to $40 (CostHelper.com 2021; Snider 2019).

8. For 2019, the CDC reported that 43.7 percent of all abortions were medical abortions: 42.3 percent occurred at nine weeks of gestation or less and 1.4 percent were carried out above nine weeks of gestation (Kortsmit et al. 2021).

9. Women Ages 15–44 by Race and Ethnicity (Number and percentage)

Reproductive age population	Total	White	Black	Asian	Hispanic
Female population 15–44 (in thousands)	62,247	35,812	9,286	3,848	12,174
Percentage of total	100.0	57.5	14.9	6.1	19.5

Source: Data from Monte and Ellis 2014.

10. According to 2019 CDC data, 38.4 percent of reported abortions were to Black women, 21.0 percent to Hispanic women, 7.2 percent to "Other," and 33.4 percent to non-Hispanic white women (Kortsmit et al. 2021).

11. The percentage of abortion patients who are unmarried has increased over time, but marriage rates have decreased as well.

12. Pregnancy "is dated from the first day of the last menstrual period (LMP) and is commonly measured by days' or weeks' gestation" (NAS 2018, 50).

13. Mifepristone "may only be dispensed by or under the supervision of a certified prescriber, or by a certified pharmacy on a prescription issued by a certified prescriber" (US Food and Drug Administration 2023b).

14. The NAS figure was taken from CDC's 2013 abortion surveillance report. When we calculated the percentage of abortions ≥14 weeks that were performed by induction for 2018, our figure was 0.54 percent (219 out of 39,979) (CDC 2021).

15. Only Alaska, Colorado, the District of Columbia, New Jersey, New Mexico, Oregon, and Vermont do not have gestational limits (Guttmacher Institute 2022g; *New York Times* 2023). For women experiencing pregnancies with fetal abnormalities only detected late in pregnancy, the options for care are extremely limited (Megas 2017).

16. In 2012, 95 percent of abortion facilities offered abortions at eight weeks of gestation, 72 percent at 12 weeks, 34 percent at 20 weeks of gestation, and 16 percent at 24 weeks (NAS 2019, 33; Jerman and Jones 2014).

17. Since 2018, self-managed abortion using mifepristone and misopristol through on-line telemedicine in the U.S. has been available via a nonprofit service called AID Access" (Aiken et al. 2022a, 2). https://aidaccess.org/en.

18. This definition modifies Meier's original definition of regulation: "any attempt by the government to control the behavior of citizens, corporations, or subgovernments" (Meier 1985, 1), expanding citizens to individuals and corporations to organizations, which includes nonprofit organizations as well as corporations.

19. Some data sources, such as NARAL Pro-Choice America, do aggregate access to reproductive health services more generally with abortion regulations. In this book, we distinguish between abortion and other reproductive health regulations.

20. In economic terms, the Hyde Amendment removes the subsidy for abortion services only.

21. Only 17 states use their own funds to pay for abortions for Medicaid-eligible women (Guttmacher Institute 2023f).

22. The cost of abortion varies greatly across the states and depends upon the length of

the pregnancy (HeyJane 2023; Knueven 2023; Planned Parenthood Federation of America 2022).

23. Low-income women may not be able to raise the funds for an abortion in time for an early abortion, which is safer and cheaper than abortions that take place later in gestation (Finer et al. 2006).

24. In economic terms, this regulation can shift the supply of abortion services inward, thus decreasing demand as the price changes.

25. As a regulatory strategy, the direct allocation of resources is fairly uncommon in the United States (Meier 1985, 2).

26. Subsidies for contraceptive services can lead to fewer unintended pregnancies, hence, lower demand for abortion.

27. Patient referrals to CPCs often occur through state-mandated counseling for women requesting abortion. States often dedicate their "Choose Life" license plates revenue to CPCs (NARAL Pro-Choice America 2014, 18).

28. Distributive policies promote, usually through subsidies, "private activities that are judged to be socially desirable. . . . This type of public policy does not have winners and losers; . . . everyone benefits equally" (Stewart et al. 2008, 59). An example would be Medicare benefits, which are not means tested.

29. Redistributive policies "distribute wealth or other valued resources in society. Essentially, these policies redistribute benefits from one group to another (e.g., welfare policy). Therefore, redistributive policy tends to be characterized by ideological concerns and often involves class conflict" (Stewart et al. 2008, 60). Nevertheless, redistributive politics tend to be more stable than regulatory politics (Smith and Larimer 2017, 33).

30. Gormley (1986) refers to civil servants as bureaucrats, a commonly used term in political science to refer to civil servants working in the federal and state bureaucracies or public agencies. *Bureaucrat*, therefore, is a neutral term here without the pejorative connotation it often has in US culture.

31. Technical detail is usually not covered, and when it is, the coverage is "often confusing, inaccurate, or misleading" (Gormley 1986, 612).

32. Unlike investigative reporting, the media in this scenario is not creating news, but instead amplifying the noncomplex messages from politicians and citizen groups (Gormley 1986, 608).

33. *Food and Drug Administration, et al. v. American College of Obstetricians and Gynecologists, et al.* (this has been discussed in the Introduction).

34. Morality policies are sometimes called social regulatory policies. In this book, we consider morality policies and social regulatory policies to be synonyms (Rose 2009; Smith 2002).

35. Policies that address morality issues are called morality policies or social regulatory policies (Smith 2002, 383).

36. Advocates often frame these issues along multiple dimensions, and they do not necessarily favor frames that emphasize moral principles over other considerations in state legislative settings (Mucciaroni et al. 2019).

37. In some cases, state legislators choose not to wait to see if the Court decided an abortion restriction was constitutional. Instead, states adopted restrictions while the constitutional context was unknown (Patton 2007, 477).

38. The structure of this section emulates the first chapter of Kenneth J. Meier's 1985 classic book, *Regulation*.

39. For example, Cooperative Congressional Election Study (2016) data reveal that nationally, 58 percent of those surveyed say that they always support allowing a woman to obtain an abortion as a matter of choice, 84 percent oppose making abortion illegal in all circumstances, and 63 percent support banning abortion after 20 weeks of pregnancy,

40. In the 2016 American National Election Studies (ANES) survey, respondents were

asked where they stood on the abortion issue on a scale from 1 to 4, where 1 is by law, abortion should never be permitted, 2 is only in the case of rape, incest, or if life of the woman is in danger, 3 allows other reasons if need is established, and 4 is by law, abortion should be a matter of personal choice. States with an average response below 2.5 include North and South Dakota, Alabama, Louisiana, Utah, Oklahoma, Kentucky, and Arkansas, and those with an average response greater than 3.5 include Vermont, Rhode Island, Oregon, Hawaii, New Hampshire, and District of Columbia. States with public opinion most opposed to abortion are also among the states with the highest average number of restrictions, averaging about 10 or more across our time period, and fewest protections. With the exception of Rhode Island, states with public opinion most supportive of abortion being a matter of personal choice have among the fewest abortion restrictions, averaging fewer than 2.4 restrictions.

41. The policy cycle approach considers sequential stages in the policy process (Stewart et al. 2008).

Chapter 2 · Setting the Parameters for State Abortion Policies

1. The count of important abortion cases adjudicated by the US Supreme Court varies by source. The American Civil Liberties Union (ACLU) counts 23, whereas NARAL counts 36. Legal databases differ as well: Westlaw with 44 and Oyez with 46. Scholars also differ, and their counts are complicated by their foci and when they published (Zeigler 2020; Zeigler 2018; McFarlane and Meier 2001; Garrow 1994). In order to provide a systematic method for choosing cases, each case mentioned by any source was included in our database. It received one point for every source that identified it as an important case. The cases reviewed in this chapter were selected by score as well as the authors' knowledge of their importance. It is included as appendix table A.1.

2. Among the best known of these cases are *Griswold v. Connecticut* (1965), *Eisenstadt v. Baird* (1972), and *U.S. v. Vuitch* (1971) (Garrow 1994). Earlier cases dealing with mandatory sterilization by the states or state institutions include *Buck v. Bell* (1927) and *Skinner v. State of Oklahoma* (1942) (NARAL Pro-Choice America 2018).

3. In 1803, the UK Parliament passed a law that made abortion before quickening a crime for the first time in English history. However, American jurisprudence did not follow suit. In 1812, for example, the Massachusetts Supreme Court dismissed charges against a man for administering an abortifacient because the pregnant woman was not yet "quick with child" (Mohr 1978, 5).

4. Fourteen states prohibited the verbal transmission of birth control or abortion information. Eleven states criminalized the possession of written instructions for pregnancy prevention. Four states authorized search and seizure for contraceptive instructions. Connecticut alone outlawed the act of controlling conception (Brodie 1994).

5. Although Kentucky had not passed anti-abortion legislation by 1900, its state courts had already outlawed the practice (Mohr 1978).

6. Attorneys relied on the right to privacy "recognized in other Supreme Court cases, especially *Griswold v. Connecticut* and *Eisenstadt v. Baird*"; meanwhile, *Roe* "held that the right to privacy 'was broad enough to encompass a woman's decision whether or not to terminate her pregnancy'" (Ziegler 2020, 22, 20).

7. *Connecticut v. Menillo* was the case that tested limiting abortion provision to physicians only within very confined conditions. Patrick Menillo had no medical training whatsoever, so the Court allowed Connecticut to apply the pre-*Roe* criminal abortion code in this case. At the time, considerable evidence showed that trained mid-level practitioners and other non-physicians could safely and effectively provide first trimester surgical abortion. Since that time, more evidence has accumulated refuting the position that only physicians can provide surgical and medical abortions (Renner et al. 2012).

8. The question of judicial standing for physicians performing abortions was also raised in the 2020 *June Medical Services v. Russo* opinions.

9. Non-therapeutic abortions are pregnancy terminations that are performed for reasons other than protecting the life or the health of the woman.

10. See McFarlane and Meier (2001, 90, Table 5-4).

11. Generally, there are three levels of scrutiny when the constitutionality of a law is challenged. Strict scrutiny, the highest level of scrutiny, requires the government to prove that "there is a *compelling state interest* behind the challenged policy, and the law or regulation is *narrowly tailored* to achieve its result" (Snider 2020). Intermediate scrutiny is less demanding; in order for a law to pass intermediate scrutiny, it must "serve an *important government objective* and be *substantially related* to achieving the objective" (Snider 2020). Rational basis review is the lowest level of scrutiny. Here the person challenging the law must show that the government has *no legitimate interest* in the law or that "there is *no reasonable, rational link* between that interest and the challenged law" (Snider 2020).

12. By "thus injecting coercive financial incentives favoring childbirth into a decision that is constitutionally guaranteed to be free from governmental intrusion, the Hyde Amendment deprives the indigent woman of her freedom to choose abortion over maternity, thereby impinging on the due process liberty right recognized in *Roe v. Wade*" (McRae, 448 U.S. 333–334) (Brennan, J., dissenting).

13. O'Connor believed that "*Roe* had struck the wrong balance between women's rights and the government's interest in fetal life" (Ziegler 2020,72).

14. In 1976, in the *Danforth* case, the Court had ruled that recordkeeping and reporting requirements were permissible if they protected a patient's confidentiality and privacy and were intended to preserve maternal health.

15. *Webster*'s public facility ban turned on Truman Medical Center in Kansas City, Missouri. In 1985, this hospital "performed 97 percent of all Missouri hospital abortions at sixteen weeks or later. Although it was a private hospital primarily staffed by private physicians, with no public funds expended on abortions performed there, it was considered a 'public facility' because it was on land leased from the state" (Mezey 2011, 222).

16. The ban on any abortions in military facilities, even with private funds, was first put into place in 1988 with an internal Department of Defense memorandum and then was signed into law by President Bush the same year (Boonstra 2010; Simon 2010).

17. Including "trespassing on or damaging clinic property, or using violence or threats of violence against clinics, their employees, or their patients" (NARAL-Pro-Choice America 2018, 8).

18. This case has exceptional language revealing the biases of the majority, not the facts of the case. No "physician uses the term 'partial birth' because the fetus is not yet viable and cannot be born and live. However, the term resonates and is very useful politically" (Goldman 2021, 91).

19. The idea of abortion regret came directly from an amicus brief filed by "the conservative and religiously inspired Justice Foundation," not from any empirical evidence (Ehrlich and Doan 2019, 123).

20. This requirement was unnecessary for patient safety and had not been applied to other facilities that provided medical services with similar low risks as abortion. It was only directed at abortion providers, dubbed a type of state regulation called a TRAP law (targeted regulation of abortion providers) (Guttmacher Institute 2022k).

21. A *per curiam* decision is "a court opinion issued in the name of the Court rather than specific judges. Most decisions on the merits by the courts take the form of one or more opinions written and signed by individual justices" (Cornell Law School 2023).

22. Justice Barrett's long-term association with the anti-abortion and anti-LGBTQ group Alliance Defending Freedom is well-documented (Burns 2020).

23. "Parties who are not satisfied with the decision of a lower court must petition the U.S. Supreme Court to hear their case. The primary means to petition the court for review is to ask it to grant a *writ of certiorari*. This is a request that the Supreme Court order a lower court to send up the record of the case for review. The Court usually is not under any obligation to hear these cases, and it usually only does so if the case could have national significance, might harmonize conflicting decisions in the federal Circuit courts, and/or could have precedential value. In fact, the Court accepts 100–150 of the more than 7,000 cases that it is asked to review each year. Typically, the Court hears cases that have been decided in either an appropriate U.S. Court of Appeals or the highest Court in a given state (if the state court decided a Constitutional issue)" (United States Courts 2022).

24. The Court ruled in the 1976 *Singleton v. Wulf* decision that providers have standing in abortion cases.

25. Oral arguments are available (*Dobbs v. Jackson Women's Health*, Oral Arguments, 2021).

26. "First, the Court examined the nature of the Court's error in the *Roe* and *Casey* decisions. . . . Second, the Court found that quality of *Roe*'s reasoning was not grounded in constitutional text, history, or precedent." Third, the Court asserted that *Casey*'s undue burden test had proved "unworkable." Fourth, the Court argued that both *Roe* and *Casey* had negatively impacted other areas of law. Finally, the Court discussed how overruling *Roe* would not upend the type of reliance issues found in any other types of holdings involving property and contractual rights, here dismissing the *Casey* decision (Lindgren 2022, 240–242).

27. A joint dissenting opinion is unusual; traditionally, "one author drafts an opinion that is signed on to by the others" (Lindgren 2022, 257).

Chapter 3 · Weakening *Roe*

1. This ban using foreign aid to support "abortion as a method of family planning," applied to international population and family planning assistance and was first adopted in 1973 (Rosoff 1975).

2. The use of federal funds for abortion was prohibited except "where the life of the mother would be endangered if the fetus were carried to term." In 1993, Congress expanded the Hyde amendment to include cases in which the pregnancy was the result of rape or incest (McFarlane and Meier 2001, 66, 73).

3. The ADF is also opposed to LBGTQ rights and works to promote religion in public institutions, including schools.

4. Affluent women were more likely to have private health insurance, the ability to travel, secure childcare, and even access to contraception.

5. *Connecticut v. Menillo* upheld allowing only physicians to provide abortion services, but it did not test the constitutionality of a state law restricting abortion provision to only physicians instead of well-trained mid-level practitioners.

6. States with post-viability laws in 1988 included Arizona, Arkansas, California, Florida, Georgia, Idaho, Illinois, Indiana, Iowa, Kentucky, Louisiana, Maine, Massachusetts, Minnesota, Missouri, Montana, Nebraska, Nevada, North Dakota, Oklahoma, Pennsylvania, Rhode Island, South Dakota, Utah, Virginia, Wisconsin, and Wyoming.

7. These data reflect NARAL reporting. There are slight differences in when state parental involvement laws are reported by NARAL and the Guttmacher Institute. Most of these difference can be attributed to the timing of state laws and what years they are counted by each source. States with parental involvement laws in 1988 included Alabama, Alaska, Arizona, California, Colorado, Delaware, Florida, Georgia, Idaho, Illinois, Indiana, Kentucky, Louisiana, Maryland, Massachusetts, Minnesota, Mississippi, Missouri, Montana,

Nebraska, Nevada, New Mexico, North Dakota, Ohio, Pennsylvania, Rhode Island, South Carolina, South Dakota, Tennessee, Utah, Washington, West Virginia, and Wyoming.

8. Common reasons for classifying state parental involvement laws as unconstitutional in 1988 were the lack of a judicial bypass for minors not wishing to inform their parent(s) or a blanket state law that did not recognize emancipated minors. In 1988, this judgment was made according to precedent in the 1983 *City of Akron v. Akron Center for Reproductive Health*.

9. The states that funded abortions for low-income women eligible for Medicaid were Alaska, California, Connecticut, Hawaii, Massachusetts, North Carolina, New Jersey, New York, Oregon, Vermont, Washington, and West Virginia. The five states that were funding abortions because "a court had invalidated restrictions that the state had imposed on funding were California, Connecticut, Massachusetts, New Jersey, and Vermont (NARAL 1989).

10. By forbidding coverage for abortions in the federally subsidized Medicaid program, a Medicaid-eligible woman has to pay full price for an abortion. If gathering the funds for the price of an abortion takes much time for a low-income woman, this policy can push women into a different price range for later term abortions.

11. In 2003, the National Abortion Rights League changed its name to NARAL-Pro-Choice America (Ziegler 2020, 171).

12. The first report, *Who Decides? A State by State Review of Abortion Rights in America* provided a status report for 1988 and was published in January 1989. These reports have been published annually, with the exception of 1990 (1989 data) and 1994 (1993 data) on the anniversary of *Roe v. Wade*. The most recent report is for 2022, which gives a 2021 update.

13. *Who Decides?* includes political information about whether governors and legislative bodies support reproductive freedom, oppose reproductive freedom, or have a mixed record on reproductive freedom. In "making the determination for state governors, NARAL Pro-Choice America evaluates each governor's stance on reproductive freedom by considering their voting and signing record, public statements, and other indications of their stance on reproductive freedom. We consider whether the governor supports the right to abortion, restrictions on abortion care, and access to contraception. For legislatures, we evaluate the likelihood that chambers will pass bills that would expand or restrict reproductive freedom. We consider the outcome of elections, bills previously passed by the chambers, and public statements to make this determination" (M. McGuirk, personal communication, April 7, 2021).

14. NARAL did not issue a report in January 2022, probably in anticipation of the *Dobbs* decision. As a result, their assessment of 2021 state abortion regulations was not reported.

15. The facility in question in the *Webster* case was the Truman Medical Center in Kansas City, Missouri, which performed 97 percent of all Missouri abortions at 16 weeks or more. Although "it was a private hospital staffed primarily by private physicians, with no public funds expended on abortions performed there, it was considered a 'public facility' because it was on land leased from the state" (Mezey 2011, 222).

16. Four states, namely, Arizona, Kentucky, North Dakota, and Pennsylvania, passed public facility bans in 1989. Louisiana enacted similar legislation in 1991.

17. In most states, public employees would be precluded by job descriptions or funding from being involved in abortions, so such a restriction would not have much effect.

18. In 1999, the total of states requiring viability testing increased to six states (Mezey 2011, 221–224; NARAL 1991, v, 94).

19. States with refusal-of-care restrictions in 1988 included Arizona, Colorado, Delaware, Idaho, Michigan, Minnesota, Missouri, Nebraska, New Jersey, New York, South Carolina, South Dakota, Virginia, Wisconsin, and Wyoming.

20. The level of scrutiny determines "how a court will go about analyzing a law and its effects" (Snider 2020). Strict scrutiny requires the *government* to prove "a compelling state interest in the challenged policy and the law or regulation is narrowly tailored to meet its result" (Snider 2020). Intermediate scrutiny is less demanding than strict scrutiny. In order for a law to pass strict scrutiny, it must "serve an important government objective" (Snider 2020) and "be substantially related to achieving the objective" (Snider 2020). The lowest form of scrutiny is the rational basis test (Snider 2020).

21. The *Casey* Court's explanation of undue burden was unclear and inconsistent, so it was applied unevenly (Freeman 2013).

22. Spousal consent had been struck down in the 1976 *Planned Parenthood v. Danforth* decision, but not under the undue burden standard.

23. The *Casey* decision stated that "this view of marriage [is] repugnant to our present understanding of marriage and of the nature of rights secured by the Constitution" (Ziegler 2020, 118). Women "do not lose their constitutionally protected liberty when they marry" (91–744 and 91–902—opinion, *Planned Parenthood of Southeastern Pennsylvania v. Casey*).

24. NARAL annual reports show that Montana had a spousal consent law on the books 1991–1994 but it was never enforced; it was struck down before the 1992 *Casey* decision.

25. Due to ongoing litigation and intermittent injunctions, Michigan moved in and out of enforcing mandatory counseling. A permanent injunction was issued in 1994, but enforced by 1997, not 1995–1996, so enforced going forward from 1997.

26. The US Supreme Court struck down an informed consent law from Akron, Ohio, in the 1983 *City of Akron v. Akron Center for Reproductive Health* decision and again struck down Pennsylvania's informed consent requirements in the 1986 *Thornburg v. ACOG* ruling.

27. By 2020, the 30 states that mandated informed consent included Alabama, Alaska, Arizona, Arkansas, Florida, Georgia, Idaho, Indiana, Iowa, Kansas, Kentucky, Louisiana, Michigan, Minnesota, Mississippi, Missouri, Nebraska, North Carolina, North Dakota, Ohio, Oklahoma, Pennsylvania, Rhode Island, South Carolina, South Dakota, Tennessee, Texas, Utah, West Virginia, and Wisconsin.

28. An exception is Medicaid-funded female sterilizations, which require a 30-day waiting period between the time a woman consents to be sterilized and the time in which she can have the surgery (Joyce et al. 2009).

29. The state of Pennsylvania's claim that the abortion reporting system provided accountability to taxpayers was disingenuous because Pennsylvania did not fund abortions for low-income women.

30. The Guttmacher Institute does have current data on the abortion reporting requirements of individual states, but these data have not been reported over time (Guttmacher Institute 2023a).

31. *Belloti v. Baird.*

32. *H.L. v. Matheson.*

33. In 1992 when the *Casey* decision was issued, one study reported that no infants born at 22 weeks survived, 15% survived at 23 weeks, 56% survived at 24 weeks, and 79% survived at 25 weeks. Sixty-nine percent of infants born at 25 weeks survived without severe abnormalities compared with 21% born at 24 weeks (Allen et al. 1993).

34. Refer to Note 6.

35. California, Connecticut, Florida, Idaho, Illinois, Massachusetts, Michigan, Minnesota, New Jersey, Oregon, Tennessee, Vermont, and West Virginia.

36. Among the facility requirements in state TRAP laws are structural standards equivalent to those for surgical centers, with procedure room size specified, corridor width specified, and maximum distance to the hospital specified (Guttmacher Institute 2022j).

37. Only Kansas, Montana, New Hampshire, Oregon, Vermont, and West Virginia had no TRAP laws (NARAL 2008).

38. The Court struck down a similar regulation from Louisiana in 2020 in *June Medical Services v. Russo.*

39. A court has blocked the Indiana requirement that mandated that the agreement with another physician who has privileges to be renewed annually and filed in every hospital in the local area (Guttmacher Institute 2022j).

40. In 1992, Dr. Mark Haskell presented data showing that dilation and extraction was, in certain instances, safer for the woman, but this information was ignored in Congress's findings of fact (Gold 2021, 89).

41. The state may not interfere with the decision of a woman to terminate a pregnancy: (1) before the fetus is viable; or (2) at any time if any abortion is necessary to protect the life or health of the woman, or the fetus is affected by genetic defect or serious deformity or abnormality (NARAL 1993, 54).

42. Other state laws mandate coverage of prescription contraception for women with health insurance. Most "of these policies include language that allows providers to opt out of the requirement because of religious or moral beliefs—conscience clause exemptions (Van Sickle-Ward and Hollis-Brusky 2013).

43. Pregnancy "begins with implantation according to medical authorities such as the USFDA, the National Institutes of Health, and the American College of Obstetricians and Gynecologists" (Trussell and Schwartz 2011, 121).

44. No California pharmacist could refuse to fill a contraceptive prescription unless "the pharmacist's employer has been notified and is able to provide a reasonable accommodation that ensures women have timely access to their prescriptions" (NARAL 2006, 4).

45. If an individual pharmacist refuses to fill a contraceptive prescription, then the pharmacy that employees that pharmacist must make sure that the prescription is filled in a timely manner (Sonfield 2005).

46. At the most extreme, states can prohibit insurance plans that participate in their health exchanges from providing any coverage for abortion. In states not proscribing abortion coverage beyond Hyde amendment exceptions, marketplace insurance plans offering abortion coverage must create separate accounts for abortion coverage premiums and premium payments for the coverage of all other health services. Women who opt for abortion coverage have to write a separate check for that coverage. The ACA "requires that at least one plan within each state insurance exchange must not offer abortion coverage beyond the narrow exceptions of the Hyde amendment" (McFarlane 2015, 56).

47. Also called pregnancy resource centers (Kimport 2020) or crisis pregnancy counseling centers (Goldman 2021).

48. Anti-abortion groups claim that there are 3,000 crisis pregnancy centers in the United States (Gaul 2021), but another study claims there about 2,000 (Bryant and Swartz 2018). At any rate, they greatly outnumber abortion providers (Swartzendruber and Lambert 2022), estimated at 1,587 in 2017 (Nash and Dreweke 2019) and declining since the *Dobbs* decision (Simmons-Duffin 2023; Kirstein et al. 2022).

49. Alabama, Alaska, Arkansas, Indiana, Iowa, Kentucky, Louisiana, Mississippi, Ohio, Oklahoma, Tennessee, Texas, and West Virginia (NARAL 2021, 15).

50. California, Hawaii, Illinois, Maryland, Massachusetts, Michigan, Minnesota, New Jersey, New Mexico, New York, Oregon, and Virginia (Jones et al. 2020).

51. An "important source of restrictive state regulations is Americans United for Life, who describe themselves as the 'legal architects of the pro-life movement'" (Goldman 2021, 99).

52. Looking at the change in restrictions and protections, we dropped 1988 from the data set because we did not have 1987 data to look at the change. Hence, our total sample size was 1,632.

53. These results do not consider the voting behavior or positions of individual legislators or governors.

54. Because of the way that laws are written and data are collected, different sources may present different counts and categories of state abortion laws. TRAP laws are a good example. NARAL reports TRAP as a binary variable. However, the Guttmacher Institute collects data on more aspects of TRAP laws.

55. Our data go through 2020 because NARAL Pro-Choice America, our principal source, did not issue an annual *Who Decides?* report in 2022 for 2021 data.

56. As of December 12, 2022 (Nash and Ephross 2022).

57. Montana voters "rejected a state measure that would have required providers to preserve the life of a fetus delivered alive after an abortion: the state already has a similar requirement in effect that applies to a viable premature infant" (Nash and Ephross 2022).

Chapter 4 · Politics across the States

1. The Squire index (Weissert and Weissert 2019; Squire 2017) compares legislative professionalization in individual state legislatures with the US Congress, including days in session, professional staffing, and per diem rates. Professionalization impacts policy decisions, among them greater investments in higher education and more ability to mediate policy disputes (Squire 2017).

2. To grant permission to a woman to have a legal abortion, the local hospital board, consisting of two physicians, had to determine that one of four conditions existed: rape, grave risk to the woman's health, incest, or the likelihood of the fetus having a grave physical or mental defect. For rape, the woman requesting the abortion had to present "an affidavit that she has been raped and that the rape has been or will be reported" to police (Sutin 1970, 614). For the woman's health rationale, the hospital board had to decide if continuation of the pregnancy would put the woman's health at grave risk. For incest, the law provided no explicit directions. For fetal defects, the board had to determine if the pregnancy were carried to term, "the child would probably have a grave physical or mental defect" (NARAL 1989, 62; Sutin 1970).

3. Also confirmed by a state court that most sections were unconstitutional (Murguia 2018).

4. The New Mexico house and senate both had Democratic majorities, and Democrat Michelle Lujan Grisham was governor.

5. A political committee with ties to a national Democratic group launched a TV ad targeting Rochetti's abortion stance. A political committee affiliated with the Republican Governors' Association launched ads critical of Lujan Grisham (Boyd 2022b).

6. For first-trimester abortion, "routine ultrasound is not considered medically necessary" (Guttmacher 2022f).

7. Gormley uses the term *citizens groups* to refer to advocacy groups with considerable grassroots involvement.

8. Of the 50 states, only Nebraska has a unicameral legislature. Included in our analysis is the District of Columbia, which also has a single legislative house, consisting of a 13-member council (Office of the City Administrator 2021).

9. Meghan McGuirk, Counsel and Manager, State Legislative Affairs, NARAL Pro-Choice America (personal communication, 2021): "*Who Decides* includes political information about whether governors and legislative bodies support reproductive freedom, oppose reproductive freedom, or have a mixed record on reproductive freedom. In making the determination for state governors, NARAL Pro-Choice America evaluates each governor's stance on reproductive freedom by considering their voting and signing record, public statements, and other indications of their stance on reproductive freedom. We consider whether the governor supports the right to abortion, restrictions on abortion care, and access to contraception. For legislatures, we evaluate the likelihood that chambers will pass bills that would expand or restrict reproductive freedom. We consider the outcome of

elections, bills previously passed by the chambers, and public statements to make this determination."

10. In Nebraska, "where the legislature is unicameral, legislators are elected on a non-partisan basis" (Center for American Women and Politics 2021).

11. This group "publishes and sends to the states a yearly briefing book suggesting language for bills. AUL Model Legislation and Legislative Guides are available on-line" (Goldman 2021, 99).

12. Lobbying tactics include testimony at legislative or agency hearings, direct contacts of legislators or other officials, informal contacts of legislators or other officials, presenting research results, working in coalitions to influence government officials, mass media, policy formation (drafting regulations, shaping policy implementation, serving on advisory commissions, and agenda-setting), constituent influence, litigation, elections, protests or demonstrations, and other tactics (Baumgartner and Leech 1998, Table 8.1, 152).

13. State-level expenditures were available for 1988–2020 for major anti-abortion interest groups (e.g., Susan B. Anthony and Right to Life or For Life organizations) and prominent pro-choice interest groups (e.g., Emily's List, NARAL Pro-Choice America, and pro-choice organizations).

14. Pew Research Center measures religiosity with an index that combines "four individual measures of religious observance—self-assessment of religion's importance in one's life, religious attendance, frequency of prayer, and belief in God. Respondents are assigned a score of 1 on each of the four measures on which they exhibit a high level of religious observance, a score of 0 on each of the measures on which they exhibit a medium level of religious observance, and a score of –1 on each measure on which they exhibit a low level of religious observance" (Lipka and Wormald 2016).

15. Only state political expenditure data for interest groups focusing on abortion policy were included in our analysis; many other broader groups donate funds and other resource to state abortion politics (Diep 2019).

Chapter 5 · After the Policymakers Go Home

1. An alternative arrangement would be an agreement with another physician who has admitting privileges at a local hospital (Guttmacher Institute 2022j).

2. Numerous "medical groups, including the American College of Obstetricians and Gynecologists, have asserted that both the ASC and the admitting privileges requirements do not have an impact on patient safety, but have as their sole purpose the closing of clinics" (Joffe 2018, 4).

3. Pennsylvania does not fund abortions for Medicaid-eligible women, except in cases of life endangerment, rape, or incest. The state "forbids health plans offered in the state's health exchange under the Affordable Care Act" to cover abortion except for life endangerment, rape, or incest, unless individuals purchase an optional rider at an additional cost. The same restrictions apply to health insurance for Pennsylvania's public employees (Guttmacher Institute 2022h).

4. Arizona's Republican attorney general also tried to enforce an 1864 pre-statehood law criminalizing most abortions, but the Arizona Court of Appeals blocked this attempt (Associated Press 2022a).

5. The CDC reported a total of 620,327 abortions for 2020, and the Guttmacher Institute reported 930,160. The CDC count was about 67 percent of the Guttmacher count. Similarly, the CDC reported a total of 612,719 abortions in 2017 and the Guttmacher Institute reported 862,320. Therefore, the CDC's count was 71.05 percent of the Guttmacher count.

6. We continue the time trend to 2020 using the 2017 provider data—the most recent consistent data available from the Guttmacher Institute.

7. Health insurance marketplaces are state or federal marketplaces, created by the Affordable Care Act, that offer health insurance plans (Kaiser Family Foundation 2013).

8. Demand restrictions include abortions banned after viability, abortions banned after a certain number of weeks, no abortion funding for low-income women, parental consent, parental notification, ban on private insurance coverage of abortion, mandatory counseling, required waiting periods, allowing medical personnel to opt out of abortion services, state health exchange forbidding abortion coverage, state funding crisis pregnancy services, abortion coverage forbidden for state employees, state requiring discussion of possibility of reversing medication abortion, bans on abortion during COVID-19, sonogram being required, and telemedicine abortion prohibited.

9. Supply restrictions include TRAP laws, TRAP laws requiring hospital privileges, TRAP laws requiring abortion be performed in a hospital, bans on certain abortion procedures, and bans on abortion sought for specific reason.

10. Protections include state requirements that private insurance cover abortion, state measures to protect providers, state funding for low-income women, abortion access protected during COVID-19, expanded roles for mid-level practitioners in provision of abortion services, expanded surgical role for mid-level practitioners in the provision of abortion services, state codified a woman's right to choose, state measures to facilitate access to emergency contraception, state constitution provides greater protection for right to choose than United States, and state supreme court has held that state constitution protects abortion separate from federal constitution.

11. This measure includes whether the state has different regulations for abortion providers than other types of medical facilities (reported as a binary variable by NARAL), whether physicians are required to have local hospital privileges (reported by Guttmacher), and whether even early abortions are restricted to hospitals or other specialized facilities.

12. Despite the substantial impact of state TRAP laws, we are unaware of any database or newsletter reports on levels of enforcement or compliance.

13. States that require ASC to perform abortions do not require other outpatient facilities offering services with comparable procedural complexity to be ASCs. The 2016 *Whole Woman* opinion noted that neither colonoscopies nor outpatient liposuction, both of which have much higher mortality rates, were required to be conducted in ASCs (Joffe 2018, 4).

Chapter 6 · How Abortion Is Regulated in Western Europe

1. The status and history of abortion in Northern Ireland is complicated. Until 2018, the practice of abortion in Northern Ireland was governed by the 1861 Offenses Against the Person Act enacted by the British Parliament. When Great Britain changed its laws to legalize abortion in 1967, the reformed law did not extend to Northern Ireland: "Successive governments in Northern Ireland never changed the 1861 law, so this arcane and draconian abortion law stayed on the books" (Glennie et al. 2021, 8–9).

In 2015, the Belfast High Court "deemed Northern Ireland's abortion law contrary to the right to respect one's private and family life under Article 8 of the European Convention on Human Rights. In 2018, the U.K. Supreme Court ruled that Northern Ireland's near-total abortion ban violated women's rights and was a breach of human rights. . . . In October 2019, abortion was decriminalized and became lawful in Northern Ireland by the force of U.K. law" (Glennie et al. 2021, 8–9). Despite the change in the law, setting up abortion services in Northern Ireland has been very slow. During the COVID-19 pandemic, the British government provided funding for women in Northern Ireland to travel to England for abortion services (McCormack 2022; Glennie et al. 2021).

2. Following "the introduction of the constitutional prohibition on abortion in 1983, anti-abortion activists began targeting groups and organizations that provided women with information about abortion clinics in Britain" (Gilmartin and Kennedy 2019, 129).

3. This estimate is based on 25 years, 1993–2018, with an estimated 6,000 Irish women a year traveling out of country, mostly to the United Kingdom, to obtain abortion services. Because annual estimates are based on women who provide Irish addresses, this is surely an undercount.

4. Thirty-Sixth Amendment of the Constitution Bill 2018 (RTE 2018).

5. The highest turnout for an Irish referendum, 70.88 percent, was for the 1972 question on joining the European Economic Community (McDonald et al. 2018).

6. Donagal voted 51.9 percent to retain the existing abortion policy (McDonald et al. 2018).

7. Over the "period 1972–2011, weekly church attendance by Irish Roman Catholics fell from 91% to 30%" (Faith Survey 2023).

8. The conclusion of medical mismanagement that led to Dr. Savita Halappanavar's death is documented in the 108-page report commissioned by the Galway Hospital and released in June 2013 (Republic of Ireland 2013).

9. Induced abortion was legalized in the Soviet Union and its allied countries well ahead of other countries (Kulczycki 2015, 176).

10. A minor was required to involve at least one parent in her decision to seek abortion (McFarlane 2015).

11. The data for most countries are from 2020, although the abortion rates from some countries are from 2018 (Denmark, Iceland, and Portugal) and 2019 (Finland, Norway, and Sweden) (Abort Report EU 2022).

12. Both age groups are available from the International Data Base of the US Census Bureau (2023b).

13. Informed consent also means that patients are told about the likely benefits of and the potential adverse effects of proposed procedures or medications.

14. In Germany, abortion counseling must be provided "quickly by specially trained professionals in state approved facilities free-of-charge. Women may obtain the required certificate, *Beratungsschein*, to show they have taken part in the counseling even if they have refused to talk about their reason(s) for the abortion" (International Planned Parenthood Federation 2019, 13).

15. By a special national agreement, there are no extra charges for abortion. This agreement includes women who reside in the country after having been denied a legal permit, making them ineligible for Norwegian national health insurance (International Planned Parenthood Federation 2019, 126).

16. Using the LMP adds about two weeks to a pregnancy because on average, ovulation and fertilization occur about two weeks after a woman's last menstrual period. For example, if the gestational limit is 12 weeks LMP, on average, a woman would have been pregnant for 10 weeks.

17. Countries can differ regarding their interpretations of what constitutes a fetal malformation: some nations restrict use to fatal fetal malformations only (International Planned Parenthood Federation 2019, 32).

18. The correlation is 0.48.

19. Here, we relied on a measure derived from the International Planned Parenthood Federation's 2019 country reports, which was whether the person filling out the country report thought that there were sufficient and willing service providers. Answers ranged from strongly agree to strongly disagree, but there were no benchmarks for helping country respondents complete that answer. Consequently, these answers can be viewed as subjective; the relationship between available service providers and the abortion rate merits further exploration.

20. Malta and Andorra are not included among the 18 because abortion is illegal in those countries.

Chapter 7 · The *Dobbs* Decision and Beyond

1. US Supreme Court. 2022. *Dobbs v. Jackson Women's Health Organization*, No. 19–1392 (597 U.S. ___ (2022).

2. Linda Greenhouse (2022) forcefully argued that religious doctrine, not the Constitution, drove the *Dobbs* decision. This argument is consistent with morality politics.

3. When serving on the Third District Court of Appeals, Judge Alito was the only judge to support the state of Pennsylvania in the *Casey* decision, which was appealed to the US Supreme Court. When serving on the district court, he was the only judge to support Pennsylvania's spousal consent requirement, a provision that was struck down by the US Supreme Court in the *Casey* decision (Ziegler 2020). Before Alito's nomination to the US Supreme Court, he had already written that the Constitution provided no right to abortion. In 2006, he was confirmed 52–48, but opposed by the American Civil Liberties Union. This was only the third time that the ACLU had opposed a nominee to the US Supreme Court (Romero 2006).

4. Chapter 4 explains that the Tennessee trigger law, for example, had a 30-day period before the law would be implemented (Farmer 2022).

5. Ectopic pregnancies are never viable and can be fatal for the woman if not treated (Mayo Clinic 2022).

6. Between April and August 2022, North Carolina had a 37 percent rise in abortions (Kelly 2023; Society of Family Planning 2023.)

7. In 2023, the federal poverty level was $14,580 for a family of one and $30,000 for a family of four (US Department of Health and Human Services 2023).

8. Assuming they have one or two children, 25 percent of abortion patients have annual household incomes between $19,720 and $60,000 (US Department of Health and Human Services 2023). Most abortion patients have lower incomes.

9. California enacted in 2022 (Beam 2022; Kyrylenko 2022). Illinois enacted in 2019 (Casetext 2022). New York enacted in 2021 (New York State Senate 2021). Oregon enacted in 2019 (Oregon State Health Authority 2023).

10. This proposed law would have criminalized health care providers who did not make every effort to save the life of an infant "born during an attempted abortion" or after labor or C-section. Doctors were concerned that the law would have limited palliative care for infants who were born but would not survive (*New York Times* 2022a).

Conclusion

1. Abortion is free of charge for some groups. German health insurance does cover the entire cost of abortion for women under a certain income level. For women in a higher economic bracket, German health insurance covers abortions only for medical indications and rape (International Planned Parenthood Federation 2019, 86).

2. Morality politics includes issues of life and death (abortion, capital punishment, and assisted suicide), gender and sexuality (transgender rights and pornography), addictive behavior (drugs and gambling), and self-determination or rights (gun policy and religious education).

3. The idea of abortion regret came directly from an amicus brief filed by "the conservative and religiously inspired Justice Foundation" (Ehrlich and Doan 2019, 123–124).

4. Emergency contraception and intrauterine devices (IUDs) are two of the methods that have been considered (Luthra 2022b).

Abort Report EU. 2022. "European Data." Excelgyn. https://abort-report.eu/europe.

ACLU (American Civil Liberties Union). 2003. "Timeline of Important Reproductive Freedom Cases Decided by the Supreme Court." https://www.aclu.org/documents/timeline-important-reproductive-freedom-cases-decided-supreme-court.

ACLU (American Civil Liberties Union). 2006. "Questions and Answers about the Supreme Court's Decision in *Ayotte v. Planned Parenthood of Northern New England, et al.*" January 19, 2006. https://www.aclu.org/documents/questions-and-answers-about-supreme-courts-decision-ayotte-v-planned-parenthood-northern-new.

ACLU (American Civil Liberties Union). 2021. "FDA Announces Long Sought-After Review of Harmful Restrictions on Medication Abortion." ACLU Press Release, May 7, 2021. https://www.aclu.org/press-releases/fda-announces-long-sought-after-review-harmful-restrictions-medication-abortion.

ACLU (American Civil Liberties Union). 2022. "About the ACLU Reproductive Freedom Project." https://www.aclu.org/other/about-aclu-reproductive-freedom-project.

ACLU Kentucky. 2023. "*EMW Women's Surgical Center v. Daniel Cameron*—Challenge to Kentucky Abortion Bans." https://www.aclu-ky.org/en/kyabortioncare.

Adam, Christian, Christoph Knill, and Emma T. Budde. 2020. "How Morality Politics Determine Morality Policy Output—Partisan Effects on Morality Policy Change." *European Journal of Public Policy* 27 (7): 1015–1033. https://doi.org/10.1080/13501763.2019.1653954.

Adams, Jill E., and Jessica Arons. 2014–2015. "A Travesty of Justice: Revisiting *Harris v. McRae.*" *William & Mary Journal of Women & Law* 21 (1): 3. https://scholarship.law.wm.edu/wmjowl/vol21/iss1/3.

Ahmed, Azizz. 2020. "Symposium: Ginsburg's Abortion Jurisprudence Prioritized Women's Health." *SCOTUS Blog* (blog), October 13, 2020. https://www.scotusblog.com/2020/10/symposium-ginsburgs-abortion-jurisprudence-prioritized-womens-health.

Aiken, Abigail R. A., Evdokia P. Romanova, Julia R. Morber, and Rebecca Gomperts. 2022a. "Safety and Effectiveness of Self-Managed Medication Abortion Provided Using Online Telemedicine in the United States: A Population Based Study." *The Lancet Regional Health - Americas* 10 (June): 1–8. https://doi.org/10.1016/j.lana.2022.100200.

Aiken, Abigail R. A., Jennifer E. Starling, Rebecca Gomperts, Mauricio Tec, James G. Scott, and Catherine E. Aiken. 2020a. "Demand for Self-Managed Online Telemedicine Abortion in the United States during the Coronavirus Disease 2019 (COVID-19) Pandemic." *Obstetrics and Gynecology* 136, no. 4 (October): 835–837. https://doi.org/10.1097/AOG.0000000000004081.

Aiken, Abigail R. A., Jennifer E. Starling, James G. Scott, and Rebecca Gomperts. 2022b. "Association of Texas Senate Bill 8 with Requests for Self-Managed Medication

Abortion." *JAMA Network Open* 5, no. 2 (February): e221122. https://doi.org/10.1001/jamanetworkopen.2022.1122.

Aiken, Abigail R. A., Jennifer E. Starling, James G. Scott, and Rebecca Gomperts. 2022c. "Requests for Self-Managed Medication Abortion Provided Using Online Telemedicine in 30 US States before and after the *Dobbs v Jackson Women's Health Organization* Decision." *JAMA* 328, no. 17 (November 1), 1768–1770. https://doi.org/10.1001/jama.2022.18865.

Aiken, Abigail R. A., Jennifer E. Starling, Alexandra van der Wal, Sascha van der Vliet, Kathleen Broussard, Dana M. Johnson, Elisa Padron, Rebecca Gomperts, and James G. Scott. 2020b. "Demand for Self-Managed Medication Abortion through an Online Telemedicine Service in the United States." *American Journal of Public Health* 110, no. 1 (January): 90–97. https://ajph.aphapublications.org/doi/10.2105/AJPH.2019.305369.

Ainsworth, Scott H., and Thad E. Hall. (2011). *Abortion Politics in Congress; Strategic Incrementalism and Policy Change.* New York: Cambridge University Press.

Alan Guttmacher Institute. 1976. "Supreme Court Says Spouse, Parent Can't Block Abortion." *Family Planning and Population Reporter* 5 (4): 1–3.

Alan Guttmacher Institute. 1977. "States Can Deny Medicaid Benefits Hospital Services for Elective Abortions." *Family Planning and Population Reporter* 6 (4): 41, 45.

Alan Guttmacher Institute. 1978. *Family Planning, Contraception, Voluntary Sterilization, and Abortion: An Analysis of Laws and Policies in the United States, Each State and Jurisdiction.* Publication No. (HSA)79–5623. Washington, DC: US Department of Health, Education, and Welfare.

Alan Guttmacher Institute. 1979. "Supreme Court Gives Judges Say in Abortion for Minors." *Washington Memo*, July 6, 1979: 1.

Alan Guttmacher Institute. 1980. "Supreme Court Upholds Hyde Amendment." *Washington Memo*, July 4, 1980: 1.

Alan Guttmacher Institute. 1983a. "Supreme Court Decisions on Abortion." *Washington Memo*, June 22, 1983: 3.

Alan Guttmacher Institute. 1983b. "Supreme Court Reaffirms Right to Abortion, Strikes Down Local Restrictions." *Washington Memo*, June 22, 1983: 1–4.

Alan Guttmacher Institute. 1986. Supreme Court Reaffirms Abortion Right, Strikes 'Baby Doe' Rule." *Washington Memo*, June 16, 1986: 1–3.

Alan Guttmacher Institute. 1990. "Further Restrictions on Minors' Right to Abortion Allowed by Supreme Court." *Washington Memo*, July 5, 1990: 1–2.

Alan Guttmacher Institute. 1991a. "Abortion Issue Tests States, Congress, as High Court Continues to Back Away." *Washington Memo*, January 18, 1991: 1–2.

Alan Guttmacher Institute. 1991b. "Title X Program Faces Major Upheaval, as High Court Okays Ban on Abortion Speech." *Washington Memo*, May 29, 1991: 1–3.

Alan Guttmacher Institute. 1992. "Bare Court Majority Reaffirms *Roe*, but Standard for Reviewing State Laws Is Relaxed." *Washington Memo*, July 2, 1992: 1–3.

Alan Guttmacher Institute. 1994a. "President to Sign FACE Bill Aimed at Deterring Abortion Violence." *Washington Memo*, May 23, 1994: 1–2.

Alan Guttmacher Institute. 1994b. "Supreme Court Unanimously Okays Use of RICO to Combat Anti-Abortion Violence." *Washington Memo*, February 2, 1994.

Alan Guttmacher Institute. 1997. "High Court Okays Fixed Buffer Zone." *Washington Memo*, March 12, 1997: 4.

Allen, Marilee C., Pamela K. Donohue, and Amy E. Dusman, 1993. "The Limit of Viability–Neonatal Outcome of Infants Born at 22 to 25 Weeks Gestation." *New England Journal of Medicine* 329, no. 22 (November): 1597–1601. https://doi.org/10.1056/nejm199311253292201.

AlmostAttorneyatLaw. 2017. "The Appeal to Repeal: Analysis on Medical Law in Ireland."

February 22, 2017. https://almostattorneyatlaw.wordpress.com/2017/02/22/the-appeal-to
-repeal-irelands-abortion-campaigns/.

Altindag, Onur, and Ted Joyce. 2017. "Judicial Bypass for Minors Seeking Abortions in
Arkansas versus Other States." *American Journal of Public Health* 107, no. 8 (August):
1266–1271. https://doi.org/10.2105/ajph.2017.303822.

American Cancer Society. 2021. "What Is Informed Consent?" https://www.cancer.org
/treatment/treatments-and-side-effects/planning-managing/informed-consent/what
-is-informed-consent.html.

American College of Obstetricians and Gynecologists (ACOG). 2020a. "ACOG Suit
Petitions Court to Remove FDA's Burdensome Barriers to Reproductive Care During
COVID-19." *Advocacy and Health Policy*, May 27, 2020. https://www.acog.org/en/News
/News%20Releases/2020/05/ACOG%20Suit%20Petitions%20the%20FDA%20to%20
Remove%20Burdensome%20Barriers%20to%20Reproductive%20Care%20During%20
COVID-19.

American College of Obstetricians and Gynecologists (ACOG). 2020b. "Medication
Abortion up to 70 Days Gestation." *Practice Bulletin* 225 (October): 1–14. https://www
.acog.org/clinical/clinical-guidance/practice-bulletin/articles/2020/10/medication
-abortion-up-to-70-days-of-gestation.

American Medical Association. 2021. "Informed Consent." https://www.ama-assn.org
/delivering-care/ethics/informed-consent.

American National Election Studies. 2016. "2016 Time Series Study." Stanford, CA: Stanford
University, and Ann Arbor, MI: University of Michigan. https://electionstudies.org
/data-center/2016-time-series-study.

American National Elections Studies. 2020. "2020 Time Series Study." Stanford, CA: Stanford University, and Ann Arbor, MI: University of Michigan. https://electionstudies.org
/data-center/2020-time-series-study.

American National Election Studies. 2022. "Pilot Study (2022)." https://electionstudies.org
/data-center.

Americans United for Life (AUL). 2010–2021. *Defending Life*. Washington, DC: Americans
United for Life. https://aul.org/defendinglife.

Arizona Daily Independent News Network. 2022. "Court of Appeals Rules 15-Week Abortion Ban Is the Law in Arizona." December 30, 2022. https://arizonadailyindependent
.com/2022/12/30/court-of-appeals-rules-15-week-abortion-ban-is-the-law-in-arizona.

Associated Press. 2021. "New Mexico Governor Signs Bill to Preserve Abortion Rights."
U.S. News and World Report, February 26, 2021. https://www.usnews.com/news/best
-states/new-mexico/articles/2021-02-26/new-mexico-governor-signs-bill-to-preserve
-abortion-rights.

Associated Press. 2022a. "Court: Abortion Doctors Can't Be Charged Under Arizona Law."
U.S. News and World Report, December 30, 2022. https://www.usnews.com/news/us
/articles/2022-12-30/court-abortion-doctors-cant-be-charged-under-arizona-law.

Associated Press. 2022b. "Oklahoma Abortion Providers Still Inundated with Texas Women."
U.S. News and World Report, February 15, 2022. https://www.usnews.com/news/us
/articles/2022-02-15/oklahoma-abortion-providers-still-inundated-with-texas-women.

Associated Press. 2022c. "Texas Abortion Provider Wants to Relocate to New Mexico."
Albuquerque Journal, July 6, 2022, A-5. https://www.abqjournal.com/news/local/texas
-abortion-provider-wants-to-relocate-to-new-mexico/article_8fa5a12c-6492-5e2d-be81
-dadfe06bc0e1.html

Associated Press. 2023. "Post-*Roe*, Native Americans Face Even More Abortion Hurdles."
Native American News, February 17, 2023. https://www.al.com/native-american-news
/2023/02/post-roe-native-americans-face-even-more-abortion-hurdles.html.

Austin, Nicole, and Sam Harper. 2017. "Assessing the Impact of TRAP Laws on Abortion and Women's Health in the USA: A Systematic Review." *BMJ Sexual and Reproductive Health* 44: 128–134. http://dx.doi.org/10.1136/bmjsrh-2017-101866.

Baker, Carrie Ann. 2022. "Texas Woman Lizelle Herrera's Arrest Foreshadows Post-*Roe* Future." *Ms.*, April 16, 2022. https://msmagazine.com/2022/04/16/texas-woman-lizelle-herrera-arrest-murder-roe-v-wade-abortion.

Ballotpedia. 2020. "New Mexico Elections 2020." https://ballotpedia.org/New_Mexico_elections,_2020

Ballotpedia. 2022. "General Election for Governor of New Mexico." https://ballotpedia.org/Michelle_Lujan_Grisham.

Ballotpedia. 2023a. "Partisan Composition of Governors." https://ballotpedia.org/Partisan_composition_of_governors.

Ballotpedia. 2023b. "Partisan Composition of State Houses." https://ballotpedia.org/Partisan_composition_of_state_houses.

Ballotpedia. 2023c. "Partisan Composition of State Senates." https://ballotpedia.org/Partisan_composition_of_state_senates.

Barnes, Robert. 2020. "Supreme Court Says Employers May Opt out of Affordable Care Act's Birth Control Mandate over Religious, Moral Objections." *Washington Post*, July 8, 2020. https://www.washingtonpost.com/politics/courts_law/supreme-court-obamacare-birth-control-mandate/2020/07/08/0b38a352-c123-11ea-b4f6-cb39cd8940fb_story.html.

Barrow, Bill, and Geoff Mulvihill. 2023. "Democratic Governors Form Alliance on Abortion Rights." *Associated Press*, February 21, 2023. https://apnews.com/article/abortion-us-supreme-court-politics-texas-gavin-newsom-5db36213df3b4de5ad94ebbb53d01d30.

Baumgartner, Frank, and Beth L. Leech. 1998. *Basic Interests: The Importance of Politics and Groups in Political Science*. Princeton, NJ: Princeton University Press.

Bazelton, Emily. 2022a. "Good Morning. Women in States with Abortion Bans Are Turning to Telemedicine." *New York Times*, November 2, 2022. https://www.nytimes.com/2022/11/02/briefing/abortion-pills.html

Bazelton, Emily 2022b. "Risking Everything to Offer Abortions across State Lines." *New York Times*, October 4, 2022. https://www.nytimes.com/2022/10/04/magazine/abortion-interstate-travel-post-roe.html?te=1&nl=the-morning&emc=edit_nn_20221102.

Beam, Adam. 2022a. "California Governor Signs Law Making Abortions Cheaper." *AP News*, March 22, 2022. https://apnews.com/article/abortion-us-supreme-court-business-health-california-d4b58d86434c9c790b8bbfcb7240f2af.

Beam, Adam. 2022b. "California Lawmakers Vote to Make Abortion Cheaper." *NBC Bay Area*, March 17, 2022. https://www.nbcbayarea.com/news/california/california-lawmakers-vote-to-make-abortions-cheaper/2840598.

Beaumont, Hillary. 2022. "Canada and Mexico Prepare to Accept Americans Seeking Abortions." *The Guardian*, May 9, 2022. https://www.theguardian.com/us-news/2022/may/09/canada-mexico-abortions-american.

Benavides, Lucia. 2019. "Malta's Fledgling Movement for Abortion Rights." *The Atlantic*, July 14, 2019. https://www.theatlantic.com/international/archive/2019/07/maltas-abortion-rights/593845.

Bennett, Christina Marie. 2014. "Arizona House Passes Bill Allowing Unannounced Inspections of Abortion Clinics." *Live Action News*, March 7, 2014. https://www.liveaction.org/news/arizona-house-passes-bill-allowing-unannounced-inspections-of-abortion-clinics.

Benson, Clea. 2010. "A New Kind of Abortion Politics." *CQ Weekly Online*, March 29, 2010, 740–746. http://library.cqpress.com/cqmagazine/weeklyreport111-000003634203.

Berer, Marge. 2009. "Provision of Abortion by Mid-Level Providers: International Policy,

Practice, and Perspectives." *Bulletin of the World Health Organization* 87: 58–63. https://doi.org/10.2471/blt.07.050138.

Bernhard, Meg. 2019. "Andorra's Abortion Rights Revolution: Push to Legalize Abortion Could Tip Country into Constitutional Crisis, Opponents Say." *Politico*, October 22, 2019. https://www.politico.eu/article/andorras-abortion-rights-revolution.

Better Wyoming. 2022. "Wyoming Legislature Passes Law to Ban Abortion if *Roe v. Wade* Is Overturned." https://betterwyo.org/2022/03/11/wyoming-legislature-passes-law-to-ban-abortion-if-roe-v-wade-is-overturned.

Bhatia, Aatish, Claire Cain Miller, and Margot Sanger-Katz. 2022. "A Surge of Overseas Abortion Pills Blunted the Effects of State Abortion Bans." *New York Times*, November 1, 2022. https://www.nytimes.com/2022/11/01/upshot/abortion-pills-mail-overseas.html?action=click&pgtype=Article&state=default&module=styln-abortion-us&variant=show&region=MAIN_CONTENT_1&block=storyline_top_links_recirc.

Bhatia, Juhie, and Hajur Naili. 2015. "Part 5: Spain's Abortion Law under Threat Despite Rescue." *Women's Enews*, February 9, 2015. http://womensenews.org/story/abortion/150208/spains-abortion-law-under-threat-despite-rescue#.VbaUMPksDv7.

Biggs, M. Antonia, Heather Gould, and Diana G. Foster. 2013. "Understanding Why Women Seek Abortions in the US." *BMC Women's Health* 13 (29): 1–13. https://doi.org/10.1186/1472-6874-13-29.

Biggs, M. Antonia, Ushma D. Upadhyay, Charles E. McCulloch, and Diana G. Foster. 2017. "Women's Mental Health and Well-Being 5 Years after Receiving or Being Denied an Abortion: A Prospective, Longitudinal Cohort Study." *JAMA Psychiatry* 74 (2): 169–178. https://doi.org/10.1001/jamapsychiatry.2016.3478.

Blackman, Josh. (2021). "SCOTUS Stays Injunction in *FDA v. ACOG*." *The Volokh Conspiracy*, January 12, 2021. https://reason.com/volokh/2021/01/12/scotus-stays-injunction-in-fda-v-acog.

Bodkin, Sarah. 2021. "New Mexico Abortion Ban Repealed: Law Comes off the Books after More than a Half-Century." *Daily Lobo.com*, March 1, 2021. https://www.dailylobo.com/article/2021/03/new-mexico-abortion-ban-repealed.

Bojovic, Neva, Jovana Stanisljevic, and Guido Giunti. 2021. "The Impact of COVID-19 on Abortion Access: Insights from the European Union and the United Kingdom." *Health Policy (Amsterdam, Netherlands)* 125 (7): 841–858. https://doi.org/10.1016/j.healthpol.2021.05.005.

Boonstra, Heather D. 2010. "Off Base: The U.S. Military's Ban on Privately Funded Abortions." *Guttmacher Policy Review*, August 12, 2010. https://www.guttmacher.org/gpr/2010/08/base-us-militarys-ban-privately-funded-abortions.

Boonstra, Heather D. 2014. "What Is Behind the Declines in Teen Pregnancy Rates?" *Guttmacher Policy Review* 17, no. 3 (Summer): 15–21. https://www.guttmacher.org/sites/default/files/article_files/gpr170315.pdf.

Boucher, David. 2022. "Michigan Supreme Court Agrees to Take up Procedural Question in Whitmer Abortion Lawsuit." *Detroit Free Press*, May 20, 2022. https://www.freep.com/story/news/politics/2022/05/20/michigan-supreme-court-whitmer-1931-abortion-lawsuit/9857162002.

Bouie, Jamelle. 2022. "The Movement That Put Alito on the Court Isn't Finished." *New York Times*, May 10, 2022. https://www.nytimes.com/2022/05/10/opinion/if-you-think-republicans-will-stop-at-overturning-roe-you-arent-paying-attention.html?referringSource=articleShare.

Boyd, Dan. 2022a. "Governor Plans to Expand Abortion Access." *Albuquerque Journal*, August 31, 2022. https://www.abqjournal.com/news/local/governor-plans-to-expand-abortion-access/article_a6a8f937-b47c-57ce-9d79-af40f56eb7b8.html.

Boyd, Dan. 2022b. "Governor's Race Sets up Abortion as a Major Issue." *Albuquerque Journal*, July 12, 2022: A1, A7. https://www.abqjournal.com/news/local/governors-race -sets-up-abortion-as-a-major-issue/article_aacfcc61-8d43-547b-b395-f155733b2334.html.

Boyd, Dan. 2022c. "Governor Signs Order Shielding Abortion Access across State." *Albu-querque Journal*, June 28, 2022: A1, A2. https://www.abqjournal.com/news/local/lujan -grisham-issues-order-aimed-at-shielding-abortion-access-in-nm/article_5c94e0dd -d668-5d06-94f9-78c989546365.html.

Boyd, Dan. 2023. "Governor Signs Bill Shielding Health Care Providers amid Simmering Debate over Abortion." *Albuquerque Journal*, April 5, 2023, Updated June 7, 2023. https:// www.abqjournal.com/news/local/governor-signs-bill-shielding-health-care-providers -amid-simmering-debate-over-abortion/article_2b97f074-f66e-5e60-951c-8447d1986d1b .html.

British Pregnancy Advisory Service. 2015. "Viability of Extremely Premature Babies." https://www.bpas.org/get-involved/campaigns/briefings/premature-babies.

Brodie, Janet Farrell. 1994. *Contraception and Abortion in Nineteenth Century America.* Ithaca, NY: Cornell University Press.

Broockman, David E., and Christopher Skovron. (2018). "Bias in Perceptions of Public Opinion among Political Elites." *American Political Science Review* 112 (3): 542–563. https://doi:10.1017/S0003055418000011.

Brown, Robert W., R. Todd Jewell, and Jeffery J. Rous. 2001. "Provider Availability, Race, and Abortion Demand." *Southern Economic Journal* 67, no. 3 (January): 656–671. https:// www.jstor.org/stable/1061456?seq=1.

Brummett, Asa. 2022. "Asa Tries a Little Nuance." *Arkansas Democrat Gazette*, May 26, 2022. https://www.arkansasonline.com/news/2022/may/26/asa-tries-a-little-nuance /?latest.

Bryant, Amy G., and Jonas J. Swartz. 2018. "Why Crisis Pregnancy Centers Are Legal but Unethical." *AMA Journal of Ethics* 20, no. 3 (March): 269–277. https://doi.org/10.1001 /journalofethics.2018.20.3.pfor1-1803.

Burgin, Eileen, and Jacqueline Bereznyak. 2013. "Compromising Partisan: Assessing Com-promise in Health Care Reform." *The Forum* 11, no. 2 (August): 209–241. https://doi.org /10.1515/for-2013-0037.

Burns, Max. 2020. "Will Amy Coney Barrett Finally Explain Her Ties to Anti-Gay Hate Group?" *Daily Beast*, October 13, 2020. https://www.thedailybeast.com/can-supreme -court-nominee-amy-coney-barrett-explain-ties-to-hate-group-that-backs-sterilizing -trans-people.

Candal, Carolina Costa. (2020). "Abortion." In *Legislating Morality in America: Debating the Morality of Controversial Laws and Policies*, edited by Donald P. Haider-Markel, 1–7. Santa Barbara, CA: ABC-CLIO.

Candelaria, Estevan. 2022. "Swift Reaction to *Roe* Ruling in New Mexico." *Albuquerque Journal*, June 25, 2022. https://www.abqjournal.com/news/local/swift-reaction-in-new -mexico-to-ruling/article_24e5397d-4f3f-5cc6-a9b2-7139012c6b20.html.

Capello, Olivia. 2020. "Surveying State Executive Orders Impacting Reproductive Health During the COVID-19 Pandemic." New York: Guttmacher Institute. https://www .guttmacher.org/article/2020/07/surveying-state-executive-orders-impacting -reproductive-health-during-covid-19.

Carnegie, Anna, and Rachel Roth. 2019. "From the Grassroots to the Oireachtas: Abortion Law Reform in the Republic of Ireland." *Health and Human Rights Journal* 21, no. 2 (December): 109–120. https://www.hhrjournal.org/2019/12/from-the-grassroots-to-the -oireachtas-abortion-law-reform-in-the-republic-of-ireland.

Camobreco, John F., and Michelle A. Barnello. 2008. "Democratic Responsiveness and

Policy Shock: The Case of State Abortion Policy." *State Politics and Policy Quarterly* 8 (1): 48–65. https://doi.org/10.1177/1532440008000800104.

Carroll, Rory. 2022. "Abortion Services in Northern Ireland Almost Nonexistent despite Legalisation." *The Guardian U.S. Edition*, May 4, 2022. https://www.theguardian.com /world/2022/may/04/abortion-services-in-northern-ireland-almost-nonexistent-despite -legalisation.

Carroll, Susan. J., and Sanbonmatsu, Kira. 2013. *More Women Can Run: Gender and Pathways to the State Legislatures*. New York: Oxford University Press.

Casetext. 2022. "Section 215 ILCS 5/356z.4a—Coverage for Abortion." Accessed June 12, 2022. https://casetext.com/statute/illinois-compiled-statutes/regulation/chapter-215 -insurance/act-5-illinois-insurance-code/article-xx-accident-and-health-insurance /section-215-ilcs-5356z4a-coverage-for-abortion.

CBS New York Team. 2022. "Connecticut Gov. Ned Lamont Signs Abortion Rights Bill Aimed at Protecting Patients and Providers." *CBS News New York*, May 10, 2022. https:// www.cbsnews.com/newyork/news/connecticut-gov-ned-lamont-to-sign-abortion-rights -bill.

CDC Foundation. 2023. "What Is Public Health?" Atlanta: CDC Foundation. https://www .cdcfoundation.org/what-public-health.

Center for American Women and Politics. 2021. "Women in State Legislatures 2021." New Brunswick, NJ: Rutgers Eagleton Institute of Politics. https://cawp.rutgers.edu/women -state-legislature-2021.

Center for Reproductive Rights. 2021. "Major Medical Groups Amicus Brief in *Dobbs v. Jackson Women's Health*." September 21, 2021. https://reproductiverights.org/major -medical-groups-amicus-brief-in-dobbs-v-jackson-womens-health.

Center for Reproductive Rights. 2022a. "*Dobbs v. Jackson Women's Health Organization*: The Case in Depth." https://reproductiverights.org/case/scotus-mississippi-abortion -ban/dobbs-jackson-womens-health.

Center for Reproductive Rights. 2022b. "Historians Amicus Brief in *Dobbs v. Jackson Women's Health*." https://reproductiverights.org/historians-amicus-brief-in-dobbs-v -jackson-womens-health.

Centers for Disease Control and Prevention. 2021. "Reproductive Health, Data and Statistics, Abortion." Atlanta: Centers for Disease Control and Prevention.

Chacon, Daniel. 2021. "Repeal of Anti-Abortion Law among First Orders of Business for New Mexico Lawmakers." *Santa Fe New Mexican*, January 20, 2021, updated January 21, 2021. https://www.santafenewmexican.com/news/legislature/repeal-of-anti-abortion -law-among-first-orders-of-business-for-new-mexico-lawmakers/article_4942ca98-5b3c -11eb-8332-1b43b1a55ca2.html.

Chavez, Nicole. 2021. "Texas Woman Died after an Unsafe Abortion Years Ago. Her Daughter Fears Same Thing May Happen Again." *CNN*, October 11, 2021. https://www .cnn.com/2021/10/11/us/texas-abortion-rosie-jimenez/index.html.

Cheung, Kylie. 2018. "It's Official: Abortion Is More Regulated than Any Other Health Care Service." *Ms.*, February 28, 2018. https://msmagazine.com/2018/02/28/abortion-is -more-regulated-than-any-other-health-care-service-according-to-study-stating-the -obvious.

Childs, Sarah, and Mona L. Krook. 2008. "Critical Mass Theory and Women's Political Representation." *Political Studies* 56 (3): 725–736. https://doi.org/10.1111/j.1467-9248 .2007.00712.x.

Childs, Sarah, and Mona L. Krook. 2009. "Analysing Women's Substantive Representation: From Critical Mass to Critical Actors." *Government Opposition* 44 (2): 125–145. https:// doi.org/10.1111/j.1477-7053.2009.01279.x.

Chotiner, Isaac. "A Supreme Court Reporter Defines the Threat to Abortion Rights." *The New Yorker*, May 14, 2019. https://www.newyorker.com/news/q-and-a/a-supreme-court-reporter-defines-the-threat-to-abortion-rights.

Cohen, David S., Greer Donelly, and Rachel Rebouche. 2022. "The New Abortion Battleground." *Columbia Law Review* 122 (1): 1–100. https://www.jstor.org/stable/27191233.

Cohen, David S., and Carole Joffe. 2020. *Obstacle Course: The Everyday Struggle to Get An Abortion in America. Berkeley, CA*: University of California Press.

Coi, Giovanna. 2022. "Abortion Laws in Europe in 4 Charts: Malta Is the Only EU Country with a Total Ban on Abortion, While Poland Controversially Imposed a Near-Total Ban in 2020." *Politico*, May 3, 2022. https://www.politico.eu/article/abortion-chart-world-map-europe-law-illegal-roe-v-wade-legislation.

Collins, Gail. 2022. "Don't Be Fooled. It's All About Women and Sex." *New York Times*, May 11, 2022. https://www.nytimes.com/2022/05/11/opinion/roe-v-wade-senate.html?referringSource=articleShare.

Colman, Silvie, and Ted Joyce. 2011. "Regulating Abortion: Impact on Patients and Providers in Texas," *Journal of Policy Analysis and Management* 30 (4): 775–797. https://doi.org/10.1002/pam.20603.

Congress.gov. 2004. *S.3—Partial-Birth Abortion Ban Act of 2003 108th Congress (2003–2004)*. https://www.congress.gov/bill/108th-congress/senate-bill/3.

Congressional Quarterly. 1993. "Ruling Favors Blockaders." *CQ Weekly*, January 16, 1993: 130. http://library.cqpress.com/cqmagazine/WR103409500.

Cooperative Congressional Election Study (CCES). 2016. Cambridge, MA: Harvard University. https://cces.gov.harvard.edu.

Cornell Law School. 2014. "*Burwell v. Hobby Lobby Stores, Inc.*" https://www.law.cornell.edu/supremecourt/text/13-354.

Cornell Law School. 2016. "*Whole Woman's Health v. Hellerstedt.*" https://www.law.cornell.edu/supct/pdf/15-274.pdf.

Cornell Law School. 2019. "*Box v. Planned Parenthood of Indiana and Kentucky, Inc.*" https://www.law.cornell.edu/supremecourt/text/18-483.

Cornell Law School. 2022. "Tenth Amendment." Legal Information Institute. https://www.law.cornell.edu/constitution/tenth_amendment.

Cornell Law School. 2023. "*per curiam.*" Legal Information Institute. https://www.law.cornell.edu/wex/per_curiam.

Costhelper.com. 2021. "Birth Control Pills Cost: How Much Do Birth Control Pills Cost?" https://health.costhelper.com/birth-control-pills.html#extres1.

Cruickhank, Saralyn. 2022. "Inside the *Dobbs* Decision: Interview with Joann Rosen." *Johns Hopkins Magazine*, July 1, 2022. https://hub.jhu.edu/2022/07/01/joanne-rosen-insight-dobbs-decision.

Dalby, Douglas. 2013a. "Irish Government Apologizes in Laundry Scandal." *New York Times*, February 19, 2013. https://www.nytimes.com/2013/02/20/world/europe/irish-government-expected-to-apologize-in-laundry-scandal.html.

Dalby, Douglas. 2013b. "Irish Premier's Apology Fails to Appease Workhouse Survivors." *New York Times*, February 5, 2013. https://www.nytimes.com/2013/02/06/world/europe/ireland-magdalene-institutions-report.html?_r=0.

Daniels, Cynthia R., Janna Ferguson, Grace Howard, and Amanda Roberti. 2016. "Informed or Misinformed Consent." *Journal of Health Politics, Policy, & Law* 41 (2): 181–209. https://doi.org/10.1215/03616878-3476105.

de Graaf, Mia Anna, Medaris Miller, and Taiyler Simone Mitchell. 2022. "Missouri Seeks to Ban Abortion for Ectopic Pregnancies, with a Penalty of up to 30 Years in Prison." *Yahoo News*, March 11, 2022. https://news.yahoo.com/missouri-seeks-ban-abortion-even-182634595.html.

Dehlendorf, Christine, Lisa H. Harris, and Tracy A. Weitz. 2013. "Disparities in Abortion Rates: A Public Health Approach." *American Journal of Public Health* 103, no. 10 (October 2013): 1772–1779. https://ajph.aphapublications.org/doi/10.2105/AJPH.2013 .301339.

Dehlendorf, Christine, and Tracy A. Weitz. 2011. "Access to Abortion Services: A Neglected Health Disparity." *Journal of Health Care for the Poor and Underserved* 22, no. 2 (May): 415–421. https://doi.org/10.1353/hpu.2011.0064.

Demirjian, Karoun. 2023. "House Narrowly Passes Defense Bill, Setting up Showdown over Social Issues." *New York Times*, July 14, 2023. https://www.nytimes.com/2023/07/14/us /politics/defense-bill-house-ndaa.html?action=click&pgtype=Article&state=default &module=styln-new-congress&variant=show&region=MAIN_CONTENT_1&block =storyline_top_links_recirc.

Democratic National Committee. 2020. "Party Platform." https://democrats.org/where-we -stand/party-platform.

Denton, Hazel. 2015. "Benefits of Family Planning." Chapter 8 in *Global Population and Reproductive Health*, edited by Deborah R. McFarlane, 199–221. Burlington, MA: Jones and Bartlett Learning.

Department of Health and Social Care. 2019. "Abortion Statistics, England and Wales: 2019." National Statistics. https://assets.publishing.service.gov.uk/government/uploads /system/uploads/attachment_data/file/891405/abortion-statistics-commentary-2019 .pdf.

Department of Health and Social Care. 2020. "Abortion Statistics, England and Wales: 2020." National Statistics. https://www.gov.uk/government/statistics/abortion-statistics -for-england-and-wales-2020.

Descano, Steve. 2022. "My Governor Can Pass Bad Abortion Laws. But I Won't Enforce Them." *New York Times*, May 31, 2022. https://www.nytimes.com/2022/05/31/opinion /prosecutor-abortion-virginia.html?referringSource=articleShare.

Diamont, Jeff, and Aleksandra Sandstrom. 2020. "Do State Laws on Abortion Reflect Public Opinion?" Washington, DC: Pew Research Center, January 21, 2020. https://www.pew research.org/fact-tank/2020/01/21/do-state-laws-on-abortion-reflect-public-opinion.

Diep, Francie. 2019. "Why Pro-Choice Groups Vastly Outspend Pro-Life Groups in Political Campaigns." *Pacific Standard*, May 23, 2019. https://psmag.com/social-justice/why-pro -choice-groups-vastly-outspend-pro-life-groups-in-political-campaigns.

Doan, Alesha. 2022. "The Kansas Abortion Vote Shows the Loudest Voices in This Debate Are Not Representative Ones." *BMJ* 378 (August): 2. https://doi.org/10.1136/bmj.o2024.

Doan, Alesha E., and Deborah R. McFarlane. 2012. "Saying No to Abstinence-Only Education: An Analysis of State Decision-Making." *Publius* 42, no. 4 (January): 613–635. https://doi.org/10.1093/publius/pjr052.

Dreweke, Joerg. 2015. "Abortion Reporting: Promoting Public Health, Not Politics." *Guttmacher Policy Review* 18 (2): 40–47. https://www.guttmacher.org/gpr/2015/06/abortion -reporting-promoting-public-health-not-politics.

Drucker, Dan. 1990. *Abortion Decisions of the Supreme Court 1973–1989: A Comprehensive Review with Historical Commentary*. Jefferson, NC: McFarland.

Durkee, Alison. 2023. "Abortion Pills: What to Know About Mifepristone as Biden Administration Defends It from Legal Attack." *Forbes*, February 24, 2023. https://www.forbes .com/sites/alisondurkee/2023/02/24/abortion-pills-what-to-know-about-mifepristone -as-biden-administration-defends-it-from-legal-attack.

Eggert, David. 2022. "Michigan Governor Sues to Secure Abortion Rights and Vacate 176-Year-Old Ban." *Los Angeles Times*, April 7, 2022. https://www.latimes.com/world-nation /story/2022-04-07/michigan-governor-sues-secure-abortion-rights.

El-Bawab, Nadine. 2022. "Tennessee 'Trigger' Law Banning Nearly All Abortions Goes into

Effect." *ABC News*, August 25, 2022. https://abcnews.go.com/US/tennessee-trigger-law
-banning-abortions-effect/story?id=88787662.

El-Sayd, Abdul. 2022. "Michigan Is Becoming the Ground Zero of Abortion Battles." *New
Republic*, May 18, 2022. https://newrepublic.com/article/166525/michigan-ground-zero
-abortion-battles.

Emba, Christine. 2022. "Abortion Feels Hyper-Polarized. But What if It's Not?" *Washington
Post*, May 15, 2022. https://www.washingtonpost.com/opinions/2022/05/13/abortion-roe
-polarization-high-conflict.

Erlich, J. Shoshanna. 2018. "Like a Withered Tree, Stripped of Its Foliage: What the *Roe*
Court Missed and Why It Matters." *Columbia Journal of Gender and Law* 35 (2): 175–227.
https://doi.org/10.7916/D8FV0355.

Erlich, J. Shoshanna, and Alesha E. Doan. 2019. *Abortion Regret: The New Attack on Reproductive Freedom*. Santa Barbara, CA: Praeger.

Espey, Eve, Sadia Haider, Joanne Stone, Cynthia Gyamfi-Bannerman, and Jody Steinauer.
2023. "Now Is The Time To Stand Up For Reproductive Justice and Abortion." *American Journal of Obstetrics and Gynecology* 228 (1): 48–52. https://doi.org/10.1016/j.ajog
.2022.07.033.

Executive Office of the Governor, Communications Division. 2022. "Governor Whitmer
Welcomes Preliminary Injunction against Michigan 1931 Law Criminalizing Abortion."
May 17, 2022. https://www.michigan.gov/whitmer/news/press-releases/2022/05/17
/governor-whitmer-welcomes-preliminary-injunction-against-michigan-1931-law
-criminalizing-abortion.

Faith Survey. n.d. "Irish Census (2016) Measuring Religious Adherence in Ireland."
Accessed April 16, 2022. https://faithsurvey.co.uk/irish-census.html.

Farmer, Blake. 2022. "What Would Happen in Tennessee If the Supreme Court Over-
turns Abortion Law?" *WKMS Morning Edition*, May 3, 2022. https://www.wkms.org
/government-politics/2022-05-03/what-would-happen-in-tennessee-if-the-supreme
-court-overturns-abortion-law.

Feminist Majority Foundation. 1993. "1993 National Clinic Violence Report." https://
feminist.org/our-work/national-clinic-access-project/monitoring-clinic-violence/1993
-national-clinic-violence-survey-report.

Feuer, Alan. 2021. "The Texas Abortion Law Creates a Kind of Bounty Hunter. Here's How
It Works." *New York Times*, September 10, 2021, updated November 1, 2021. https://www
.nytimes.com/2021/09/10/us/politics/texas-abortion-law-facts.html.

Finer, Lawrence B., Lori F. Frohwirth, Lindsay A. Dauphinee, Susheela Singh, and Ann M.
Moore. 2005. "Reasons U.S. Women Have Abortions: Quantitative and Qualitative
Perspectives." *Perspectives in Sexual and Reproductive Health* 37, no. 3 (September):
110–118. https://doi.org/10.1363/psrh.37.110.05.

Finer, Lawrence B., Lori F. Frohwirth, Lindsay A. Dauphinee, Susheela Singh, and Ann M.
Moore. 2006. "Timing of Steps and Reasons for Delays in Obtaining Abortions in the
United States." *Contraception* 74 (4): 334–344. https://doi.org/0.1016/j.contraception
.2006.04.010.

Finer, Lawrence B., and Stanley K. Henshaw. 2003. "Abortion Incidence and Services in the
United States in 2000." *Perspectives in Sexual and Reproductive Health* 35, no. 1 (January/
February): 6–15. https://doi.org/10.1111/j.1931-2393.2003.tb00079.x.

Finer, Lawrence B., and Stanley K. Henshaw. 2007. "Disparities in Rates of Unintended
Pregnancy in the United States, 1994 and 2001." *Perspectives on Sexual and Reproductive
Health* 38, no. 2 (January/February): 90–96. https://doi.org/10.1363/3809006.

Finer, Lawrence B., and Mia Zolna. 2016. "Declines in Pregnancy in the United States, 2008–
2011." *New England Journal of Medicine* 374, no. 9 (March 3): 843–852. https://www.nejm
.org/doi/10.1056/NEJMsa1506575.

Fontaine, Andie Sophia. 2019. "Iceland's New Abortion Law Goes into Effect Today." *Reykjavik Grapevine*, September 2, 2019. https://grapevine.is/news/2019/09/02/icelands -new-abortion-law-goes-into-effect-today.

Forman-Rabinovici, Aliza, and Udi Sommer. 2018. "An Impediment to Gender Equality?: Religion's Influence on Development and Reproductive Policy." *World Development* 105 (May): 48–58. https://doi.org/10.1016/j.worlddev.2017.12.024.

Foster, Diana Greene. 2020. *The Turnaway Study: Ten Years, a Thousand Women, and the Consequences of Having–or Being Denied–an Abortion.* New York: Scribner.

Fox, Dov, and Erin Cole. 2021. "The Supreme Court's Abortion Exceptionalism—Judicial Deference, Medical Science, and Mifepristone Access." *New England Journal of Medicine* 384, no. 24 (April): e94(1)–e94(2). https://doi.org/10.1056/nejmp2104461.

Frontera Fund. 2023. "About Us." Accessed June 28, 2023. https://fronterafundrgv.org /about-us.

Galea, Sandro, and Roger D. Vaughn. 2019. "Editorial: Public Health, Politics, and the Creation of Meaning: A Public Health of Consequence." *American Journal of Public Health* 109 (7): 966–967. https://doi.org/10.2105/AJPH.2019.305128.

Gallup. 2021. "Supreme Court." https://news.gallup.com/poll/4732/Supreme-Court.aspx.

Garcia-Ditta, Alexa. 2015. "Reckoning with Rosie." *Texas Observer*, November 3, 2015. https://www.texasobserver.org/rosie-jimenez-abortion-medicaid.

Garrow, David J. 1994. *Liberty and Sexuality: The Right to Privacy and the Making of Roe v. Wade.* New York: Macmillan.

Gaul, Moira. 2021. "Fact Sheet: Pregnancy Centers – Serving Women and Saving Lives (2020 Study)." Arlington, VA: Charlotte Lozier Institute. https://lozierinstitute.org /fact-sheet-pregnancy-centers-serving-women-and-saving-lives-2020.

Gerber, Brian J., and Paul Teske. 2000. "Regulatory Policymaking in the American States: A Review of Theories and Evidence." *Political Research Quarterly* 53, no. 4 (December): 849–866. https://doi.org/10.2307/449263.

Gerstein, Josh. 2022. "Conservative Lawyers Hail Alito for Abortion Ruling." *Politico*, November 11, 2022. https://www.politico.com/news/2022/11/11/alito-abortion-federalist -society-00066443.

Gerstein, Josh, and Alexander Ward. 2022. "Supreme Court Has Voted to Overturn Abortion Rights, Draft Opinion Shows." *Politico*, May 2, 2022. https://www.politico.com /news/2022/05/02/supreme-court-abortion-draft-opinion-00029473.

Gilmartin, Mary, and Sinead Kennedy. 2019. "A Double Movement: The Politics of Reproductive Mobility in Ireland." Chapter 5 in *Abortion across Borders*, edited by Christabelle Sethna and Gayle Davis, 123–143. Baltimore: Johns Hopkins University Press.

Githens, Marianne, and Dorothy E. McBride. 1996. *Abortion Politics: Public Policy in Cross Cultural Perspective.* New York: Routledge.

Gius, Mark. 2019. "Using the Synthetic Control Method to Determine the Effect of Ultrasound Laws on State-Level Abortion Rates." *Atlantic Economic Journal* 47, no. 2 (June): 205–215. https://doi.org/10.1007/s11293-019-09619-4.

Glennie, Madison, Lily Milwit, and Julie Zuckerbrod. 2021. "The World's Abortion Laws." Chapter 1 in *Who's Choice Is It? Abortion, Medicine, and the Law.* 7th ed., edited by David F. Walbert and J. Douglas Butler, 1–75. Chicago: American Bar Association.

Glenza, Jessica. 2022. "Oklahoma Republican-Led Legislature Passes Nation's Strictest Abortion Ban." *The Guardian*, May 19, 2022. https://www.theguardian.com/us-news /2022/may/19/oklahoma-abortion-ban-strictest.

Gold, Rachel Benson, and Elizabeth Nash. 2007. "State Abortion Counseling Policies and the Fundamental Principles of Informed Consent." *Guttmacher Policy Review* 10 (4): 6–13. https://www.guttmacher.org/sites/default/files/article_files/gpr100406.pdf.

Goldberg, Michelle. 2022. "An America Without *Roe v. Wade* Will Be a Dark Place." *New*

York Times, May 3, 2022. https://www.nytimes.com/2022/05/03/opinion/roe-v-wade
-america-future.html?action=click&module=RelatedLinks&pgtype=Article.

Goldman, Edward B. 2021. "Abortion Law in the United States." Chapter 2 in *Who's Choice Is It? Abortion, Medicine, and the Law*. 7th ed., edited by David F. Walbert and J. Douglas Butler, 77–119. Chicago: American Bar Association.

Gonzalez, Fidel, Troy Quast, and Alex Venanzi. 2020. "Factors Associated with the Timing of Abortions." *Health Economics* 29, 223–233. https://doi.org/10.1002/hec.3981.

Gormley, William T, Jr. 1986. "Regulatory Issue Networks in a Federal System." *Polity* 18, no. 4 (Summer): 595–620. https://doi.org/10.2307/3234884.

Government of Ireland. 2013. "Report of the Inter-Departmental Committee to Establish the Facts of State Involvement with the Magdalen Laundries." Dublin, Ireland: Department of Justice. February 5, 2013, last updated August 9, 2021. https://www.gov.ie/en /collection/a69a14-report-of-the-inter-departmental-committee-to-establish-the-facts -of/?referrer=http://www.justice.ie/en/JELR/Pages/MagdalenRpt20.

Government of Ireland. 2022. "Eighth Amendment of the Constitution Act, 1983." Dublin, Ireland: Office of the Attorney General. https://www.irishstatutebook.ie/eli/1983/ca/8 /schedule/enacted/en/html#sched-part1.

Grammich, Clifford, Kirk Hadaway, Richard Houseal, Dale E. Jones, Alexei Krindatch, Richie Stanley, and Richard H. Taylor. 2012. *2010 U.S. Religion Census: Religious Congregations & Membership Study*. Association of Statisticians of American Religious Bodies (ASARB). Kansas City, MO: Nazarene Publishing House. http://www.usreligion census.org/images/2010_US_Religion_Census_Introduction.pdf.

Grammich, Clifford, Kirk Hadaway, Richard Houseal, Dale E. Jones, Alexei Krindatch, Richie Stanley, and Richard H. Taylor. 2019. "Longitudinal Religious Congregations and Membership File, 1980–2010 (State Level)." https://www.thearda.com/Archive/Files /Descriptions/RCMSMGST.asp.

Greenhouse, Linda. 1999. "Justice Blackmun, Author of Abortion Right, Dies." *New York Times*, March 5, 1999. https://www.nytimes.com/1999/03/05/us/justice-blackmun-author -of-abortion-right-dies.html.

Greenhouse, Linda. 2022. "Religious Doctrine, Not the Constitution, Drove the *Dobbs* Decision." *New York Times*, July 22, 2022. https://www.nytimes.com/2022/07/22/opinion /abortion-religion-supreme-court.html?smid=nytcore-ios-share&referringSource =articleShare.

Grossman, Daniel, Kari White, Lisa Harris, Matthew Reeves, Paul D. Blumenthal, Beverly Winikoff, and David A. Grimes. 2015. "Continuing Pregnancy after Mifepristone and 'Reversal' of First-Trimester Medical Abortion: A Systematic Review." *Contraception* 92, no. 3 (September): 206–212. https://doi.org/10.1016/j.contraception.2015.06.001.

Guttmacher Institute. 2017. "Targeted Regulation of Abortion Providers." *State Laws and Policies* (as of December 1, 2017). Washington, DC: Guttmacher Institute.

Guttmacher Institute. 2019. "Unintended Pregnancy in the United States." *Fact Sheet*. https://www.guttmacher.org/fact-sheet/unintended-pregnancy-united-states.

Guttmacher Institute. 2021a. "Abortion Bans in Cases of Race or Sex Selection or Fetal Anomaly." *State Laws and Policies* (as of October 1). https://www.guttmacher.org/state -policy/explore/abortion-bans-cases-sex-or-race-selection-or-genetic-anomaly.

Guttmacher Institute. 2021b. "Abortion Reporting Requirements." *State Laws and Policies* (as of July 1). https://www.guttmacher.org/state-policy/explore/abortion-reporting -requirements.

Guttmacher Institute. 2021c. "Contraceptive Use in the United States by Method." *Fact Sheet* (as of May 21). https://www.guttmacher.org/fact-sheet/contraceptive-method -use-united-states.

Guttmacher Institute. 2022a "Abortion Policy in the Absence of *Roe*." *State Laws and*

Policies, April 4, 2022. https://www.guttmacher.org/state-policy/explore/abortion -policy-absence-roe.

Guttmacher Institute. 2022b. "'Choose Life' License Plates." *State Laws and Policies*, December 1, 2022. https://www.guttmacher.org/state-policy/explore/choose-life-license -plates.

Guttmacher Institute. 2022c. "Counseling and Waiting Periods for Abortion." *State Laws and Policies* (as of December 1). https://www.guttmacher.org/state-policy/explore /counseling-and-waiting-periods-abortion.

Guttmacher Institute. 2022d. "Countries." *Data Center*. https://data.guttmacher.org /countries.

Guttmacher Institute. 2022e. "An Overview of Consent to Reproductive Health Services by Young People." *State Laws and Policies* (as of December 1). https://www.guttmacher.org /state-policy/explore/overview-minors-consent-law.

Guttmacher Institute. 2022f. "Requirements for Ultrasound." *State Laws and Policies*. https://www.guttmacher.org/state-policy/explore/requirements-ultrasound.

Guttmacher Institute. 2022g. "State Bans on Abortion throughout Pregnancy." *State Laws and Policies*. https://www.guttmacher.org/state-policy/explore/state-policies-later -abortions.

Guttmacher Institute. 2022h. "State Facts about Abortion: Pennsylvania." *Fact Sheet* (June). https://www.guttmacher.org/fact-sheet/state-facts-about-abortion-pennsylvania.

Guttmacher Institute. 2022i. "State Facts about Abortion: Tennessee." *Fact Sheet* (January). https://www.guttmacher.org/fact-sheet/state-facts-about-abortion-tennessee.

Guttmacher Institute. 2022j. "Targeted Regulation of Abortion Providers." *State Laws and Policies*. https://www.guttmacher.org/state-policy/explore/targeted-regulation-abortion -providers.

Guttmacher Institute. 2023a. "Abortion Reporting Requirements." *State Laws and Policies* (as of January 1). https://www.guttmacher.org/state-policy/explore/abortion-reporting -requirements

Guttmacher Institute. 2023b. "Emergency Contraception." *State Laws and Policies* (as of January 1). https://www.guttmacher.org/state-policy/explore/emergency-contraception.

Guttmacher Institute. 2023c. "Medication Abortion." *State Laws and Policies* (as of June 1). https://www.guttmacher.org/state-policy/explore/medication-abortion.

Guttmacher Institute. 2023d. "An Overview of Abortion Laws," *State Laws and Policies* (as of June 1). https://www.guttmacher.org/state-policy/explore/overview-abortion-laws

Guttmacher Institute. 2023e. "Regulating Insurance Coverage of Abortion." *State Laws and Policies* (as of June 1). https://www.guttmacher.org/state-policy/explore/regulating -insurance-coverage-abortion.

Guttmacher Institute. 2023f. "State Funding of Abortion under Medicaid." *State Laws and Policies* (as of March 1, 2022). https://www.guttmacher.org/state-policy/explore/state -funding-abortion-under-medicaid.

Haas-Wilson, Deborah. 1993. "The Economic Impact of State Restrictions on Abortion: Parental Consent and Notification Laws and Medicaid Funding Restrictions." *Journal of Policy Analysis and Management* 12 (3): 498–511. https://doi.org/10.2307/3325303.

Haider-Markel, Donald P. 2020. *Legislating Morality in America: Debating the Morality of Controversial Laws and Policies*. Santa Barbara, CA: ABC-CLIO.

Hakim, Danny, and Douglas Dalby. 2015. "Ireland Votes to Approve Gay Marriage, Putting Country in Vanguard." *New York Times*, May 23, 2015. https://www.nytimes.com/2015 /05/24/world/europe/ireland-gay-marriage-referendum.html.

Halva-Neubauer, Glen A. 1990. "Abortion Policy in the Post-*Webster* Age." *Publius* 20, no. 3 (Summer), 27–44.

Hargis, Cydney, and Gideon Taaffe. 2022. "Fox News is downplaying the effects of over-

turning *Roe v. Wade.*" *Media Matters to America*, May 4, 2022. https://www.media
matters.org/fox-news/fox-news-downplaying-effects-overturning-roe-v-wade.

Harrison, Shane. 2013. "How Savita Halappanavar's Death Called Attention to Irish Abortion Law." *BBC News*, April 19, 2013. http://www.bbc.com/news/world-europe-22204377.

Harvard Law Review. 2018. *"National Institute of Family & Life Advocates v. Becerra*, Leading Case: 138 S. Ct. 2361." *Harvard Law Review* 132 (2018): 347–356. https://harvardlaw
review.org/2018/11/national-institute-of-family-life-advocates-v-becerra.

Henderson, Nia-Malika. 2014. "How Justice Ginsburg's *Hobby Lobby* Dissent Helps Shape
the Debate about Reproductive vs. Religious Rights." *Washington Post*, July 1, 2014.
https://www.washingtonpost.com/blogs/she-the-people/wp/2014/07/01/how-justice
-ginsburgs-hobby-lobby-dissent-helps-shape-the-debate-about-reproductive-and
-religious-rights.

Henshaw, Stanley K. 1998a. "Abortion Incidence and Services in the United States, 1995–
1996." *Family Planning Perspectives* 30 (6): 263–270, 287. https://doi.org/10.2307/2991501.

Henshaw, Stanley K. 1998b. "Unintended Pregnancy in the United States." *Family Planning
Perspectives* 30 (1): 24–29, 46.

Henshaw, Stanley K., Jacqueline D. Forrest, and Jennifer Van Vort. 1987. "Abortion Services
in the United States, 1984 and 1985." *Family Planning Perspectives* 19, no. 2 (March/
April): 63–70. https://pubmed.ncbi.nlm.nih.gov/3595820.

Henshaw, Stanley K., and Kathryn Kost. 2008. *Trends in the Characteristics of Women
Obtaining Abortions, 1974–2004.* New York: Guttmacher Institute. https://www.gutt
macher.org/sites/default/files/report_pdf/trendswomenabortions-wtables.pdf.

Henshaw, Stanley K., and Jennifer Van Vort. 1990. "Abortion Services in the United States,
1987 and 1988." *Family Planning Perspectives* 22 (2): 102–108, 142. https://www.jstor.org
/stable/2135639.

Henshaw, Stanley K., and Jennifer Van Vort. 1994. "Abortion Services in the United States,
1991 and 1992." *Family Planning Perspectives* 26 (3): 100–106, 112. http://www.jstor.org
/stable/2136033.

Hern, Warren. 2021. "Late Abortion: Clinical and Ethical Issues." Chapter 20 in *Who's
Choice Is It? Abortion, Medicine, and the Law.* 7th ed., edited by David F. Walbert and
J. Douglas Butler, 537–553. Chicago: American Bar Association.

HeyJane. 2023. "How Much Does an Abortion Cost in My State?" Accessed June 27, 2023.
https://www.heyjane.com/cost-of-abortion.

Hing, Anna K., Asha Hassan, and Rachel R. Hardeman. 2022. "Advancing the Measure-
ment of Structural Racism through the Lens of Antiabortion Policy." *American Journal
of Public Health* 112 (11): 1529–1531. https://doi.org/10.2105/AJPH.2022.307091.

Howe, Amy. 2021. "Court to Weigh in on Mississippi Abortion Ban Intended to Challenge
Roe v. Wade." *SCOTUS Blog* (blog), May 17, 2021. https://www.scotusblog.com/2021/05
/court-to-weigh-in-on-mississippi-abortion-ban-intended-to-challenge-roe-v-wade.

Htun, Mala, and S. Laurel Weldon. 2018. *Logics of Gender Justice: State Action on Women's
Rights Around the World.* Cambridge, UK: Cambridge University Press.

Idelson, Holly. 1994. "Supreme Court: Abortion Clinics Can Use RICO to Fight Violence."
CQ Weekly, January 29, 1994, 175. http://library.cqpress.com.libproxy.unm.edu/cq
magazine/WR103403454.

Institute of Medicine. 1988. "The Future of Public Health." Washington, DC: National
Academy Press.

International Planned Parenthood Federation. 2012. *Abortion Legislation in Europe.* Brussels, Belgium: IPPF European Network. http://www.ippfen.org/NR/rdonlyres/BB5E8
C4F-66B0-405E-9DD5-7E0614A5651C/0/Final_Abortionlegislation_May2012.pdf.

International Planned Parenthood Federation. 2019. *Abortion Legislation in Europe.*
Brussels, Belgium: IPPF European Network. https://europe.ippf.org/resource/ippf

-en-partner-survey-abortion-legislation-and-its-implementation-europe-and-central
-asia.

International Planned Parenthood Federation. 2020. "COVID-19 Pandemic Cuts Access to
Sexual and Reproductive Healthcare for Women Around the World." https://www.ippf
.org/news/covid-19-pandemic-cuts-access-sexual-and-reproductive-healthcare-women
-around-world.

Iones, Ellen. 2023. "How To Understand Competing Medication Abortion Rulings." *Vox*,
April 19, 2023. https://www.vox.com/2023/4/8/23675237/abortion-pill-mifepristone
-kacsmaryk-contradictory-rulings.

Jacobson, Mireille, and Heather Royer. 2011. "Aftershocks: The Impact of Clinic Violence
on Abortion Services." *American Economic Journal* 3 (1): 189–223. https://doi.org/10
.1257/app.3.1.189.

Joffe, Carole. 2013. "The Politicization of Abortion and the Evolution of Abortion Counseling." *American Journal of Public Health* 103, no. 1 (January): 57–65. https://doi.org/10
.2105/AJPH.2012.301063.

Joffe, Carole. 2018. "Abortion Providers and the New Regulatory Regime: The Impact of
Extreme Reproductive Governance on Abortion Care in the United States." *Revue De
Recherche En Civilisation Americaine* 8: 1–17. https://journals.openedition.org/rrca/977.

Jones, Bonnie S., Sara Daniel, and Lindsay K. Cloud. 2018. "State Law Approaches to Facility Regulation of Abortion and other Office Interventions." *American Journal of
Public Health* 108 (4): 486–492.

Jones, Jeffrey M. 2021. "Confidence in U.S. Supreme Court Sinks to Historic Low." GALLUP,
September 23, 2021. https://news.gallup.com/poll/354908/approval-supreme-court-down
-new-low.aspx.

Jones, Kelly, and Mayra Pineda-Torres. 2021. "TRAP'd Teens: Impacts of Abortion Provider
Regulations on Fertility & Education." Discussion Paper No. 14837. Bonn, Germany:
IZA Institute of Labor Economics. https://www.iza.org/publications/dp/14837/trapd
-teens-impacts-of-abortion-provider-regulations-on-fertility-education.

Jones, Rachel K., Lawrence. B. Finer, and Susheela Singh. 2010. *Characteristics of U.S. Abortion Patients, 2008*. New York: Guttmacher Institute.

Jones, Rachel K., and Jenna Jerman. 2014. "Abortion Incidence and Service Availability in
the United States, 2011." *Perspectives in Sexual and Reproductive Health* 46 (1): 3–14.
https://doi.org/10.1363/46e0414.

Jones, Rachel K., and Jenna Jerman. 2017a. "Abortion Incidence and Service Availability in
the United States, 2014." *Perspectives on Sexual and Reproductive Health* 49 (1): 17–27.
https://doi.org/10.1363/psrh.12015.

Jones, Rachel K., and Jenna Jerman. 2017b. "Characteristics and Circumstances of U.S.
Women Who Obtain Very Early and Second-Trimester Abortions." *PLoS ONE* 12 (1):
e0169969. https://doi.org/10.1371/journal.pone.0169969.

Jones, Rachel K., and Jenna Jerman. 2017c. "Population Group Abortion Rates and Lifetime
Incidence of Abortion: United States, 2008–2014." *American Journal of Public Health*
107 (12): 1904–1909. https://doi.org/10.2105%2FAJPH.2017.304042.

Jones, Rachel K., Marielle Kirstein, and Jesse Philbin. 2022a. "Abortion Incidence and
Service Availability in the United States, 2020." *Perspectives in Sexual and Reproductive
Health* 54: 128–141. https://doi.org/10.1363/psrh.12215.

Jones, Rachel K., and Kathryn Kooistra. 2011. "Abortion Incidence and Access to Services
in the United States, 2008." *Perspectives in Sexual and Reproductive Health* 43 (1): 41–50.
https://doi.org/10.1363/4304111.

Jones, Rachel K., Laura Lindberg, and Elizabeth Witwer. 2020. "COVID 19 Abortion Bans
and Their Implications for Public Health." *Perspectives on Sexual and Reproductive
Health* 52 (2): 65–68. https://doi.org/10.1363/psrh.12139.

Jones, Rachel K., Elizabeth Nash, Lauren Cross, Jesse Philbin, and Marielle Kirstein. 2022b. "Medication Abortion Now Accounts for More than Half of All US Abortions." New York: Guttmacher Institute. https://www.guttmacher.org/article/2022/02/medication-abortion-now-accounts-more-half-all-us-abortions.

Jones, Rachel K., Jesse Philbin, Marielle Kirstein, Elizabeth Nash, and Kimberley Lufkin. 2022c. "Long-Term Decline in US Abortions Reverses, Showing Rising Need for Abortion as Supreme Court Is Poised to Overturn *Roe v. Wade*." *Policy Analysis*, June 15, 2022. https://www.guttmacher.org/article/2022/06/long-term-decline-us-abortions-reverses-showing-rising-need-abortion-supreme-court.

Jones, Rachel K., Elizabeth Witwer, and Jenna Jerman. 2019. "Abortion Incidence and Service Availability in the United States, 2017." New York: Guttmacher Institute. https://doi.org/10.1363/2019.30760.

Jones, Rachel K., Mia R. S. Zolna, Stanley K. Henshaw, and Lawrence B. Finer. 2008. "Abortion in the United States: Incidence and Access to Services, 2005." *Perspectives in Sexual and Reproductive Health* 40 (1): 6–16. https://doi.org/10.1363/4000608.

Joyce, Ted. 2010. "Parental Consent for Abortion and the Judicial Bypass Option in Arkansas: Effects and Correlates." *Perspectives in Sexual and Reproductive Health* 42 (3): 1688–1175. https://doi.org/10.1363/4216810.

Joyce, Theodore. 2011. "The Supply-Side Economics of Abortion." *New England Journal of Medicine* 365, no. 16 (October): 1466–1469. https://doi.org/10.1056/NEJMp1109889.

Joyce, Theodore J., Stanley K. Henshaw, Amanda Dennis, Lawrence B. Finer, and Kelly Blanchard. 2009. "The Impact of State Mandatory Counseling and Waiting Period Laws on Abortion: A Literature Review." New York: Guttmacher Institute. https://www.guttmacher.org/report/impact-state-mandatory-counseling-and-waiting-period-laws-abortion-literature-review.

Joyce, Theodore J., Robert Kaestner, and Silvie Colman. 2006. "Changes in Abortions and Births and the Texas Parental Notification Law." *New England Journal of Medicine* 354: 1031–1038. https://doi.org/10.1056/NEJMsa054047.

Kaiser Family Foundation. 2013. "Summary of the Affordable Care Act." Publication No. 8061-02. https://www.kff.org/health-reform/fact-sheet/summary-of-the-affordable-care-act.

Kaiser Family Foundation. 2020. "Percentage of Legal Abortions Obtained by Out-of-State Residents: State Health Facts." https://www.kff.org/womens-health-policy/state-indicator/abortions-by-out-of-state-residents.

Kaiser Family Foundation. 2021. "Median Household Income. Demographics and the Economy: State Health Facts." https://www.kff.org/other/state-indicator/median-annual-income.

Kaiser Family Foundation. 2022. "Abortion in the U.S. Dashboard." July 1, 2022. https://www.kff.org/womens-health-policy/press-release/abortion-in-the-united-states.

Kaiser Family Foundation. 2023a. "Health Insurance Coverage of the Total Population (CPS): State Health Facts." https://www.kff.org/other/state-indicator/health-insurance-coverage-of-the-total-population-cps.

Kaiser Family Foundation. 2023b. "The Availability and Use of Medication Abortion." *Women's Health Policy*. June 1. 2023 https://www.kff.org/womens-health-policy/fact-sheet/the-availability-and-use-of-medication-abortion.

Kamenitsa, Lynn. 2001. "Abortion Debates in Germany." In *Abortion Politics, Women's Movements, and the Democratic State: A Comparative Study of State Feminism*, edited by Dorothy McBride Stetson. New York: Oxford University Press.

Kapp, Nathalie, Elisabeth Eckersberger, Antonella Lavelanet, and Maria Isabel Rodriguez. 2018. "Medical Abortion in the Late First Trimester: A Systematic Review." *Contraception* 99 (2): 77–86. https://doi.org/10.1016/j.contraception.2018.11.002.

Kassam, Ashifa. 2014. "Spain's Prime Minister, Mariano Rajoy, Said It Would Have Been Wrong to Introduce a Law that the Next Government Would Have Changed." *The Guardian*, September 23, 2014. http://www.theguardian.com/world/2014/sep/23/spain-abandons-plan-introduce-tough-new-abortion-laws.

Kaufman, Amanda. 2022. "Missouri Abortion Bill That Includes Ectopic Pregnancies Is One of the Many Aggressive Anti-Abortion Bills under Consideration." *Boston Globe*, March 17, 2022. https://www.msn.com/en-us/news/us/missouri-abortion-bill-that-includes-ectopic-pregnancies-is-one-of-many-aggressive-anti-abortion-measures-under-consideration.

Kavanagh, Erin K., Lee A. Hasselbacher, Brittany Betham, Sigrid Tristan, and Melissa L. Gilliam. 2012. "Abortion-Seeking Minors' Views on the Illinois Parental Notification Law: A Qualitative Study." *Perspectives on Sexual and Reproductive Health* 44 (3): 159–166. https://doi.org/10.1363/4415912.

Keating, Christopher. 2022. "Connecticut's New Abortion Law Offers Protections for Patients, Providers: How Does It Work?" *Hartford Courant*, May 3, 2022. https://www.courant.com/politics/hc-pol-abortion-clarifying-breakdown-20220503-qcndqq4m4bcu5fjrhc34udos5q-story.html.

Kelly, Janet, and Emma Welch. 2018. "Ethical Decision-Making Regarding Infant Viability: A Discussion." *Nursing Ethics* 25 (7): 897–905. https://doi.org/10.1177/0969733016677869.

Kelly, Kate. 2023. "How the Fall of *Roe* Turned North Carolina into an Abortion Destination." *New York Times*, March 4, 2023. https://www.nytimes.com/2023/03/04/us/abortion-north-carolina.html.

Kirstein, Marielle, Joerg Dreweke, Rachel K. Jones, and Jesse Philbin. 2022. "100 Days Post-*Roe*: At Least 66 Clinics across 15 US States Have Stopped Offering Abortion Care." Guttmacher Institute. https://www.guttmacher.org/2022/10/100-days-post-roe-least-66-clinics-across-15-us-states-have-stopped-offering-abortion-care.

Kitchener, Caroline. 2022. "Murder Charges to Be Dropped for Texas Woman Arrested over Abortion: The District Attorney's Office Overseeing the Case Said this Was 'Not a Criminal Matter.'" *Washington Post*, April 10, 2022. https://www.washingtonpost.com/politics/2022/04/10/texas-abortion-murder-arrest.

Kitchener, Caroline, Kevin Schaul, N. Kirkpatrick, Daniela Santamariña, and Lauren Tierney. 2023. "States where Abortion is Legal, Banned or under Threat." *Washington Post*, May 26, 2023. https://www.washingtonpost.com/politics/2022/06/24/abortion-state-laws-criminalization-roe.

Klibanoff, Eleanor. 2022. "How Reproductive Rights Groups Sounded the Alarm after a South Texas Woman Was Charged with Murder for an Abortion." *Texas Tribune*, April 13, 2022. https://www.texastribune.org/2022/04/13/abortion-murder-lizelle-herrera-texas.

Knueven, Liz. 2023. "This Is How Much an Abortion Costs." *U.S. News and World Report Money*, January 12, 2023. https://money.usnews.com/money/personal-finance/family-finance/articles/this-is-how-much-an-abortion-costs.

Kortsmit, Katherine, Tara C. Jatlaoui, Michele G. Mandel, Jennifer A. Reeves, Titilope Oduyebo, Emily Petersen, and Maura K. Whiteman. 2020. "Abortion Surveillance—United States, 2018." *MMWR Surveillance Summary* 69 (SS-7): 1–29. https://www.cdc.gov/mmwr/volumes/69/ss/ss6907a1.htm.

Kortsmit, Katherine, Michele G. Mandel, J. A. Reeves, Elizabeth Clark, H. Pamela Pagano, Antoinette Nguyen, Emily E. Petersen, Maura K. Whiteman. 2021. "Abortion Surveillance—United States, 2019." *MMWR Surveillance Summary* 70 (SS-9): 1–29. https://www.cdc.gov/mmwr/volumes/70/ss/ss7009a1.htm.

Kortsmit, Katherine, Antoinette T. Nguyen, Michele G. Mandel, Elizabeth Clark, Lisa M. Hollier, Jessica Rodenhizer, Maura K. Whiteman. 2022. "Abortion Surveillance—United

States, 2020." *MMWR Surveillance Summary* 71 (SS-10): 1–27. http://dx.doi.org/10.15585/mmwr.ss7110a1.

Kreitzer, Rebecca J. 2015. "Politics and Morality in State Abortion Policy." *State Politics & Policy Quarterly* 15 (1): 41–66. https://doi.org/10.1177/1532440014561868.

Kreitzer, Rebecca J., Kellen A. Kane, and Christopher Z. Mooney. 2019. "The Evolution of Morality Policy Debate: Moralization and Demoralization." *The Forum* 17 (1): 3–24. https://doi.org/10.1515/for-2019-0003.

Kulczycki, Andrzej. 2015. "Abortion and Reproductive Health." Chapter 7 in *Global Population and Reproductive Health*, edited by D. R. McFarlane. Burlington, MA: Jones and Bartlett.

Kyrylenko, Veronika. 2022. "California Eliminates Out of Pocket Abortion Fees." *New American*, March 25, 2022. https://thenewamerican.com/california-eliminates-out-of-pocket-abortion-fees.

Lauter, David. 2023. "Abortion Issue Still a Major Force Boosting Democrats in Swing-State Races." *Los Angeles Times*, February 24, 2023. https://www.latimes.com/politics/newsletter/2023-02-24/abortion-issue-still-major-force-boosting-democrats-in-swing-state-races-essential-politics.

Lazzarini, Zita. 2008. "South Dakota's Abortion Script—Threatening the Physician–Patient Relationship." *New England Journal of Medicine* 359, no. 21 (November): 2189–2191. https://www.nejm.org/doi/full/10.1056/NEJMp0806742.

Lee, Jongkon. 2020. "Different Policies, Different Voices: Gender and Legislative Coordination in the United States Congress." *Policy Studies* 43 (4): 659–675. https://doi.org/10.1080/01442872.2020.1803254.

Legal Information Institute. 2022. *"per curiam* (definition)." Cornell Law School. https://www.law.cornell.edu/wex/per_curiam

Levels, Mark, Roderick Sluiter, and Ariana Need. 2014. "A Review of Abortion Laws in Western-European Countries: A Cross-National Comparison of Legal Developments between 1960 and 2010." *Health Policy* 118 (95): 104. https://doi.org/10.1016/j.healthpol.2014.06.008.

Levin, Bess. 2022. "Idaho's Uniquely Evil Abortion Bill Gives Rapists' Families a Say." *Vanity Fair*, March 14, 2022. https://www.vanityfair.com/news/2022/03/idaho-abortion-bill-rapist-families.

Library of Congress. 2022. "Tenth Amendment, Constitution of the United States." In *Constitution Annotated: Analysis and Interpretation of the U.S. Constitution*. Washington, DC: Library of Congress. https://constitution.congress.gov/constitution/amendment-10.

Lindgren, Yvonne. 2022. *"Dobbs v. Jackson Women's Health* and the Post-*Roe* Landscape." *Journal of the American Academy of Matrimonial Lawyers* 35 (1): 235–283.

Lipka, Michael, and Benjamin Wormald. 2016. "How Religious Is Your State?" Pew Research Center, February 29, 2016. https://www.pewresearch.org/fact-tank/2016/02/29/how-religious-is-your-state.

Liptak, Adam. 2020. "Supreme Court Upholds Trump Administration Regulation Letting Employers Opt out of Birth Control Coverage." *New York Times*, July 8, 2020. https://www.nytimes.com/2020/07/08/us/supreme-court-birth-control-obamacare.html.

Liptak, Adam. 2021a. "Supreme Court to Hear Abortion Case Challenging *Roe v. Wade*." *New York Times*, May 17, 2021. https://www.nytimes.com/2021/05/17/us/politics/supreme-court-roe-wade.html.

Liptak, Adam. 2021b. "Supreme Court Revives Abortion-Pill Restriction." *New York Times*, January 12, 2021. https://www.nytimes.com/2021/01/12/us/supreme-court-abortion-pill.html.

Litman, Leah. 2021. "The Supreme Court Won't Explain Why It Just Greenlit New Abortion Restrictions." *Slate*, January 14, 2021. https://slate.com/news-and-politics/2021/01/the-supreme-court-abortion-pill-order.html.

Llamas, Alyssa, Liz Borkowski, and Susan F. Wood. 2018. "Public Health Impacts of State-Level Abortion Restrictions: Overview of Research & Policy in the United States." In *Bridging the Divide: A Project of the Jacobs Institute of Women's Health*. Washington, DC: Jacobs Institute of Women's Health. https://publichealth.gwu.edu/sites/default/files/downloads/projects/JIWH/Impacts_of_State_Abortion_Restrictions.pdf.

Lozada, Carlos. 2022. "How Three Major Abortion Rulings Reveal a Fractured Culture." *Washington Post*, July 1, 2022. https://www.washingtonpost.com/outlook/2022/07/01/roe-casey-dobbs-abortion-supreme-court.

Lujan Grisham, Michelle. 2021. "Gov. Lujan Grisham Signs Senate Bill 10, a Victory for Reproductive Rights." Press Release, February 26, 2021. https://www.governor.state.nm.us/2021/02/26/gov-lujan-grisham-signs-senate-bill-10-a-victory-for-reproductive-rights.

Luker, Kristin (1984). *Abortion and the Politics of Motherhood*. Berkeley, CA: University of California Press.

Luthra, Shefali. 2022a. "Oklahoma Abortion Clinics Were Briefly a Haven for People Needing Care—Now New Bans Loom." *The Guardian*, April 25, 2022. https://www.theguardian.com/world/2022/apr/25/oklahoma-abortion-clinics-texas-new-bans.

Luthra, Shefali. 2022b. "Right-Wing Lawmakers Are Eyeing Restrictions on Contraception Like IUDs." *Truthout*, May 25, 2022. https://truthout.org/articles/right-wing-lawmakers-are-eyeing-restrictions-on-contraception-like-iuds.

Madden, Richard L. 1973. "Mail to Javits and Buckley Dominated by Letters from the Foes of Abortion." *New York Times*, March 10, 1973, 15.

Mangan, Dan. 2016. "Trump: I'll Appoint Supreme Court Justices to Overturn *Roe v. Wade* Abortion Case." *CNBC*, October 19, 2016. https://www.cnbc.com/2016/10/19/trump-ill-appoint-supreme-court-justices-to-overturn-roe-v-wade-abortion-case.html.

Marcus, Ruth. 2021. "The Rule of Six: A Newly Radicalized Supreme Court Is Poised to Reshape the Nation." *Washington Post*, November 28, 2021, updated December 2, 2021. https://www.washingtonpost.com/opinions/2021/11/28/supreme-court-decisions-abortion-guns-religious-freedom-loom.

Marmor, Ted, Richard Freeman, and Kieke Okma. 2005. "Comparative Perspectives and Policy Learning in the World of Health Care." *Journal of Comparative Policy Analysis* 7 (4): 331–348. https://doi.org/10.1080/13876980500319253.

Martinez, Fidel. 2022. "LatinX File: The Troubling Case of Lizelle Herrera." *Los Angeles Times*, April 14, 2022. https://www.latimes.com/world-nation/newsletter/2022-04-14/latinx-files-lizelle-herrera-release-latinx-files.

Masci, David. 2018. "American Religious Groups Vary Widely in Their Views of Abortion." *FactTank: News in Numbers*. Philadelphia: Pew Research Center. https://www.pewresearch.org/fact-tank/2018/01/22/american-religious-groups-vary-widely-in-their-views-of-abortion.

Mayo Clinic. 2021. "Medical Abortion." *Mayo Clinic Tests and Procedures*. https://www.mayoclinic.org/tests-procedures/medical-abortion/about/pac-20394687.

Mayo Clinic. 2022. "Ectopic Pregnancy." *Diseases and Conditions*. https://www.mayoclinic.org/diseases-conditions/ectopic pregnancy/symptoms-causes/syc-20372088.

Mazmanian, Daniel A. and Paul A. Sabatier. 1989. *Implementation and Public Policy, with a New Postscript*. Lanham, MD: University Press of America.

McBride, Dorothy E. 2001. *Abortion Politics, Women's Movements, and the Democratic State: A Comparative Study of State Feminism*. New York: Oxford University Press.

McCammon, Sarah. 2023a. "Kentucky High Court Upholds State Abortion Bans while Case Continues." *NPR*, February 16, 2023. https://www.npr.org/2023/02/16/1156192879 /abortion-kentucky-supreme-court-bans-roe-dobbs.

McCammon, Sarah. 2023b. "With Abortion Pill Access Uncertain, States Strike Deals to Stock Up." *NPR Politics*, April 11, 2023. https://www.npr.org/2023/04/10/1162182382 /california-strikes-deal-to-stock-up-on-abortion-pills.

McCormack, Jayne. 2022. "Abortion in NI: Timeline of Key Events." *BBC News*, June 8, 2022. https://www.bbc.com/news/uk-northern-ireland-politics-56041849.

McCullough, Jolie. 2022. "NM Abortion Clinic Fields Calls from Texas; Schedules 'About 4 Weeks Out.'" *Albuquerque Journal*, July 2, 2022. https://www.abqjournal.com/news /local/nm-abortion-clinic-fields-calls-from-texas-schedules-about-4-weeks-out/article _712e2be4-a477-5c1b-9a15-01c443a45a6c.html.

McDonald, Henry, Emma Graham-Harrison, and Sinead Baker. 2018. "Ireland Votes by Landslide to Legalise Abortion." *The Guardian US Edition*, May 26, 2018. https://www .theguardian.com/world/2018/may/26/ireland-votes-by-landslide-to-legalise-abortion.

McFarlane, Deborah R. 2006. "Reproductive Health Policies in President Bush's Second Term: Old Battles and New Fronts in the U.S. and Internationally." *Journal of Public Health Policy* 27 (4): 405–426. https://doi.org/10.1057/palgrave.jphp.3200099.

McFarlane, Deborah R. 2015. "The Affordable Care Act and Abortion: Comparing the U.S. and Western Europe." *Politics and the Life Sciences* 34 (2): 52–70. https://doi.org/10.1017 /pls.2015.12.

McFarlane, Deborah R., and Kenneth J. Meier. 2001. *The Politics of Fertility Control: Family Planning and Abortion Policies in the States*. New York: Chatham House Publishers of Seven Bridges Press.

McGinley, Laurie, and Katie Shepherd. 2021. "FDA Eliminates Key Restriction on Abortion Pill as Supreme Court Weighs Case that Challenges *Roe v. Wade*." *Washington Post*, December 16, 2021. https://www.washingtonpost.com/health/2021/12/16/abortion-pill -fda.

McKay, Dan. 2022a. "Officials Ask Judge to Dismiss Abortion Suit." *Albuquerque Journal*, August 5, 2022, A6–A7. https://www.abqjournal.com/news/local/nm-officials-ask-judge -to-reject-abortion-suit/article_6b0710c0-a23e-56ef-a6a2-4b07e3555d21.html.

McKay, Dan. 2022b. "NM Lawmakers Preparing for New Debate on Abortion Rights." *Albuquerque Journal*, December 14, 2022. https://www.abqjournal.com/2557259/nm -lawmakers-prepare-for-debate-on-abortion-rights-in-2023-session-exce.html.

McKay, Dan. 2023. "AG Torrez Challenges Local Abortion Bans." *Albuquerque Journal*, January 24, 2023. https://www.abqjournal.com/2567053/ag-torrez-challenges-legality -of-local-abortion-bans.html.

McKetta, Sarah C., and Katherine M. Keyes. 2019. "Health Consequences of State-Level Restrictive Abortion Legislation." *Paper presented at the Annual Meeting of the Population Association of America, Austin, Texas, April 10–13, 2019.*

Medoff, Marshall H. 2002. The Determinants and Impact of State Abortion Restrictions." *American Journal of Economics & Sociology* 61 (2): 481–493. https://doi.org/10.1111/1536 -7150.00169.

Medoff, Marshall H., and Christopher Dennis. 2011. "TRAP abortion laws and partisan political party control of state government." *American Journal of Economics & Sociology* 70 (4): 951–97. https://doi.org/10.1111/j.1536-7150.2011.00794.x.

Megas, Natalia. 2017. "The Agony of Ending a Wanted Late-term Pregnancy: Three Women Speak Out." *The Guardian*, April 18, 2017. https://www.theguardian.com/society/2017 /apr/18/late-term-abortion-experience-donald-trump.

Meier, Kenneth J. 1985. *Regulation, Bureaucracy, and Economics*. New York: St. Martin's Press.

Meier, Kenneth J., Donald P. Haider-Markel, Anthony Stanislawski, and Deborah R. McFarlane. 1996. "The Impact of Post-*Webster* Restrictions on Abortion." *Demography* 33, no. 3 (August): 307–312. https://doi.org/10.2307/2061763.

Meier, Kenneth J., and Deborah R. McFarlane. 1993. "The Politics of Funding Abortion: State Responses to the Political Environment." *American Politics Quarterly* 21 (1): 81–101. https://doi.org/10.1177/1532673X9302100106.

Meier, Kenneth J., and Deborah R. McFarlane. 1994. "State Family Planning and Abortion Expenditures: Their Effect on Public Health." *American Journal of Public Health* 84, no. 9 (September): 1468–1472. https://doi.org/10.2105/AJPH.84.9.1468.

Mezey, Susan Gluck. 2009a. "Freedom of Access to Clinic Entrances Act of 1994." In *First Amendment Encyclopedia*, edited by John R. Vile, David L. Hudson, and David A. Schultz. Washington, DC: CQ Press. https://mtsu.edu/first-amendment/article/1080/freedom-of-access-to-clinic-entrances-act-of-1994.

Mezey, Susan Gluck. 2009b. "*Scheidler v. National Organization for Women* (2006)." In *First Amendment Encyclopedia*, edited by John R. Vile, David L. Hudson, and David A. Schultz. Washington, DC: CQ Press. https://mtsu.edu/first-amendment/article/11/scheidler-v-national-organization-for-women.

Mezey, Susan Gluck. 2011. *Elusive Equality: Women's Rights, Public Policy, and the Law.* 2nd ed. Boulder, CO: Lynne Rienner.

Miller, Mira. 2022. "Research Shows Texas Abortion Ban Didn't Stop People from Seeking Abortion Care." *VeryWellHealth*, March 16, 2022. https://www.verywellhealth.com/texas-ban-did-not-stop-abortion-care-5222203.

Mohr, James. 1978. *Abortion in America: The Origins and Evolution of National Policy.* New York: Oxford University Press.

Montanaro, Domenico. 2023. "Poll: Two-thirds Oppose Banning Medication Abortion." *NPR Politics*, April 24, 2023. https://www.npr.org/2023/04/24/1171352545/poll-two-thirds-oppose-banning-medication-abortion.

Mooney, Christopher Z. 2001. "The Public Clash of Private Values." Chapter 1 in *The Public Clash of Private Values*, edited by C. Z. Mooney, 3–18. New York: Chatham House.

Mooney, Christopher, and Mei-Hsien Lee. 1995. "Legislative Morality in the American States: The Case of Pre-*Roe* Abortion Regulation Reform." *American Journal of Political Science* 39 (3) 599–627. https://doi.org/10.2307/2111646.

Morone, James A. 1998. *The Democratic Wish: Popular Participation and the Limits of American Government.* New Haven, CT: Yale University Press.

Morone, James A. 2003. *Hellfire Nation: The Politics of Sin in American History.* New Haven, CT: Yale University Press.

Mucciaroni, Gary, Kathleen Ferraiolo, and Meghan E. Rubado. 2019. "Framing Morality Policy Issues: State Legislative Debates on Abortion Restrictions." *Policy Sciences* 52 (2): 171–189. http://dx.doi.org/10.1007/s11077-018-9336-2.

Mukpo, Ashoka. 2020. "TRAP Laws Are the Threat to Abortion Rights You Don't Know About." *ACLU News and Commentary*, March 3, 2020. https://www.aclu.org/news/reproductive-freedom/trap-laws-are-the-threat-to-abortion-rights-you-dont-know-about.

Mulvihill, Geoff, and Linley Sanders. 2023. "Few Adults Support Full Abortion Bans." *Albuquerque Journal*, July 13, 2023, A-2. https://abqjournal.pressreader.com/article/281535115458338.

Murguia, Sophie. 2018. "New Mexico May Finally Repeal Its Archaic Abortion Ban." *Mother Jones*, August 21, 2018. https://www.motherjones.com/politics/2018/08/new-mexico-archaic-abortion-ban.

Murphy, Sean. 2022. "Oklahoma Passes Strictest Abortion Ban; Services to Stop." *AP*, May

19, 2022. https://apnews.com/article/abortion-us-supreme-court-politics-texas-legislature -a43f7f21c1b8e07a383b120d1bdbc695.

Myers, Caitlin Knowles. 2017. "The Power of Abortion Policy: Reexamining the Effects of Young Women's Access to Reproductive Control." *Journal of Political Economy* 125 (6): 2178–2224. https://doi.org/10.1086/694293.

Myers, Caitlin, Rachel Jones, and Ushma Upadhyay. 2019. "Predicted Changes in Abortion Access and Incidence in a Post-*Roe* World." *Contraception* 100, no. 5 (November): 367–373. https://doi.org/10.1016/j.contraception.2019.07.139.

Myers, Megan. 2023. "Troops Can Take Three Weeks Off to Travel for Abortions, IVF Treatment." *Military Times*, February 16, 2023. https://www.militarytimes.com/news /your-military/2023/02/16/troops-can-take-three-weeks-off-to-travel-for-abortions -ivf-treatment.

Naftulin, Julia. 2022. "Tennessee Plans to Make the Mail-Order Abortion Pill Illegal—and Other Red States Are Expected to Try the Same If *Roe v. Wade* Falls." *Insider*, May 10, 2022. https://www.insider.com/abortion-pills-mail-order-could-become-illegal -tennessee-red-states-2022-5.

NARAL. 1989–2002. *Who Decides?* Washington, DC: NARAL and NARAL Foundation.

NARAL Pro-Choice America. 2003–2022. *Who Decides?* Washington, DC: NARAL Pro-Choice America and NARAL Pro-Choice America Foundation. https://www .prochoiceamerica.org/report/2020_who-decides.

NARAL Pro-Choice America. 2018. "U.S. Supreme Court Decisions Concerning Reproductive Rights, 1927–2018." https://www.prochoiceamerica.org/report/u-s-supreme-court -decisions-concerning-reproductive-rights-1927-2018.

NARAL Pro-Choice America. 2021. "Issues." https://www.prochoiceamerica.org/issues.

NARAL Pro-Choice America. 2022. "The State of Legal Abortion: States Poised to Ban Abortion If *Roe* Falls." https://www.prochoiceamerica.org/wp-content/uploads/2022 /01/WHODecides2022-LEGAL-STATE-OF-ABORTION-REPORT-011722-1.pdf.

NAS (National Academies of Sciences, Engineering, and Medicine). 2018. *The Safety and Quality of Abortion Care in the United States*. Washington, DC: National Academies Press. https://www.nap.edu/catalog/24950/the-safety-and-quality-of-abortion-care -in-the-united-states.

Nash, Elizabeth, and Lauren Cross. 2022. "26 States Are Certain or Likely to Ban Abortion without *Roe*: Here's Which Ones and Why." *Policy Analysis*, April 19, 2022. https://www .guttmacher.org/article/2021/10/26-states-are-certain-or-likely-ban-abortion-without -roe-heres-which-ones-and-why.

Nash, Elizabeth, and Joerg Dreweke. 2019. "The U.S. Abortion Rate Continues to Drop: Once Again, State Abortion Restrictions Are Not the Main Driver." *Guttmacher Policy Review* 22: 41–48. https://www.guttmacher.org/gpr/2019/09/us-abortion-rate-continues -drop-once-again-state-abortion-restrictions-are-not-main.

Nash, Elizabeth, and Peter Ephross. 2022. "State Policy Trends 2022: In a Devastating Year, US Supreme Court's Decision to Overturn *Roe* Leads to Bans, Confusion and Chaos." *Policy Analysis*, December 2022. https://www.guttmacher.org/2022/12/state-policy -trends-2022-devastating-year-us-supreme-courts-decision-overturn-roe-leads.

National Council of State Legislatures. 2022. "State Partisan Composition." https://www .ncsl.org/research/about-state-legislatures/partisan-composition.aspx.

National Network of Abortion Funds. 2011. "Remembering Rosie Jimenez through Our Work." https://abortionfunds.org/remembering-rosie.

National Women's Health Network. 2017. *How Much Do Different Kinds of Birth Control Cost Without Insurance?* Washington, DC: National Women's Health Network. https:// nwhn.org/much-different-kinds-birth-control-cost-without-insurance.

Nearns, Jodi. 2009. "Health Insurance Coverage and Prescription Contraceptive Use

Among Young Women at Risk for Unintended Pregnancy." *Contraception* 79 (2): 105–10. https://doi.org/10.1016/j.contraception.2008.08.004.

New England Journal of Medicine, The Editors. 2022. "Lawmakers v. The Scientific Realities of Human Reproduction." *New England Journal of Medicine* 387 (July): 367–368. https://doi.org/10.1056/NEJMe2208288.

New York State Senate. 2021. "Assembly Bill A7573." https://www.nysenate.gov/legislation /bills/2021/A7573.

New York Times. 2022a. "Abortion on the Ballot." *New York Times*, December 20, 2022. https://www.nytimes.com/interactive/2022/11/08/us/elections/results-abortion.html.

New York Times. 2022b. "The Ruling Overturning Roe Is an Insult to Women and the Judicial System." Editorial Board Opinion, *New York Times*, June 24, 2022. https:// www.nytimes.com/2022/06/24/opinion/dobbs-ruling-roe-v-wade.html.

New York Times. 2023. "Tracking the States Where Abortion Is Now Banned." *New York Times*, June 26, 2023. https://www.nytimes.com/interactive/2022/us/abortion-laws-roe -v-wade.html.

Nippita, Siripanth, and Maureen Paul. 2018. "Abortion." Chapter 25 in *Contraceptive Technology*. 21st ed., edited by Robert A. Hatcher, Anita L. Nelson, James Trussell, Carrie Cwiak, Patty Cason, Michael S. Policar, Alison B. Edelman, Abigail R.A. Aiken, Jeanne M. Marrazzo, and Deborah Kowal, 779–827. New York: Ayer. www.contraceptive technology.com.

Nir, Sarah Maslin, and Kate Zernike. 2022. "Connecticut Moves to Blunt Impact of Other States' Anti-Abortion Laws." *New York Times*, April 30, 2022. https://www.nytimes.com /2022/04/30/nyregion/connecticut-texas-abortion-law.html.

Norrander, Barbara, and Wilcox, Clyde. 1999. "Public Opinion and Policymaking in the States: The Case of Post-Roe Abortion Policy." *Policy Studies Journal* 27: 707–722. https:// doi.org/10.1111/j.1541-0072.1999.tb01998.x.

Ollstein, Alice Miranda, and Megan Messerly. 2022. "Missouri Wants to Stop Out-of-State Abortions. Other States Could Follow." *Politico*, March 19, 2022. https://www.politico .com/news/2022/03/19/travel-abortion-law-missouri-00018539.

On the Issues. 2022. "John Roberts on Abortion." *On the Issues: Every Political Leader on Every Issue*. https://ontheissues.org/Court/John_Roberts_Abortion.htm.

Oregon State Health Authority. 2023. "Reproductive Health Equity Act." https://www .oregon.gov/oha/ph/healthypeoplefamilies/reproductivesexualhealth/Pages/repro ductive-health-equity-act.aspx.

Outshoorn, Judith. 1996. "The Stability of Compromise: Abortion Politics in Western Europe." Chapter 7 in *Abortion Politics: Public Policy in Cross-Cultural Perspective*, edited by Marianne Githens and Dorothy McBride Stetson, 141–164. New York: Routledge.

Palmer, Elizabeth A. 2000. "Supreme Court Abortion Ruling Complicates GOP Efforts to Craft 'Partial Birth' Ban." *CQ Magazine*, July 1, 2000: 1612. https://library.cqpress.com /cqmagazine/document.php?id=weeklyreport106-000000108378&type=hitlist&num =4&PHPSESSID=9aaiv4glrf1iq7igjlmut3h5jj.

Parasidis, Efthimios. 2019. "Reclaiming the First Amendment." *American Journal of Public Health* 109, no. 3 (March): 352–353. https://doi.org/10.2105/AJPH.2018.304938.

Patton, Dana. 2007. "The Supreme Court and Morality Policy Adoption in the American States: The Impact of Constitutional Context." *Political Research Quarterly* 60, no. 3 (September): 468–488. https://doi.org/10.1177/1065912907303844.

Paul, Maureen, and Tara Stein. 2011. "Abortion." Chapter 24 in *Contraceptive Technology*, edited by Robert A. Hatcher, James Trussell, Anita L. Nelson, Willard Cates Jr., Deborah Kowal, and Michael S. Policar, 695–736. New York: Ardent Media.

Pennsylvania Department of Health. 2020. "2019 Abortion Statistics." HD0344P. https:// www.health.pa.gov/topics/HealthStatistics/HealthStatisticsAtoZ/Pages/Abortions.aspx.

Permoser, Julia M. 2019. "What Are Morality Policies? The Politics of Values in a Post-Secular World." *Policy Studies Review* 0 (0): 1–6. https://doi.org/10.1177/1478929918816538.

Perreira, Krista M., Emily M. Johnston, Adele Shartzer, and Sophie Yin. "Perceived Access to Abortion Among Women in the United States in 2018: Variation by State Abortion Policy Context." *American Journal of Public Health* 110 (7): 1039–1045. https://doi.org/10.2105/AJPH.2020.30 5659.

Perine, Keith. 2006. "Abortion Cases: A Key to the Court." *CQ Weekly*, October 30, 2006: 2848. Accessed March 4, 2019. http://library.cqpress.com/cqweekly/document.php?id=weeklyreport109-000002395335&type=hitlist&num=0.

Perine, Keith. 2007. "Supreme Court Upholds Abortion Ban." *CQ Weekly*, April 23, 2007: 1204. Accessed March 4, 2019. http://library.cqpress.com/cqweekly/weeklyreport110-000002494586.

Petchesky, Rosalind Pollack. 1980. "Beyond the Right to Choose." *Signs* 5 (4): 661–685. https://www.jstor.org/stable/3173835?seq=1#metadata_info_tab_contents.

Pew Research Center. 2022a. "Majority of Public Disapproves of Supreme Court's Decision to Overturn *Roe v. Wade*." https://www.pewresearch.org/politics/2022/07/06/majority-of-public-disapproves-of-supreme-courts-decision-to-overturn-roe-v-wade.

Pew Research Center. 2022b. "Public Opinion on Abortion: Views on Abortion 1995–2022." https://www.pewforum.org/fact-sheet/public-opinion-on-abortion.

Pew Research Center. 2022c. "Public's Views of Supreme Court Turned More Negative before News of Breyer's Retirement." https://www.pewresearch.org/politics/2022/02/02/publics-views-of-supreme-court-turned-more-negative-before-news-of-breyers-retirement.

Planned Parenthood Federation of America. 2022. "How Much Does an Abortion Cost?" Last modified November 2022. https://www.plannedparenthood.org/learn/ask-experts/how-much-does-an-abortion-cost.

Pluta, Rick. 2023. "MI Supreme Court Dismisses Whitmer Abortion Rights Case." January 21, 2023. *Michigan Radio NPR*. https://www.michiganradio.org/criminal-justice-legal-system/2023-01-21/mi-supreme-court-dismisses-whitmer-abortion-right-case.

Pomerantz, Jennifer L. 2019. "Abortion Disclosure Laws and the First Amendment: The Broader Public Health Implications of the Supreme Court's Becerra Decision." *American Journal of Public Health* 109, no. 3 (March): 412–418. https://doi.org/10.2105/AJPH.2018.304871.

Population Reference Bureau. 2011. *Population Handbook*. Washington, DC: Population Reference Bureau. https://www.prb.org/wp-content/uploads/2011/09/prb-population-handbook-2011.pdf.

Prebeck, Nicole. 2022. "Tennessee Abortion Laws." FindLaw. https://www.findlaw.com/state/tennessee-law/tennessee-abortion-laws.html.

Press, Eyal. 2022. "In Medicine, a Lack of Courage Has Helped Put *Roe* in Jeopardy." *New York Times*, January 21, 2022. https://www.nytimes.com/2022/01/21/opinion/roe-v-wade-abortion-doctors-violence.html?action=click&module=RelatedLinks&pgtype=Article.

Rakich, Nathaniel, and Amelia Thomson-Deveaux. 2022. "Democrats Want to Put Abortion on the Ballot—But Many States Won't Let Them." *FiveThirtyEight*, December 13, 2022. https://fivethirtyeight.com/features/democrats-want-to-put-abortion-on-the-ballot-but-many-states-wont-let-them.

Ralph, Lauren, Diana G. Foster, Sarah Raifman, M. Antonia Biggs, Goleen Samari, Ushma Upadhyay, Caitlin Gerdts, and Daniel Grossman. 2020. "Prevalence of Self-Managed Abortion among Women of Reproductive Age in the United States." *JAMA Network Open* 3:12: e2029245. https://doi.org/10.1001/jamanetworkopen.2020.29245.

Ranji, Usha, and Alina Salganicoff. 2010. "Access to Abortion and Health Reform." *Focus on Health Reform.* Menlo Park, CA: Henry J. Kaiser Foundation. https://kaiserfamily foundation.files.wordpress.com/2013/01/8021.pdf.

Raymond, Elizabeth G., and David A. Grimes. 2012. "The Comparative Safety of Legal Induced Abortion and Childbirth in the United States." *Obstetrics and Gynecology.* 119 (2 Pt 1): 215–219. https://doi.org/10.1097/AOG.0b013e31823fe923.

Reagan, Leslie J. 2022. *When Abortion Was a Crime: Women, Medicine, and the Law in the United States, 1867–1973.* Berkeley, CA: University of California Press.

Rebouche, Rachel. 2021. "Assuring Access to Abortion." Chapter 17 in *COVID-19 Policy Playbook: Legal Recommendations for a Safer, More Equitable Future,* edited by S. Burris, S. de Guia, L. Gable, D. E. Levin, W. E. Parmet, and N. P. Terry, 108–112. Boston: Public Health Law Watch.

Reed, Anna. 2021. "A Future from the Past: Self-Managed Abortions with Ancient Care and Modern Medicines." Chapter 7 in *Who's Choice Is It? Abortion, Medicine, and the Law.* 7th ed., edited by David F. Walbert and J. Douglas Butler. Chicago: American Bar Association, 231-281.

Reed, Naida. 2020 April. *Beyond Medicalization: Midwives & Maternity Care in America.* Pittsburgh: Jewish Healthcare Foundation. https://www.jhf.org/publications-videos /pub-and-vids/roots.

Reed, Rachel. 2022. "Harvard Law School professors call potential abortion rights rollback 'unprecedented.'" *Harvard Law Today,* May 16, 2022. https://today.law.harvard.edu /harvard-law-school-professors-call-potential-abortion-rights-rollback-unprecedented.

Renner, R. M., D. Brahmi, and N. Kapp. 2012. "Who Can Provide Effective and Safe Termination of Pregnancy Care? A Systematic Review." *BJOG: An International Journal of Obstetrics and Gynaecology 120* (August): 23–31. https://doi.org/10.1111/j.1471-0528.2012 .03464.x.

Republican National Committee. 2016. "Republican Platform." https://prod-static.gop.com /media/Resolution_Platform.pdf.

Republic of Ireland, Health Service Executive. 2013. "Investigation of Incident 50278 from Time of Patient's Self-Referral to Hospital on the 21st of October 2012 to the Patient's Death on the 28th of October 2012." https://www.hse.ie/eng/services/news/nimtreport 50278.pdf.

Rice, Thomas. 2013. "Markets and Politics in Health Care." Chapter 2 in *Health Politics and Policy.* 4th ed., edited by James A. Morone and Daniel C. Ehlke, 4–25. Stamford, CT: Cengage Learning.

Rich, Miriam. 2016. "The Curse of Civilised Woman: Race, Gender and the Pain of Childbirth in Nineteenth-Century American Medicine." *Gender and History* 28 (1): 57–76. https://doi.org/10.1111/1468-0424.12177.

Richards, Cecile. 2016. "Protecting and Expanding Access to Birth Control." *New England Journal of Medicine* 374 (9): 801–803. https://doi.org/10.1056/nejmp1601150.

Richardson, L. Anita. 1992. "Parsing *Roe v. Wade*: Will the Court Reaffirm the Right to Choose But Make It Easier for States to Regulate." *Preview of United States Supreme Court Cases 1991* 9 (May): 297–303.

Rolnick, Joshua A., and John S. Vorhies. 2012. "Legal Restrictions and Complications of Abortion: Insights from Data on Complication Rates in the United States." *Journal of Public Health Policy* 33 (3): 348–362. https://doi.org/10.1057/jphp.2012.12.

Romero, Anthony D. 2006. "Testimony of the American Civil Liberties Union on the Nomination of Judge Samuel A. Alito, Jr. Senate Judiciary Committee before the Senate Judiciary Committee." Washington, DC: Washington Legislative Office of the American Civil Liberties Union. https://www.aclu.org/sites/default/files/field_document/asset _upload_file975_23535.pdf.

Rose, Melody. 2005. "Divided Government and the Rise of Social Regulation." *Policy Studies Journal* 29, no. 4 (July): 611–626. https://doi.org/10.1111/j.1541-0072.2001.tb02113.x.

Rosenblatt, Roger. 1992. *Life Itself: Abortion in the American Mind.* New York: Random House.

Rosoff, Jeannie I. 1973. "Constitutional Amendments on Abortion." *Memorandum, Part III.* Washington, DC: Planned Parenthood World Population.

Rosoff, Jeannie I. 1975. "1974 Actions Offer Clues to Direction of 1975 Federal Family Planning and Population Laws and Policies." *Planned Parenthood-World Population Washington Memo W-1* (January 15): 2. Washington, DC: Alan Guttmacher Institute.

RTE (Raidió Teilifís Éireann). 2018. "Referendum: The Paper Ballot Explained." *Raidió Teilifís Éireann,* May 17, 2018. https://www.rte.ie/news/newslens/2018/0517/964134-referendum-the-ballot-paper-explained.

Sahagian, Sarah. 2019. "When *Roe v. Wade* Is Overturned, America Can't Rely on Canada for Abortion Care." *The Establishment,* January 11, 2019. https://theestablishment.co/when-roe-v-wade-is-overturned-america-cant-rely-on-canada-for-abortion-care/index.html.

Salganicoff, Alina, Adara Beamesderfer, Nisha Kurani, and Laura Sobel. 2014. "Coverage for Abortion Services and the ACA." *Issue Brief,* September 19, 2014. http://kff.org/womens-health-policy/issue-brief/coverage-for-abortion-services-and-the-aca.

Salganicoff, Alina, and Laurie Sobel. 2015 "Abortion Coverage in Marketplace Plans." *Issue Brief,* January 21, 2015. Menlo Park, CA: Kaiser Family Foundation. https://www.kff.org/womens-health-policy/issue-brief/abortion-coverage-in-marketplace-plans-2015/

Sanchez, Mary, and Cody Boston. 2022 "Abortion in Spotlight on August Ballot in Kansas." *Flatland.* Television program. Kansas City, KS PBS (9 minutes). https://flatlandkc.org/news-issues/abortion-in-spotlight-on-august-ballot-in-kansas.

Sanger-Katz, Margot, and Claire Cain Miller. 2022. "Legal Abortions Fell around 6 Percent in Two Months after End of *Roe.*" *New York Times,* October 30, 2022. https://www.nytimes.com/2022/10/30/upshot/legal-abortions-fall-roe.html.

Saul, Rebekah. 1998. "Abortion Reporting in the United States: An Examination of the Federal-State Partnership." *Perspectives on Sexual and Reproductive Health* 30 (5): 244–247. https://www.jstor.org/stable/2991612.

Sciubba, Jennifer Dabbs. 2010. *Future Faces of War: Population and National Security.* Santa Barbara, CA: Praeger.

SCOTUSblog. 2020. "*Trump v. Pennsylvania.*" *SCOTUS Blog* (blog), August 10, 2020. https://www.scotusblog.com/case-files/cases/trump-v-pennsylvania.

Sedgh, Gilda, Susheela Singh, Iqbal H. Shah, Elisabeth Åhman, Stanley K. Henshaw, and Akinrinola Bankole. 2012. "Induced Abortion: Incidence and Trends Worldwide from 1995 to 2008." *Lancet* 379 (2012): 625–632. https://doi.org/10.1016/S0140-6736(11)61786-8.

Seitz, Amanda. 2014. "Nearly All of Ohio Abortion Clinics Unlicensed." *Dayton Daily News,* August 23, 2014. https://www.daytondailynews.com/news/nearly-all-ohio-abortion-clinics-unlicensed/5Ovn7hUgSu23Yol4EgjO5K.

Shane, Leo, III. 2022. "Lawmakers Press DOD to Provide Troops Access to Abortion if *Roe v. Wade* Is Overturned." *Military Times,* May 12, 2022. https://www.militarytimes.com/news/pentagon-congress/2022/05/12/lawmakers-press-dod-to-provide-troops-access-to-abortion-if-roe-v-wade-is-overturned.

Shear, Michael, and Adam Liptak. 2022. "Leaked Supreme Court Draft Would Overturn *Roe v. Wade.*" *New York Times,* May 2, 2022. https://www.nytimes.com/live/2022/05/02/us/roe-v-wade-abortion-supreme-court#roe-v-wade-abortion-supreme-court.

Sheeran, Patrick J. 1987. *Women, Society, the State, and Abortion: A Structuralist Analysis.* New York: Praeger.

Sieg, Stina. 2014. "How Abortion Providers Are Inspected in Arizona." March 19, 2014.

KJZZ Radio. https://kjzz.org/content/22837/how-abortion-providers-are-inspected -arizona.

Siegel, Reva. 2007. "The New Politics of Abortion: An Equality Analysis of Woman-Protective Abortion Restrictions." *University of Illinois Law Review* 2007 (3): 991–1054. https://law.yale.edu/sites/default/files/documents/pdf/Faculty/SiegelTheNewPolitics ofAbortion2.pdf.

Simmons-Duffin, Selena. 2023. "Why an Economics Professor Mapped All the Abortion Providers Across the Country." *NPR Morning Edition*, 2-minute interview with Professor Caitlin Myers, June 22, 2023. https://www.npr.org/2023/06/22/1183653550/how -opening-and-closing-of-abortion-clinics-affect-how-many-people-could-reach-t.

Simon, Amanda. 2010. "Fact vs. Fiction on the Military's Abortion Ban." *ACLU News and Commentary*, June 10, 2010. https://www.aclu.org/news/reproductive-freedom/facts-vs -fiction-militarys-abortion-ban.

Simon, Sarah K. 2021. "Is the Church Amendment Constitutional?" *University of Cincinnati Law Review*, April 8, 2021. https://uclawreview.org/2021/04/08/is-the-church-amendment -constitutional/#_ftn1.

Skelley, Geoffrey, Holly Fuong, and Humera Lohdi. 2022. "We Asked Americans to Explain Their 2022 Votes—And How They're Thinking About 2024." *Five-Thirty-Eight*, December 12, 2022. https://fivethirtyeight.com/features/we-asked-americans-to-explain-their -2022-votes-and-how-theyre-thinking-about-2024.

Slavin, Peter. 2022. "A New Abortion Battleground, in South Dakota." *New Yorker*, March 25, 2022. https://www.newyorker.com/news/dispatch/a-new-abortion-battleground-in -south-dakota.

Slusky, David. 2022. "The Cost of Restricting Abortion Access." *Intereconomics* 57 (3): 199– 200. https://doi.org/10.1007/s10272-022-1055-4.

Smith, Jack C. 1970. *Abortion Surveillance Report, Hospital Abortions, Annual Summary 1969*. Atlanta: US Department of Health, Education, and Welfare, Public Health Service, Health Services and Mental Health Administration, National Communicable Disease Center.

Smith, Jack C., and Judith P. Bourne. 1973. "Abortion Surveillance Program of the Center for Disease Control." *Health Services Reports* 88 (3): 255–259. https://www.jstor.org /stable/pdf/4594778.pdf.

Smith, Kevin B. 2002. "Typologies, Taxonomies, and the Benefits of Policy Classification." *Policy Studies Journal* 30 (3): 379–395. https://doi.org/10.1111/j.1541-0072.2002.tb02153.

Smith, Kevin B., and Christopher W. Larimer. 2017. *The Public Policy Theory Primer*. 3rd ed. Boulder, CO: Westview Press.

Smyth, Julie Carr. 2022. "Explainer: Abortion Landscape under State 'Heartbeat' Laws." *AP News*, June 29, 2022. https://apnews.com/article/abortion-us-supreme-court-health-ohio -tennessee-0056dcfb4e5fe1590f07b5993c52078a.

Snider, Brett. 2020. "What Are the Levels of Scrutiny?" *FindLaw*, January 27, 2014, updated May 12, 2020. https://www.findlaw.com/legalblogs/law-and-life/challenging-laws-3 -levels-of-scrutiny-explained.

Snider, Sussanah. 2019. "The Cost of Birth Control." *U.S. News and World Report*, May 2, 2019. https://money.usnews.com/money/personal-finance/family-finance/articles/the -cost-of-birth-control.

Sobel, Laurie, Amrutha Ramaswamy, and Alina Salganicoff. 2020. "Abortion at SCOTUS: A Review of Potential Cases this Term and Possible Rulings." *Women's Health Policy*, October 30, 2020. https://www.kff.org/womens-health-policy/issue-brief/abortion-at -scotus-a-review-of-potential-cases-this-term-and-possible-rulings.

Sobel, Laurie, Amrutha Ramaswamy, and Alina Salganicoff. 2022a. "Policies on Access to Medication Abortion via Telehealth." *Women's Health Policy*, February 7, 2022. https://

www.kff.org/womens-health-policy/issue-brief/the-intersection-of-state-and-federal
-policies-on-access-to-medication-abortion-via-telehealth.

Sobel, Laurie, Alina Salganicoff, and Amrutha Ramaswamy. 2022b. "State Actions to Protect and Expand Access to Abortion Services." *Women's Health Policy*, May 16, 2022. https://www.kff.org/womens-health-policy/issue-brief/state-actions-to-protect-and -expand-access-to-abortion-services.

Society of Family Planning. 2023. "#WeCount." https://societyfp.org/research/wecount.

Solazzo, Alexa L. 2018. "Different and Not Equal: The Uneven Association of Race, Poverty, and Abortion Laws on Abortion Timing." *Social Problems* 2019 (66): 519–547. https://doi .org/10.1093/socpro/spy015.

Squire, Peverill. 2017. "A Squire Index Update." *State Politics & Policy Quarterly* 17 (4): 361– 371. https://doi.org/10.1177/1532440017713314.

Stack, Liam. 2015. "A Brief History of Deadly Attacks on Abortion Providers." *New York Times*, November 29, 2015. https://www.nytimes.com/interactive/2015/11/29/us/30 abortion-clinic-violence.html.

Staman, Jennifer A., and Jon O. Shimabukuro. 2022. "Medication Abortion: A Changing Legal Landscape." *Congressional Research Service Legal Sidebar*, October 5, 2022. https:// crsreports.congress.gov/product/pdf/LSB/LSB10706.

State of California. 2023. "California Abortion Access." Official Website of the State of California. https://abortion.ca.gov.

Stewart, Felicia H., and James Trussell. 2000. "Prevention of Pregnancy Resulting from Rape: A Neglected Preventive Health Measure." *American Journal of Preventive Medicine* 19 (4): 228–229. https://doi.org/10.1016/s0749-3797(00)00243-9.

Stewart, Joseph, Jr., David M. Hedge, and James P. Lester. 2008. *Public Policy: An Evolutionary Approach.* 3rd ed. Boston: Wadsworth.

Stracqualursi, Veronica. 2022a. "Federal Judge Temporarily Blocks New Kentucky Abortion Law from Being Enforced." *CNN Politics*, April 21, 2022. https://www.cnn.com/2022/04 /21/politics/kentucky-abortion-law-planned-parenthood/index.html.

Stracqualursi, Veronica. 2022b. "Kentucky Legislature Approves Sweeping Abortion Bill, Sending it to Governor's Desk." *CNN Politics*, March 30, 2022. https://www.cnn.com /2022/03/30/politics/kentucky-omnibus-abortion-bill/index.html.

Stracqualursi, Veronica, and Caroline Kelly. 2020. "Tennessee Lawmakers Pass Fetal Heartbeat Abortion Bill Backed by Governor." *CNN Politics*, June 19, 2020. https://www.cnn .com/2020/06/19/politics/tennessee-abortion-heartbeat-bill/index.html.

Stracqualursi, Veronica, and Amanda Musa. 2022. "Kentucky Legislature Overrides Governor's Veto of Sweeping Abortion Bill." *CNN Politics*, April 14, 2022. https://www.cnn .com/2022/04/13/politics/kentucky-abortion-bill-legislature-override-veto/index.html.

Strickland, Ruth A., and Marcia L. Whicker. 1992. "Political and Socioeconomic Indicators of State Restrictiveness Toward Abortion." *Policy Studies Journal* 20 (4): 598–617. https:// doi.org/10.1111/j.1541-0072.1992.tb00185.x.

Stuenkel, Cynthia A., and JoAnn E. Manson. 2021. "Women's Health—Traversing Medicine and Public Policy." *New England Journal of Medicine* 384 (June): 2073–2076. https://doi .org/10.1056/NEJMp2105292.

Supreme Court of the United States. 2021. *Oral Argument, Audio and Transcript. Dobbs v. Jackson Women's Health.* Docket Number: 19-1392. Date Argued: December 1, 2021. https://www.supremecourt.gov/oral_arguments/audio/2021/19-1392.

Supreme Court of the United States. 2022. "A Reporter's Guide to Applications Pending Before the Supreme Court of the United States. Prepared by the Public Information Office of the United States Supreme Court." https://www.supremecourt.gov/publicinfo /reportersguide.pdf.

Sutin, Jonathan B. 1970. "New Mexico's 1969 Criminal Abortion Law." *Natural Resources Journal* 10 (3): 591–614. https://digitalrepository.unm.edu/nrj/vol10/iss3/8.

Swartzendruber, Andrea, and Danielle Lambert. 2022. *Crisis Pregnancy Center Map*. Athens, GA: University of Georgia. https://crisispregnancycentermap.com/about-us.

Talbot, Margaret. 2022. "Amy Coney Barrett's Long Game." *New Yorker Annals of Law*, February 7, 2022. https://www.newyorker.com/magazine/2022/02/14/amy-coney-barretts-long-game.

Taylor, Diana, Barbara Safriet, Beth Kruse, Grayson Dempsey, and Lisa Summers. 2018. *Abortion Provider Toolkit*. San Francisco: University of California at San Francisco Bixby Center for Global Reproductive Health. https://aptoolkit.org.

Tennessee Advocates for Planned Parenthood. 2022. "Let's Talk About Tennessee's Trigger Laws." *Blog*, February 14, 2022. https://www.plannedparenthoodaction.org/tennessee-advocates-planned-parenthood/blog/lets-talk-about-tennessees-trigger-laws.

Tesler, Michael. 2022. "For The First Time in Years, Democrats Are More Concerned about Abortion than Republicans Are." *Five-Thirty-Eight*, May 25, 2022. https://fivethirtyeight.com/features/for-the-first-time-in-years-democrats-are-more-concerned-about-abortion-than-republicans-are.

Thomson-DeVeaux, Amelia, and Sophia Lebowitz. 2022. "Where Americans Voted to Protect Abortion Rights in the Midterms." *FiveThirtyfEight*, December 5, 2022. https://fivethirtyeight.com/videos/where-americans-voted-to-protect-abortion-rights-in-the-midterms.

Timms, Mariah. 2020. "Moments after Gov. Lee Signed It, Court Halts Tennessee's Restrictive Abortion Law." *Tennessean.com*, July 13, 2020. https://www.tennessean.com/story/news/local/2020/07/13/tennessee-abortion-ban-judge-halts-new-law-signed-gov-bill-lee/5428635002.

Timms, Mariah. 2021. "Tennessee's Strict New Abortion Law Will Remain Blocked, Federal Appeals Court Rules." *Tennessean.com*, December 1, 2021. https://www.tennessean.com/story/news/politics/2021/12/01/tennessees-strict-new-abortion-law-go-before-full-6th-circuit-court-appeals/8826966002.

Tobin-Tyler, Elizabeth. 2022. "A Grim New Reality: Intimate Partner Violence after *Dobbs* and *Bruen*." *New England Journal of Medicine* 387 (14): 1247–1249. https://doi.org/10.1056/nejmp2209696.

Todd, Annie. 2022. "South Dakota Gov. Kristi Noem Bans Abortions via Telemedicine, Restricts Abortion Pills." *Argus Leader*, March 23, 2022. https://www.argusleader.com/story/news/2022/03/23/governor-noem-signs-south-dakota-telemedicine-abortion-pills-coercion-laws/7146043001.

Tribe, Laurence H. 1992. *Abortion: The Clash of Absolutes*. New York: Norton.

Trussell, James. 2011. "Contraceptive Failure in the United States." *Contraception* 83 (5): 397–404. https://pubmed.ncbi.nlm.nih.gov/21477680.

Trussell, James, and Eleanor Bimla Schwartz. 2011. "Emergency Contraception." Chapter 11 in *Contraceptive Technology*. 20th ed., edited by Robert A. Hatcher, James Trussell, Anita L. Nelson, Willard Cates Jr., Deborah Kowal, and Michael S. Policar, 113–145. New York: Ardent Media.

United Nations Population Division. 2021. "World Contraceptive Use." https://www.un.org/development/desa/pd/data/world-contraceptive-use.

United States Census Bureau. 2021a. "History: Pop Culture 1800." https://www.census.gov/history/www/through_the_decades/fast_facts/1800_fast_facts.html.

United States Census Bureau. 2021b. "2019 Population Estimates by Age, Sex, Race and Hispanic Origin." https://www.census.gov/newsroom/press-kits/2020/population-estimates-detailed.html.

United States Census Bureau. 2023a. "American Community Survey Data." https://www
.census.gov/programs-surveys/acs/data.html.

United States Census Bureau. 2023b. "International Data Base." https://www.census.gov
/data-tools/demo/idb/#/country?COUNTRY_YEAR=2023&COUNTRY_YR_ANIM
=2023.

United States Courts. 2022. "Supreme Court Procedures." https://www.uscourts.gov/about
-federal-courts/educational-resources/about-educational-outreach/activity-resources
/supreme-1.

Upadhyay, Ushma D., Sheila Desai, Vera Zlidar, Tracy A. Weitz, Daniel Grossman, Patricia
Anderson, and Diana Taylor. 2015. "Incidence of Emergency Department Visits and
Complications after Abortion." *Obstetrics and Gynecology* 125 (1): 175–183. https://doi
.org/10.1097/AOG.0000000000000603.

US Department of Health and Human Services. 2021. "Conscience and Religious Freedom."
https://www.hhs.gov/conscience/conscience-protections/index.html.

US Department of Health and Human Services. 2023. *HHS Poverty Guidelines for 2023.*
Washington, DC: Office of the Assistant Secretary for Planning and Evaluation. https://
aspe.hhs.gov/topics/poverty-economic-mobility/poverty-guidelines.

US Food and Drug Administration. 2023a. "Approved Risk and Mitigation Strategies
(REMS)." https://www.accessdata.fda.gov/scripts/cder/rems/index.cfm?event=Rems
Details.page&REMS=390.

US Food and Drug Administration. 2023b. "Information about Mifepristone for Medical
Termination of Pregnancy Through Ten Weeks Gestation." https://www.fda.gov/drugs
/postmarket-drug-safety-information-patients-and-providers/information-about
-mifepristone-medical-termination-pregnancy-through-ten-weeks-gestation.

Vaida, Bara. 2016. "Abortion." *CQ Researcher.* August 9, 2016. https://library.cqpress.com
/cqresearcher/document.php?id=cqr_ht_abortion_2016.

Van Sickle, Rachel, and Amanda Hollis-Brusky. 2013. "An (Un)clear Conscience Clause:
The Causes and Consequences of Statutory Ambiguity in State Contraceptive Mandates." *Journal of Health Politics, Policy, and Law* 38, no. 4 (August): 683–708. https://
doi.org/10.1215/03616878-2208576.

Vilda, Dovile, Maeve E. Wallace, Clare Daniel, Melissa Goldin Evans, Charles Stoecker, and
Katherine P. Theall. 2021. "State Abortion Policies and Maternal Death in the United
States, 2015–2018." *American Journal of Public Health* 111 (9):1696–1704. https://ajph
.aphapublications.org/doi/full/10.2105/AJPH.2021.306396.

Watson, Eleanor. 2023. "GOP Sen. Tuberville's Hold On Nominations Could Cause Armed
Forces To 'Lose Talent,' Nominee for Top Military Officer Says." *CBS News*, July 11, 2023.
https://www.cbsnews.com/news/tommy-tuberville-military-nominations-hold-charles
-q-brown-senate-armed-forces-committee.

Webber, Miriam. 2020. "How Coronavirus Is Changing Access to Abortion." *Politico*, May
21, 2020. https://www.politico.com/news/2020/05/21/how-coronavirus-is-changing
-access-to-abortion-273193.

Weissert, William, and Carol Weissert. 2019. *Governing Health: The Politics of Health Policy.*
5th ed. Baltimore: Johns Hopkins University Press.

Weitz, Tracy, Patricia Anderson, and Diana Taylor. 2009. "Advancing the Scope of Practice
for Advanced Practice Clinicians: More than a Matter of Access." *Contraception* 80 (2):
105–107. https://doi.org/10.1016/j.contraception.2009.04.013.

Weschler, Lawrence. 2018. "How the Supreme Court Lost Its Legitimacy." *The Nation*, September 17, 2018. https://www.thenation.com/article/archive/how-the-us-supreme-court
-lost-its-legitimacy.

White, Kari, Asha Dane'el, Elsa Vizcarra, Laura Dixon, Klaira Lerma, Anitra Beasley,
Joseph E. Potter, and Tony Ogburn. 2022. "Out-of-State Travel for Abortion Following

Implementation of Texas Senate Bill 8." *Research Brief.* Austin, TX: University of Texas at Austin. http://sites.utexas.edu/txpep/files/2022/03/TxPEP-out-of-state-SB8.pdf.

Wight, Patty. 2019. "Newly Blue, Maine Expands Access to Abortion." *NPR Shots: Health News from NPR,* July 2, 2019, 3 minutes.

Williams, Pete. 2019. "Supreme Court Upholds Indiana Abortion Law Requiring Fetal Remains Be Buried or Cremated." *NBC News Digital,* May 28, 2019. https://www.nbc news.com/politics/supreme-court/supreme-court-upholds-indiana-abortion-law -requiring-fetal-remains-be-n1010736.

Williamson, Vanessa. 2022. "The War on Abortion Drugs Will Be Just as Racist and Classist." *Brookings FIXGOV* (blog), May 9, 2022. https://www.brookings.edu/blog /fixgov/2022/05/09/the-war-on-abortion-drugs-will-be-just-as-racist-and-classist.

Wilson, Joshua C. 2020. "Striving to Rollback or Protect *Roe*: State Legislation and the Trump-Era Politics of Abortion." *Publius* 50 (3): 370–397. https://doi.org/10.1093 /publius/pjaa015.

Wolf, Richard, and Shari Rudavsky. 2019. "Supreme Court Upholds Part of Indiana Anti-Abortion Law Requiring Disposal of Fetal Remains by Burial or Cremation." *IndyStar,* May 28, 2019. https://www.indystar.com/story/news/2019/05/28/indiana-abortion-law -supreme-court-rules-fetal-remains-law/1256953001.

Wong, Joseph. 2014. "Comparing Europe and North America." In *Comparative Policy Studies,* edited by Isabelle Engeli and Christine Rothmayr Allison, 163–184. New York: Palgrave Macmilllan.

World Health Organization. 2022. "Recommendations and best practice statements across the continuum of abortion care." Chapter 3 in *Medical Management of Induced Abortion: Recommendations,* 27–30 (3.4.2). Washington, DC: World Health Organization. https://www.who.int/publications/i/item/9789240039483.

Yi, Jean, and Amelia Thomson-DeVeaux. 2022. "Where Americans Stand on Abortion in 5 Charts." *FiveThirtyEight,* May 6, 2022. https://fivethirtyeight.com/features/where -americans-stand-on-abortion-in-5-charts.

Zernike, Kate. 2022. "The New Landscape of the Abortion Fight." *New York Times,* December 11, 2022. https://www.nytimes.com/2022/12/10/us/abortion-roe-wade.html.

Zettler, Patricia J., and Ameet Sarpatwari.2021. "State Restrictions on Mifepristone Access—The Case for Federal Preemption." *New England Journal of Medicine* 386 (8): 705–707. https://doi.org/10.1056/NEJMp2118696.

Ziegler, Mary. 2015. *After Roe: The Lost History of the Abortion Debate.* Cambridge, MA: Harvard University Press.

Ziegler, Mary. 2020. *Abortion and the Law in America: Roe v. Wade to the Present.* Cambridge, UK: Cambridge University Press.

Ziegler, Mary. 2022. "Lizelle Herrera's Texas Arrest Is a Warning: Even Mistakes Quickly Resolved or Retracted Can Have a Chilling Effect." *NBC News Think: Opinion, Analysis, Essays,* April 16, 2022. https://www.nbcnews.com/think/opinion/lizelle-herreras-texas -abortion-arrest-warning-rcna24639.